WITHDRAWN

D1429381

BURNLEY MACKENZIE
HEALTHCARE LIBRARY
TU11082

Quality Improvement

Editors

MUNISH GUPTA
HEATHER C. KAPLAN

CLINICS IN PERINATOLOGY

www.perinatology.theclinics.com

Consulting Editor
LUCKY JAIN

September 2017 • Volume 44 • Number 3

ELSEVIER

1600 John F. Kennedy Boulevard • Suite 1800 • Philadelphia, Pennsylvania, 19103-2899

http://www.theclinics.com

CLINICS IN PERINATOLOGY Volume 44, Number 3
September 2017 ISSN 0095-5108, ISBN-13: 978-0-323-54564-8

Editor: Kerry Holland
Developmental Editor: Casey Potter

Clinics in Perinatology (ISSN 0095-5108) is published quarterly by Elsevier Inc., 360 Park Avenue South, New York, NY 10010-1710. Months of issue are March, June, September, and December. Business and Editorial Offices: 1600 John F. Kennedy Blvd., Ste. 1800, Philadelphia, PA 19103-2899. Customer Service Office: 3251 Riverport Lane, Maryland Heights, MO 63043. Periodicals postage paid at New York, NY and additional mailing offices. Subscription prices are $299.00 per year (US individuals), $532.00 per year (US institutions), $350.00 per year (Canadian individuals), $651.00 per year (Canadian institutions), $433.00 per year (international individuals), $651.00 per year (international institutions), $100.00 per year (US students), and $195.00 per year (Canadian and international students). International air speed delivery is included in all Clinics subscription prices. All prices are subject to change without notice. **POSTMASTER:** Send address changes to *Clinics in Perinatology*, Elsevier Health Sciences Division, Subscription Customer Service, 3251 Riverport Lane, Maryland Heights, MO 63043. **Customer Service: Telephone: 1-800-654-2452** (U.S. and Canada); **1-314-447-8871** (outside U.S. and Canada). **Fax: 1-314-447-8029. E-mail: journalscustomerservice-usa@elsevier.com** (for print support); **journalsonlinesupport-usa@elsevier.com** (for online support).

Reprints. For copies of 100 or more, of articles in this publication, please contact the Commercial Reprints Department, Elsevier Inc., 360 Park Avenue South, New York, NY 10010-1710. Tel. 212-633-3874; Fax: 212-633-3820; E-mail: reprints@elsevier.com.

Clinics in Perinatology is also pubilshed in Spanish by McGraw-Hill Interamericana Editores S.A., P.O. Box 5-237, 06500 Mexico D.F., Mexico.

Clinics in Perinatology is covered in *MEDLINE/PubMed (Index Medicus) Current Contents, Excepta Medica, BIOSIS and ISI/BIOMED.*

Printed in the United States of America.

Contributors

CONSULTING EDITOR

LUCKY JAIN, MD, MBA
Richard W. Blumberg Professor and Interim Chairman, Emory University School of Medicine, Department of Pediatrics, Executive Medical Director and Interim Chief Academic Officer, Children's Healthcare of Atlanta, Atlanta, Georgia

EDITORS

MUNISH GUPTA, MD, MMSc
Instructor in Pediatrics, Harvard Medical School, Department of Neonatology, Beth Israel Deaconess Medical Center, Boston, Massachusetts

HEATHER C. KAPLAN, MD, MSCE
Associate Professor, Department of Pediatrics, Perinatal Institute, James M. Anderson Center for Health Systems Excellence, Cincinnati Children's Hospital Medical Center, The University of Cincinnati College of Medicine, Cincinnati, Ohio

AUTHORS

KATHRYN C. ADAIR, PhD
Department of Psychiatry, Duke University School of Medicine, Duke Patient Safety Center, Duke University Health System, Durham, North Carolina

MAYA BALAKRISHNAN, MD, CSSBB
Associate Professor, Division of Neonatology, Department of Pediatrics, University of South Florida Morsani College of Medicine, Tampa, Florida

ANN E.B. BORDERS, MD, MSc, MPH
Department of Obstetrics and Gynecology, Evanston Hospital, Pritzker School of Medicine, NorthShore University HealthSystem, Clinical Assistant Professor, University of Chicago, Evanston, Illinois; Department of Medical Social Sciences, Executive Director and Obstetric Lead, Illinois Perinatal Quality Collaborative, Center for Healthcare Studies, Adjunct Assistant Professor, Northwestern University Feinberg School of Medicine, Chicago, Illinois

CARL LEWIS BOSE, MD
Professor of Pediatrics, University of North Carolina at Chapel Hill School of Medicine, Chapel Hill, North Carolina

MADGE E. BUUS-FRANK, DNP, APRN-BC, FAAN
Executive Vice President, Director of Quality Improvement and Education, Vermont Oxford Network, Geisel School of Medicine and University of Vermont, Burlington, Vermont

WALDEMAR CARLO, MD
Edwin M. Dixon Professor of Pediatrics, Director, Division of Neonatology, The University of Alabama at Birmingham, Birmingham, Alabama

AARON B. CAUGHEY, MD, PhD
Professor and Chair, Department of Obstetrics and Gynecology, Associate Dean, Women's Health Research & Policy, Oregon Health & Science University, Portland, Oregon

JOANNA F. CELENZA, MA, MBA
March of Dimes/CHaD ICN Family Support Specialist, Children's Hospital at Dartmouth-Hitchcock, Lebanon, New Hampshire

DMITRY DUKHOVNY, MD, MPH
Assistant Professor, Department of Neonatology, Department of Pediatrics, Oregon Health & Science University, Portland, Oregon

DANIELLE YERDON EHRET, MD, MPH
Assistant Professor of Pediatrics, The Robert Larner, M.D. College of Medicine, University of Vermont, Burlington, Vermont

MUNISH GUPTA, MD, MMSc
Instructor in Pediatrics, Harvard Medical School, Department of Neonatology, Beth Israel Deaconess Medical Center, Boston, Massachusetts

JAMES I. HAGADORN, MD, MS
Associate Professor, Department of Pediatrics, University of Connecticut School of Medicine, Farmington, Connecticut; Division of Neonatology, Connecticut Children's Medical Center, Hartford, Connecticut

TIMMY HO, MD, MPH
Instructor, Department of Neonatology, Beth Israel Deaconess Medical Center, Harvard Medical School, Boston, Massachusetts

JEFFREY D. HORBAR, MD
Chief Executive and Scientific Officer, Vermont Oxford Network, Jerold F. Lucey Professor of Neonatal Medicine, University of Vermont, Burlington, Vermont

KENDALL R. JOHNSON, MD
Assistant Professor, Department of Pediatrics, University of Connecticut School of Medicine, Farmington, Connecticut; Division of Neonatology, Connecticut Children's Medical Center, Hartford, Connecticut

HEATHER C. KAPLAN, MD, MSCE
Associate Professor, Department of Pediatrics, Perinatal Institute, James M. Anderson Center for Health Systems Excellence, Cincinnati Children's Hospital Medical Center, The University of Cincinnati College of Medicine, Cincinnati, Ohio

WANNASIRI LAPCHAROENSAP, MD
Assistant Professor, Department of Pediatrics, Oregon Health & Science University, Portland, Oregon

HENRY C. LEE, MD, MS
Associate Professor, Department of Pediatrics, Chief Medical Officer, California Perinatal Quality Care Collaborative, Stanford University, Stanford, California

PATRICIA ANN LEE KING, PhD, MSW
State Project Director, Feinberg School of Medicine of Northwestern University, Chicago, Illinois

SCOTT A. LORCH, MD, MSCE
Associate Professor, Pediatrics, Perelman School of Medicine, Senior Scholar, Leonard Davis Institute for Health Economics, Division of Neonatology, Center for Perinatal and Pediatric Health Disparities Research, and PolicyLab, The Children's Hospital of Philadelphia, University of Pennsylvania, Philadelphia, Pennsylvania

KRISTIN R. MELTON, MD
Associate Professor, Division of Neonatology, Department of Pediatrics, Cincinnati Children's Hospital Medical Center, Cincinnati, Ohio

YIZHAO NI, PhD
Instructor, Division of Biomedical Informatics, Department of Pediatrics, Cincinnati Children's Hospital Medical Center, Cincinnati, Ohio

PATOULA G. PANAGOS, MD
Attending Neonatologist, Quality Improvement Director, Nemours Delaware Valley, Division of Neonatology, Nemours Alfred I. duPont Hospital for Children, Wilmington, Delaware; Nemours Neonatology, Thomas Jefferson University Hospital, Clinical Assistant Professor, Pediatrics, Sidney Kimmel School of Medicine, Thomas Jefferson University, Philadelphia, Pennsylvania; Assistant Professor of Pediatrics, Director of Neonatal Quality Improvement, Rush University Children's Hospital, Chicago, Illinois

ALOKA L. PATEL, MD
Associate Professor of Pediatrics, Research Director, Section of Neonatology, Rush University Children's Hospital, Chicago, Illinois

JACQUELYN KNUPP PATTERSON, MD
Fellow of Neonatal-Perinatal Medicine, University of North Carolina School of Medicine, Chapel Hill, North Carolina

STEPHEN A. PEARLMAN, MD, MSHQS
Clinical Professor of Pediatrics, Sidney Kimmel School of Medicine, Thomas Jefferson University, Philadelphia, Pennsylvania; Attending Neonatologist, Quality and Safety Officer, Division of Neonatology, Women and Children's Services, Christiana Care Health System, Newark, Delaware

ALAN PETER PICARILLO, MD
Maine Neonatology Associates, Barbara Bush Children's Hospital, Maine Medical Center, Portland, Maine

JOCHEN PROFIT, MD, MPH
Lucile Packard Children's Hospital, Palo Alto, California; Perinatal Epidemiology and Health Outcomes Research Unit, Neonatology, Division of Neonatal and Developmental Medicine, Department of Pediatrics, Stanford University School of Medicine, Stanford University, California Perinatal Quality Care Collaborative, Stanford, California

DEWAYNE M. PURSLEY, MD, MPH
Associate Professor, Department of Neonatology, Beth Israel Deaconess Medical Center, Harvard Medical School, Boston, Massachusetts

AARTI RAGHAVAN, MD
Assistant Professor, Division of Neonatology, Department of Pediatrics, UIC Hospital, University of Illinois College of Medicine at Chicago, Chicago, Illinois

BETHANY A. SABOL, MD
Department of Obstetrics and Gynecology, Oregon Health & Science University, Portland, Oregon

PATRICK D. SCHNEIDER, MD
Maternal-Fetal Medicine, NorthShore University HealthSystem, University of Chicago, Evanston, Illinois

JOHN BRYAN SEXTON, PhD
Department of Psychiatry, Duke University School of Medicine, Duke Patient Safety Center, Duke University Health System, Durham, North Carolina

JEAN M. SILVESTRI, MD
Professor of Pediatrics, Pediatric Vice Chair, Safety, Quality and Clinical Effectiveness, Rush University Children's Hospital, Chicago, Illinois

DAVID W. SINK, MD
Assistant Professor, Department of Pediatrics, University of Connecticut School of Medicine, Farmington, Connecticut; Division of Neonatology, Connecticut Children's Medical Center, Hartford, Connecticut

ALAN R. SPITZER, MD
Emeritus Director of Research, Education, and Quality, Pediatrix Medical Group, MEDNAX, Inc., Sunrise, Florida

GAUTHAM K. SURESH, MD, DM, MS
Professor, Division of Neonatology, Professor, Department of Pediatrics, Texas Children's Hospital, Baylor College of Medicine, Houston, Texas

DANIEL S. TAWFIK, MD
Division of Pediatric Critical Care Medicine, Department of Pediatrics, Stanford University School of Medicine, Stanford, California; Lucile Packard Children's Hospital, Palo Alto, California

HEATHER L. TUBBS-COOLEY, PhD, RN
Assistant Professor, Research in Patient Services, Division of Nursing, Cincinnati Children's Hospital Medical Center, Cincinnati, Ohio

KATHLEEN E. WALSH, MD, MSc
Associate Professor, Department of Pediatrics, James M. Anderson Center for Health Systems Excellence, Cincinnati Children's Hospital Medical Center, Cincinnati, Ohio

DENISE ZAYACK, RN, MPH
Collaboratives Coordinator and Coach, Vermont Oxford Network, Burlington, Vermont

JOHN A.F. ZUPANCIC, MD, ScD
Associate Professor, Department of Neonatology, Beth Israel Deaconess Medical Center, Harvard Medical School, Boston, Massachusetts

Contents

Foreword: Quality Improvement: The Journey Continues! xv

Lucky Jain

Preface: Improving Quality Improvement in Neonatal-Perinatal Care xvii

Munish Gupta and Heather C. Kaplan

Has Quality Improvement Really Improved Outcomes for Babies in the Neonatal Intensive Care Unit? 469

Alan R. Spitzer

During the past decade, the emergence of outcome measurement and quality improvement in the neonatal intensive care unit, far more than the introduction of new research approaches or novel therapies, has had a profound effect on improving outcomes for premature neonates. Collection of outcome data, review of those data, and strategies to identify and resolve problems using continuous quality improvement methods can dramatically improve patient outcomes. It is likely that further initiatives in quality improvement will continue to have additional beneficial effects for the neonate.

National Quality Measures in Perinatal Medicine 485

Scott A. Lorch

There are numerous measures of perinatal quality endorsed by national agencies such as the National Quality Forum (NQF). The sheer number of metrics may lead to confusion about what these measures truly assess, and how to interpret variation in these measures across hospitals, health care systems, and geographic regions. This article presents a conceptual model for the numerous validated measures, an overview of the types of measures endorsed for perinatal quality by NQF in 2016, and potential measures absent from endorsement by these national bodies.

The Hard Work of Improving Outcomes for Mothers and Babies: Obstetric and Perinatal Quality Improvement Initiatives Make a Difference at the Hospital, State, and National Levels 511

Patrick D. Schneider, Bethany A. Sabol, Patricia Ann Lee King, Aaron B. Caughey, and Ann E.B. Borders

Quality improvement efforts are an increasingly expanding focus for perinatal care providers across the United States. From successful hospital-level initiatives, there has been a growing effort to use and implement quality improvement work in substantive and meaningful ways. This article summarizes the foundations of maternal-focused, birth-focused, and neonatal-focused quality improvement initiatives to highlight the underpinnings and potential future directions of current state-level perinatal quality care collaboratives.

Eliminating Undesirable Variation in Neonatal Practice: Balancing Standardization and Customization 529

Maya Balakrishnan, Aarti Raghavan, and Gautham K. Suresh

Consistency of care and elimination of unnecessary and harmful variation are underemphasized aspects of health care quality. This article describes the prevalence and patterns of practice variation in health care and neonatology; discusses the potential role of standardization as a solution to eliminating wasteful and harmful practice variation, particularly when it is founded on principles of evidence-based medicine; and proposes ways to balance standardization and customization of practice to ultimately improve the quality of neonatal care.

Context in Quality of Care: Improving Teamwork and Resilience 541

Daniel S. Tawfik, John Bryan Sexton, Kathryn C. Adair, Heather C. Kaplan, and Jochen Profit

Quality improvement in health care is an ongoing challenge. Consideration of the context of the health care system is of paramount importance. Staff resilience and teamwork climate are key aspects of context that drive quality. Teamwork climate is dynamic, with well-established tools available to improve teamwork for specific tasks or global applications. Similarly, burnout and resilience can be modified with interventions such as cultivating gratitude, positivity, and awe. A growing body of literature has shown that teamwork and burnout relate to quality of care, with improved teamwork and decreased burnout expected to produce improved patient quality and safety.

Family Involvement in Quality Improvement: From Bedside Advocate to System Advisor 553

Joanna F. Celenza, Denise Zayack, Madge E. Buus-Frank, and Jeffrey D. Horbar

Video content accompanies this article at: http://www.perinatology.theclinics.com.

Family involvement in newborn intensive care quality improvement dates to the 1980s. In recent years, there has been an evolution of support for family partnerships at the bedside, transforming parents from being passively present to being active and engaged caregivers and team members. Through those same efforts, a transformational understanding of the power of the family perspective in system design and improvement has occurred. Even with the progression and deepening of this involvement, opportunities exist to learn from families and to improve the quality of neonatal care as a result of the unique family perspective.

Improving Neonatal Care: A Global Perspective 567

Danielle Yerdon Ehret, Jacquelyn Knupp Patterson, and Carl Lewis Bose

Each year, approximately 2.7 million infants die during the neonatal period; more than 90% of these deaths occur in developing countries, largely from preventable causes. The known, evidence-based, simple, low-cost interventions that may improve neonatal survival often have low or unknown baseline coverage rates. Gaps in coverage of essential interventions and in quality of care may be amenable to improvement strategies. However, often these gaps are not easily identified. A variety of international organizations have recommended key indicators of quality and established roadmaps for improving neonatal outcomes. Quality improvement at the facility level is an area for future investment.

Using Health Information Technology to Improve Safety in Neonatal Care: A Systematic Review of the Literature **583**

Kristin R. Melton, Yizhao Ni, Heather L. Tubbs-Cooley, and Kathleen E. Walsh

Health information technology (HIT) interventions may improve neonatal patient safety but may also introduce new errors. The objective of this article was to evaluate the evidence for use of HIT interventions to improve safety in neonatal care. Evidence for improvement exists for interventions like computerized provider order entry in the neonatal population, but is lacking for several other interventions. Many unique applications of HIT are emerging as technology and use of the electronic health record expands. Future research should focus on the impact of these interventions in the neonatal population.

Improving Value in Neonatal Intensive Care **617**

Timmy Ho, John A.F. Zupancic, DeWayne M. Pursley, and Dmitry Dukhovny

Work within the US health care system has sought to improve outcomes, decrease costs, and improve the patient experience. Combining those 3 elements leads to value-added care. Quality improvement within neonatology has focused primarily on the improvement of clinical outcomes without explicit consideration of cost. Future improvement efforts in neonatology should consider opportunities to decrease or eliminate waste, and improve outcomes. Consideration of how a change affects all stakeholders reveals potential cost-saving opportunities, and developing aims with value in mind facilitates understanding and goal setting with senior administrative leaders.

Using Statistical Process Control to Drive Improvement in Neonatal Care: A Practical Introduction to Control Charts **627**

Munish Gupta and Heather C. Kaplan

Quality improvement (QI) is based on measuring performance over time, and variation in data measured over time must be understood to guide change and make optimal improvements. Common cause variation is natural variation owing to factors inherent to any process; special cause variation is unnatural variation owing to external factors. Statistical process control methods, and particularly control charts, are robust tools for understanding data over time and identifying common and special cause variation. This article provides a practical introduction to the use of control charts in health care QI, with a focus on neonatology.

Creating a Highly Reliable Neonatal Intensive Care Unit Through Safer Systems of Care **645**

Patoula G. Panagos and Stephen A. Pearlman

Neonates requiring intensive care are at high risk for medical errors due to their unique characteristics and high acuity. Designing a safer work environment begins with safe processes. Creating a culture of safety demands the involvement of all organizational levels and an interdisciplinary approach. Adverse events can result from suboptimal communication and lack of a shared mental model. This article describes tools to promote better patient safety in the neonatal intensive care unit through monitoring adverse events, improving communication, and using information technology. Unplanned extubation is an example of a neonatal safety concern that can be reduced by using quality improvement methodology.

Tackling Quality Improvement in the Delivery Room 663

Wannasiri Lapcharoensap and Henry C. Lee

Implementation of standardized practices in the delivery room fosters a safe environment to ensure that newborn infants are cared for optimally, whether or not they require extensive resuscitation. Quality improvement (QI) is an excellent methodology for implementation of standardized practices due to the multidisciplinary nature of the delivery room, complexity of tasks involved, and opportunities to track processes and outcomes. This article discusses how the delivery room is a unique environment and presents examples on how to approach delivery room QI. Key areas of potential focus for teams pursuing delivery QI include thermal regulation, optimizing respiratory support, and facilitating team communication.

Reducing Incidence of Necrotizing Enterocolitis 683

Aloka L. Patel, Patoula G. Panagos, and Jean M. Silvestri

Necrotizing enterocolitis (NEC) is a multifactorial disease that occurs when multiple risk factors and/or stressors overlap, leading to profound inflammation and intestinal injury. Because of its multifactorial nature, there has been much uncertainty in identifying clear strategies for prevention of NEC. Despite these obstacles, the incidence of NEC has gradually been decreasing over the past 10 years, in part due to quality improvement (QI) initiatives to prevent NEC. Current QI strategies primarily target the various predisposing conditions. This article reviews the evidence on which QI interventions to prevent NEC have been based and provides examples of successful QI interventions.

Using Quality Improvement Tools to Reduce Chronic Lung Disease 701

Alan Peter Picarillo and Waldemar Carlo

Rates of chronic lung disease (CLD) in very low birthweight infants have not decreased at the same pace as other neonatal morbidities over the past 20 years. Multifactorial causes of CLD make this common morbidity difficult to reduce, although there have been several successful quality improvement (QI) projects in individual neonatal intensive care units. QI projects have become a mainstay of neonatal care over the past decade, with an increasing number of publications devoted to this topic. A specific QI project for CLD must be based on best available evidence in the medical literature and expert recommendations, or based on work by previous QI initiatives.

Alarm Safety and Alarm Fatigue 713

Kendall R. Johnson, James I. Hagadorn, and David W. Sink

Clinical alarm systems have received significant attention in recent years following warnings from hospital accrediting and health care technology organizations regarding patient harm caused by unsafe practices. Alarm desensitization or fatigue from frequent, false, or unnecessary alarms has led to serious events and even patient deaths. Other concerns include settings inappropriate to the patient population or condition, inadequate staff training, and improper use or disabling. Research on human factors in alarm response and of functionality of medical devices will help clinicians develop appropriate policies, practices, and device settings for clinical alarms in neonatal intensive care units.

PROGRAM OBJECTIVE

The goal of *Clinics in Perinatology* is to keep practicing perinatologists, neonatologists, obstetricians, practicing physicians and residents up to date with current clinical practice in perinatology by providing timely articles reviewing the state of the art in patient care.

TARGET AUDIENCE

Perinatologists, neonatologists, obstetricians, practicing physicians, residents and healthcare professionals who provide patient care utilizing findings from *Clinics in Perinatology.*

LEARNING OBJECTIVES

Upon completion of this activity, participants will be able to:

1. Review concepts in teamwork and resilience in quality improvement.
2. Discuss quality improvement in the emergency and delivery rooms, among other departments.
3. Recognize efforts in improving outcomes in neonatal intensive care units.

ACCREDITATION

The Elsevier Office of Continuing Medical Education (EOCME) is accredited by the Accreditation Council for Continuing Medical Education (ACCME) to provide continuing medical education for physicians.

The EOCME designates this enduring material for a maximum of 15 *AMA PRA Category 1 Credit*(s)™. Physicians should claim only the credit commensurate with the extent of their participation in the activity.

All other healthcare professionals requesting continuing education credit for this enduring material will be issued a certificate of participation.

DISCLOSURE OF CONFLICTS OF INTEREST

The EOCME assesses conflict of interest with its instructors, faculty, planners, and other individuals who are in a position to control the content of CME activities. All relevant conflicts of interest that are identified are thoroughly vetted by EOCME for fair balance, scientific objectivity, and patient care recommendations. EOCME is committed to providing its learners with CME activities that promote improvements or quality in healthcare and not a specific proprietary business or a commercial interest.

The planning committee, staff, authors and editors listed below have identified no financial relationships or relationships to products or devices they or their spouse/life partner have with commercial interest related to the content of this CME activity:

Kathryn C. Adair, PhD; Maya Balakrishnan, MD, CSSBB; Ann E.B. Borders, MD, MSc, MPH; Carl Lewis Bose, MD; Waldemar Carlo, MD; Dmitry Dukhovny, MD, MPH; Danielle Yerdon Ehret, MD, MPH; Anjali Fortna; Munish Gupta, MD, MMSc; James I. Hagadorn, MD, MS; Timmy Ho, MD, MPH; Kerry Holland; Lucky Jain, MD, MBA; Kendall R. Johnson, MD; Heather C. Kaplan, MD, MSCE; Wannasiri Lapcharoensap, MD; Henry C. Lee, MD, MS; Patricia Ann Lee King, PhD, MSW; Scott A. Lorch, MD, MSCE; Kristin R. Melton, MD; Yizhao Ni, PhD; Patoula G. Panagos, MD; Aloka L. Patel, MD; Jacquelyn Knupp Patterson, MD; Stephen A. Pearlman, MD,MSHQS; Alan Peter Picarillo, MD; Jochen Profit, MD, MPH; DeWayne M. Pursley, MD, MPH; Aarti Raghavan, MD; Bethany A. Sabol, MD; Patrick D. Schneider, MD; J. Bryan Sexton, PhD; Jean M. Silvestri, MD; David W. Sink, MD; Gautham K. Suresh, MD, DM, MS; Daniel S. Tawfik, MD; Heather L. Tubbs-Cooley, PhD, RN; Subhalakshmi Vaidyanathan; Kathleen E. Walsh, MD, MSC; Katie Widmeier; Amy Williams; John AF Zupancic, MD, ScD.

The planning committee, staff, authors and editors listed below have identified financial relationships or relationships to products or devices they or their spouse/life partner have with commercial interest related to the content of this CME activity:

Madge E. Buus-Frank, DNP, APRN-BC, FAAN has an employment affiliation with Vermont Oxford Network.

Aaron B. Caughey, MD, PhD is a consultant/advisor for Celmatix Inc. and MindChild Medical, Inc.

Joanna F. Celenza, MA, MBA has an employment affiliation with Mary Hitchcock Memorial Hospital.

Jeffrey D. Horbor, MD has an employment affiliation with Vermont Oxford Network.

Alan R. Spitzer, MD is a consultant/advisor for Medolac and Mallinckrodt Pharmaceuticals, has stock ownership in Mednax Services, Inc and Medolac, and had an employment affiliation with Mednax Services, Inc.

Denise Zayack, RN, MPH is a consultant/advisor for Vermont Oxford Network.

UNAPPROVED/OFF-LABEL USE DISCLOSURE

The EOCME requires CME faculty to disclose to the participants:

1. When products or procedures being discussed are off-label, unlabelled, experimental, and/or investigational (not US Food and Drug Administration [FDA] approved); and
2. Any limitations on the information presented, such as data that are preliminary or that represent ongoing research, interim analyses, and/or unsupported opinions. Faculty may discuss information about pharmaceutical agents that is outside of FDA-approved labelling. This information is intended solely for CME and is not intended to promote off-label use of these medications. If you have any questions, contact the medical affairs department of the manufacturer for the most recent prescribing information.

TO ENROLL

To enroll in the *Clinics in Perinatology* Continuing Medical Education program, call customer service at 1-800-654-2452 or sign up online at http://www.theclinics.com/home/cme. The CME program is available to subscribers for an additional annual fee of $235 USD.

METHOD OF PARTICIPATION

In order to claim credit, participants must complete the following:

1. Complete enrolment as indicated above.
2. Read the activity.
3. Complete the CME Test and Evaluation. Participants must achieve a score of 70% on the test. All CME Tests and Evaluations must be completed online.

CME INQUIRIES/SPECIAL NEEDS

For all CME inquiries or special needs, please contact elsevierCME@elsevier.com.

CLINICS IN PERINATOLOGY

FORTHCOMING ISSUES

December 2017
Minimally Invasive Neonatal Surgery
Mark Wulkan and Hanmin Lee, *Editors*

March 2018
Endocrinology
Andrew Muir and Susan Rose, *Editors*

June 2018
Perinatal Interventions to Improve Neonatal Outcomes
Ravi Mangal Patel and Tracy A. Manuck, *Editors*

RECENT ISSUES

June 2017
Delivery in the Periviable Period
Brian M. Mercer and Keith J. Barrington, *Editors*

March 2017
Human Milk for Preterm Infants
Francis B. Mimouni and Berthold Koletzko, *Editors*

December 2016
Non-Invasive Ventilation
Bradley Yoder and Haresh Kirpalani, *Editors*

ISSUE OF RELATED INTEREST

Pediatric Clinics of North America, April 2016 (Vol. 63, Issue 2)
Quality of Care and Information Technology
Srinivasan Suresh, *Editor*
Available at: www.pediatric.theclinics.com

Foreword

Quality Improvement: The Journey Continues!

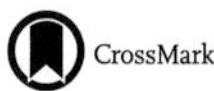

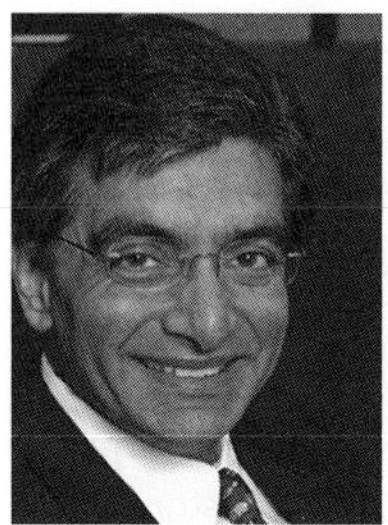

Lucky Jain, MD, MBA
Consulting Editor

If W. Edwards Deming[1] were alive today, he (and other stalwarts of the quality improvement [QI] movement) would have been delighted to see the gains we have made in health care by embracing methodologies originally developed for the manufacturing industry. One such success story from our own institution is shown in **Fig. 1**.[2] Deming, who died in 1993, developed the System of Profound Knowledge[1] that he took to Japan after the Second World War and started a quality movement at institutions like Toyota. He is also credited for further refining the statistical approach to QI developed by Walter A. Shewhart and others and applying it to process improvement through the PDSA (Plan, Do, Study, Act) cycle.[3] Deming did us another huge favor: he was a strong believer in the philosophy that defects originate in systems and should not be viewed as human errors. In health care, this laid the foundation for establishment of a fair and just culture within our institutions and a movement away from "*whose fault is it*."

The *Science of Improvement* continues to evolve and has now become inextricably woven into our health care fabric.[4] Broad principles of this science include simple steps such as starting with a focused aim, creating an effective feedback mechanism to assess improvements, developing ideas for change, testing them before implementation, and, finally, knowing when and how to make a change sustainable. Quality-related data have also become increasingly more reliable and transparent. Indeed, hospital systems are extending the pioneering perinatal quality work done by consortiums such as the Vermont Oxford Network (VON) that relied on rigorously collected data and regular feedback.[5] The NIC/Q (Quality Improvement Collaborative for Neonatology) Project began in 1995 as the first formal quality-improvement project by the VON applying methods of collaborative improvement and benchmarking to improve neonatal intensive care.[5]

Clin Perinatol 44 (2017) xv–xvi
http://dx.doi.org/10.1016/j.clp.2017.06.003
0095-5108/17/© 2017 Published by Elsevier Inc.

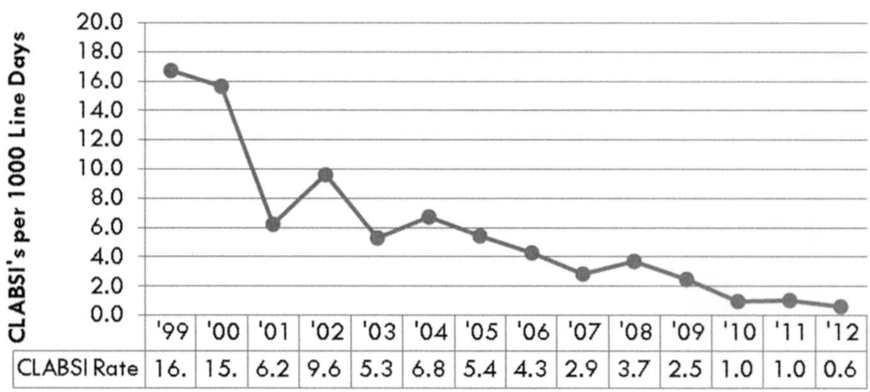

	'99	'00	'01	'02	'03	'04	'05	'06	'07	'08	'09	'10	'11	'12
CLABSI Rate	16.	15.	6.2	9.6	5.3	6.8	5.4	4.3	2.9	3.7	2.5	1.0	1.0	0.6

Fig. 1. Experience over time with central line–associated blood stream infections (CLABSI) at a single institution from 1999-2012. NICU, neonatal intensive care unit. EG, Egleston. (*From* Jain L. Necrotizing enterocolitis prevention: art or science? Clin Perinatol 2013;40:xiv; with permission.)

There is much still to learn about QI. In this issue of the *Clinics in Perinatology*, Drs Gupta and Kaplan have assembled an impressive array of articles highlighting many of these important concepts; they also point to gaps in our approach and understanding. We hope that these writings will stimulate further discussion and efforts about novel ways of improving the quality of care and long-term outcomes of patients who put their trust in us.

Lucky Jain, MD, MBA
Department of Pediatrics
Emory University School of Medicine
Children's Healthcare of Atlanta
2015 Uppergate Drive
Atlanta, GA 30322, USA

E-mail address:
ljain@emory.edu

REFERENCES

1. Jain L. Necrotizing enterocolitis prevention: art or science? Clin Perinatol 2013;40: xiii–xv.
2. Harolds J. Quality and safety in health care, Part I: five pioneers in quality. Clin Nucl Med 2015;40:660–2.
3. Clark DM, Silvester K, Knowles S. Lean management systems: creating a culture of continuous quality improvement. J Clin Pathol 2013;66:638–43.
4. Perla RJ, Provost LP, Parry GJ. Seven propositions of the science of improvement: exploring foundations. Qual Manag Health Care 2013;22:170–86.
5. Horbar JD. The Vermont Oxford Network: evidence-based quality improvement for neonatology. Pediatrics 1999;103:350–9.

Has Quality Improvement Really Improved Outcomes for Babies in the Neonatal Intensive Care Unit?

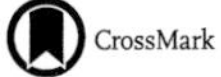

Alan R. Spitzer, MD

KEYWORDS

• Quality improvement • Neonatal intensive care unit • Outcomes • Babies • NICU

KEY POINTS

- During the past decade, the emergence of outcome measurement and quality improvement in the neonatal intensive care unit, far more than the introduction of new research approaches or novel therapies, has had a profound effect on improving outcomes for premature neonates.
- Collection of outcome data, review of those data, and strategies to identify and resolve problems using continuous quality improvement methods can dramatically improve patient outcomes.
- It is likely that further initiatives in quality improvement will continue to have additional beneficial effects for the neonate.

In the neonatal intensive care unit (NICU), as in other areas of medical practice, the provision of high-quality care is universally acknowledged as a mandatory aspect of patient treatment. No clinician, whether physician, nurse, respiratory therapist, physical therapist, nutritionist, or any other clinical provider, interacts with patients with the thought in mind that he or she intends to deliver only adequate care or the minimum necessary to treat an individual. Such thinking is contrary to the most basic tenet of medical practice in which the clinician strives to provide the best possible treatment of patients. Even the finest clinician, however, is still only human and sometimes faces overwhelming clinical circumstances or external demands that can detract from their

The author of this article has no known conflicts of interest that would affect the materials contained within this article. The author currently has the following related issues within the medical field, none of which are pertinent to this article: (1) stock in MEDNAX, Inc as a component of his former employment with that company, (2) is a consultant to Mallinckrodt, Inc, and (3) is a board member for Medolac, Inc.

MENDAX, Inc, Pediatrix Medical Group, 1301 Concord Terrace, Sunrise, FL 33323, USA
E-mail address: alan.spitzer@gmail.com

Clin Perinatol 44 (2017) 469–483
http://dx.doi.org/10.1016/j.clp.2017.04.005
0095-5108/17/

ability to always do the absolute best for their patients. The reality of health care is that despite best efforts and best intentions, at times, high-quality care is not achieved.

WHAT IS QUALITY?

Although there is always an effort to provide the best possible care, it is unclear how often that goal is achieved. Furthermore, one of the great difficulties that exists in making this assessment is the determination of what constitutes quality in health care. To patients, quality may mean nothing more than someone taking the time to listen to their complaint and its associated details. For a physician, provision of quality care might mean something quite different, focusing on the achievement of a certain health outcome. For a hospital or health care system, quality may center on avoidance of errors or adverse events. For a community, quality health care may be defined by appropriate access and insurance coverage for its population.

It is often fascinating to ask patients what they think about a physician who they think is a wonderful doctor. Their responses may be so vague ("She has a great bedside manner." or "He spent an entire hour with me.") as to be undefinable and unmeasurable, yet they exist as an essential component of quality for that individual patient. In contrast, a clinician may have spectacular measured outcome results, but if he or she is abrupt with patients, patients may think that treatment has not been entirely successful, even if clinical improvement is apparent and the problem is resolved. Some patients may not receive optimal care until their story is heard, evaluated, and dissected in detail, often requiring an in-depth assessment of a variety of factors that may not even be apparent to patients, yet are critical to resolving the issue at hand. Until all appropriate concerns are identified and addressed, the outcome may be poor and no one, patient or clinician, will think that quality care was delivered.

It is, therefore, safe to state that quality in health care means different things from different perspectives; understanding the issue of quality care requires thoughtful appreciation of many complex and distinct aspects of medical practice. In recognition of this complexity in defining quality, the Institute for Healthcare Improvement (IHI) has developed its Triple Aim, which attempts in a very simple way to define health care quality as inclusively as possible.[1] In the Triple Aim, there are 3 fundamental goals:

1. Improving the overall patient care experience (for the neonate, this must include the family's experience as well)
2. Enhancing population health (which means continuing to improve outcomes)
3. Achieving the first two provisions in the Triple Aim with the least possible cost to the health care system

Traditionally, the health care system has not been concerned about such issues. Providers treated patients based on what was learned during training, focusing on the individual patient in a specific clinical situation, with limited consideration of costs of care or outcomes of populations of patients. Prospective, randomized clinical trials were the core of medical practice change and improvement, and measurement of outcomes was uncommon except in research programs. The use of large patient databases to measure population-based outcomes and support improvements and advances was not thought to be terribly relevant and was not a critical component of the health care system.[2–4]

This view on improvement in medical practice has been changing. This change was likely first driven by collaborating groups that began to demonstrate that large databases and a specific focus on outcome improvement could address certain issues that might not necessarily be answered by prospective trials. For example, in pediatrics, the Children's Oncology Group, using well-defined protocols and data collection, demonstrated dramatic clinical improvement in a variety of children's cancers.[5] The Cystic Fibrosis Foundation, initially founded by patients and families, developed a robust network of specialized cystic fibrosis (CF) centers across the country and used sharing of data, organized in a detailed patient registry, to identify variations in practices and outcomes and drive dramatic improvements in outcomes for patients with CF.[6] In neonatal medicine, the Vermont-Oxford Collaborative has had a profound effect on neonatal practice, altering the approach to many common neonatal problems, while continuously assessing outcomes, especially for the low birth weight infant.[7] Pediatrix Medical Group (now MEDNAX, Inc) developed a Clinical Data Warehouse (CDW) to examine the outcomes for its neonatal practices, which has resulted in more than 100 publications to date.[8]

This approach of using large, collaborative patient registries to measure outcomes and support practice improvements has distinct potential benefits as compared with the traditional randomized control trial paradigm, including (1) assessing outcomes over large populations that could allow for novel analyses and comparisons with greater statistical power; (2) incorporating large numbers of clinical providers in diverse geographic and practice settings; (3) comparing variations in practices and outcomes among centers and providers; (4) comparing variations in outcomes among different populations; and (5) ongoing monitoring of safety considerations and adverse events. Increasing attention has been paid to the collection and evaluation of data in large patient populations; now, many similar networks exist throughout pediatrics and medicine. Although the potential impact of these networks and this type of large data collection is substantial, the question of what actual improvements in outcomes have been seen can still be asked. In particular, has big data improved the quality of care in the NICU?

THE PATH TO QUALITY IMPROVEMENT

Traditionally, improvement in medicine was driven by research. Specific efforts to address quality and safety by practitioners focused on a backward-looking approach, whereby adverse events or outcomes were reviewed in morbidity and mortality rounds or clinical-pathologic conferences, and lessons learned from those reviews were used to inform future care. In general, clinical providers focused on this historical review system of safety, and allowed research laboratories to drive change through new discoveries and innovations. For decades, this research-driven approach led to dramatic improvements in the practice of medicine, as new drug therapies, new diagnostic modalities, and new surgical techniques led to significant enhancements of both life expectancy and quality of life.

At the start of this millennium, however, several highly visible organizations in medicine began to question this system and argued that much more could be done to enhance not only the outcome for a single patient but also for populations of patients. In 2001, the Institute of Medicine (now the Health and Medicine Division of the National Academies of Science, Engineering, and Medicine) published a critical document, entitled "Crossing the Quality Chasm."[9] In this document, they pointed out several disturbing aspects of health care in the United States: (1) the health care delivery system did not provide consistent, high-quality care to all people; (2) health care had grown increasingly complex and subspecialized; as a result, (3) the health care system was poorly organized to meet the needs of the public, which was now living longer; and (4) various health care groups, including physicians, hospitals, and other entities, essentially worked in silos, failing to share information and data that would ensure care that is appropriate, effective, timely, and safe. In addition to advocating for a marked reorganizational effort in American medicine, they also stated that "carefully designed, evidence-based care processes, supported by automated clinical information and decision-support systems, offer the greatest promise of achieving the best outcomes from care."[9] Furthermore, they urged a fundamental change in the traditional approach to reimbursement for care. Historically, physicians and hospitals have been reimbursed on a fee-for-service basis; if you treated a patient, you were paid for providing the service, and the patient's outcome was irrelevant to the reimbursement (though clearly not to the patient). This document proposed instead that physicians and hospitals should be reimbursed based on patient outcomes and not on the traditional fee-for-service approach. They urged the alignment of payment policy with quality improvement at all levels within the health care system. This document and these recommendations—though still in a process of evolution even today—nonetheless initiated the march toward quality and quality improvement throughout medicine in this country.

Shortly after the publication and dissemination of this document, the American Board of Medical Specialties also began urging its members to rethink their recertification processes to include quality improvement awareness as a vital part of ongoing Maintenance of Certification.[10] Although a controversial step in many medical specialties, it did serve as a factor in enhancing physician and practitioner awareness of the growing role of data collection and quality improvement in basic medical practice.

QUALITY IMPROVEMENT IN NEONATAL MEDICINE

As a specialty, neonatal medicine is quite young. One can point to the death of Patrick Bouvier Kennedy, born to President John F. Kennedy in August 1963, as the event that was primarily responsible for the development of the NICU in the United States.[11] Patrick Kennedy's death demonstrated that even the infant son of the President of the United States could not be appropriately treated and expect to survive with the technology available at that time. Shortly afterward, a series of NICUs began to appear across the country, first in the largest medical centers (notably at Yale, Vanderbilt, and Stanford) and then more broadly throughout the country over the ensuing decades. The neonate remained, however, a novel type of patient in most pediatricians' experience, whose treatment was uncertain at best and whose outcome was essentially unknown. Consequently, people caring for this new category of intensive care patients were intensely interested in the outcome of care; few specialties in medicine were as ideally set up for quality improvement as neonatology. In neonatal medicine, from the very infancy of the specialty, outcome measurement was a key component of care, primarily in research programs at first and more recently as a part of large-scale quality improvement efforts.

As might be expected, though, with a new patient population, the neonate, there were a variety of therapeutic approaches to management, a rapid development of new treatment strategies, and the introduction of new medications and types of equipment, all at such a rapid pace that by the time one could assess what happened to patients treated in a specific manner, much had already changed in NICU practice. Attempts at evaluating neonatal care practices using traditional research modalities had limitations; most evaluations were single-center based, and even those studies that were multicenter often had confounding variables that were difficult to incorporate into the trial. For example, the HiFi trial that first studied the role of high-frequency ventilation in neonatal management specifically outlined how the high-frequency ventilator should be used; but other practices varied significantly between participating centers, including the use of conventional ventilation, delivery room care, and fluid and nutritional management.[12] Whether the prospective randomized trial was as truly immaculate in its design as hoped for was, therefore, always a question.

The practice of neonatology consequently lurched forward in a somewhat haphazard manner but with solid evidence of significant progress. By the early 1980s, 2 decades after the death of President Kennedy's son, survival of an infant that size and gestation (34 weeks) was essentially a given and the benefits of NICUs were readily demonstrated by a dramatic decrease in infant mortality both in this country and around the world (**Fig. 1**).

As with improvements seen in many other branches of medicine, by the year 2000, this improvement in neonatal survival gave rise to a sense of self-satisfaction and accomplishment among neonatologists when they retrospectively examined how far the specialty had come during the prior 4 decades. About this time, however, several elements changed in neonatal practice. First, the early torrential pace of innovation in the NICU began to slow. It became possible to observe patient outcomes over months to years, allowing more meaningful assessment of comparative interventions. Second, advances in computer technology made the collection of large volumes of patient data and the statistical evaluation of that data much simpler than had ever been the case previously. The importance of the electronic database, or data warehouse, using data from different centers, added immeasurably to the robust nature of collections of what has been referred to as big data. Finally, external pressure from society and payers to bridge the quality chasm combined with these other changes to compel neonatologists to examine their outcomes and to search for improvement methodology with novel approaches.

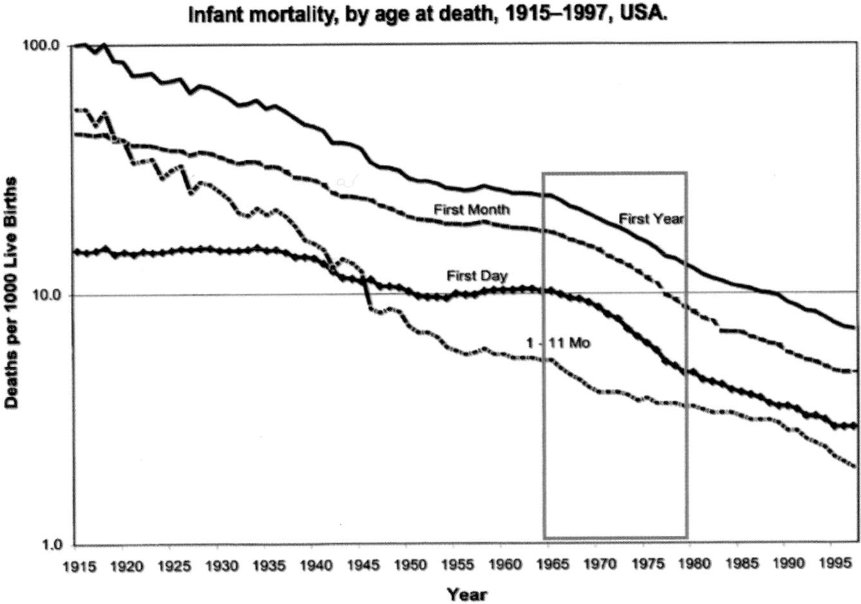

Fig. 1. Infant mortality by age at death, 1915 to 1997. The bracketed area demonstrates the rapid decline in infant mortality in the 15 years following the establishment of neonatal intensive care in the United States. (*Modified from* Wegman ME. Infant mortality in the 20th century. J Nutrition 2001;131:401S–8S; with permission.)

OUTCOMES AND IMPROVEMENT: THE STANDARD FOR THE TWENTY-FIRST CENTURY

Sensing the new capability of defining better neonatal outcomes, several organizations took up the challenge of understanding how NICU patients could be best managed. Although there are now several outstanding groups dedicated to quality outcomes in neonatal medicine, perhaps 4 can be singled out as the early leaders in this regard.

The Vermont-Oxford Network

Founded in 1988, the Vermont-Oxford Network (VON) began collecting data in 1989 and now includes more than 1000 international NICUs that submit outcome data to the network.[13] They have more than 2 million infants in their database and more than 63 million patient days of information, used in support of their mission "to improve the quality and safety of medical care for newborn infants and their families through a coordinated program of research, education, and quality improvement projects." Since its inception, VON has served as the gold standard used by many institutions to assess how their neonates are doing based on the outcome data collected and shared through VON. Although VON initially collected data only on very-low-birth-weight infants (<1500 g), they have expanded their data collection to all infants, if desired by an institution, and have published numerous articles related to outcomes as well as supporting prospective clinical comparative outcome trials and collaborative quality improvement efforts.

California Perinatal Quality Care Collaborative

As has often been the case, the state of California was one of the first to acknowledge the importance of examining outcomes for its NICU infants. In the 1990s, there was both state and payer activity to promote outcome reporting in California, giving rise to the California Perinatal Quality Care Collaborative (CPQCC).[14] At present, more than 90% of NICU infants have data reporting on their outcomes, which are used by enrolling institutions, payers, and the state to monitor NICU success. On their Web site are many toolkits designed to enhance care and outcomes, and they have also established ongoing collaboratives to share and disseminate ideas (www.cpqcc.org). CPQCC has also published outcome data on a variety of neonatal issues.

The Eunice Kennedy Shriver National Institute of Child Health and Human Development Neonatal Network

The Neonatal Network was organized in 1986. It was "established to conduct multi-center clinical trials and observational studies in neonatal medicine to reduce infant morbidity and mortality and to promote healthy outcomes."[15] Membership in the Neonatal Network is competitive and is primarily confined to some of the major academic programs in the United States. The network has not traditionally collected data on all infants admitted to the participating NICUs, but that has now been expanded in some units. The hallmark of the Neonatal Network is the publication of their findings, which have had a profound effect on improving neonatal practice; as of September 2016, 323 publications were listed on the Eunice Kennedy Shriver National Institute of Child Health and Human Development (NICHD) Web site.

MEDNAX, Inc (Pediatrix Medical Group)

MEDNAX is a unique entity among this group of outcome-oriented organizations. MEDNAX (originally Pediatrix Medical Group) was formed in 1979 by Dr Roger Medel, who began to recruit neonatal practices to join this private practice organization, eventually reaching more than 225 practices in 34 states plus Puerto Rico. Presently, practices in MEDNAX care for nearly 25% of NICU patients in the Unites States each year, providing an extraordinary patient volume for outcome assessment and quality improvement. In 1996, MEDNAX began its development of a proprietary electronic health record, which subsequently progressed into the larger MEDNAX CDW, which allows clinical evaluation and research using data from patients in each of the now 300+ NICUs in the company. More than 130 articles related to NICU outcomes have been published by MEDNAX physicians since the year 2000.

Although these 4 organizations may be considered among the first organizations focused on neonatal-perinatal outcomes research and improvement, there are now several other neonatal-perinatal collaboratives, with similar goals, active at state, regional, and national levels. State-based perinatal quality collaboratives, in particular, have assumed significant roles in using structured quality improvement methods to advance population-level outcome improvements for mothers and babies.[16]

INFLUENCING OUTCOMES IN NEONATAL PRACTICE: THE ROLE OF BIG DATA

Each of the 4 organizations noted have had extensive data collection as the centerpiece of their efforts to improve neonatal outcomes, developing new approaches to paper or electronic data abstraction and storage that are typically expensive and time consuming. Obviously, the organizations supporting these efforts think that the expense is worthwhile and that the information gained is essential in improving neonatal outcomes for the infants in their charge. But has that been effectively shown to date?

To answer this question, one first needs to establish some ground rules for distinguishing continuous quality improvement (CQI) from research, the other method widely acknowledged for enhancing outcomes. Although there is some overlap in methodology, research and quality improvement are quite different. Research refers to the testing of a novel idea, method, drug, device, or surgical approach in the treatment of a patient. *Novel* is the key word, as the researcher is examining something new. During research, measurement of carefully collected outcome data is a cardinal part of the process. In contrast, CQI, which also relies heavily on outcome data, involves the application of *already established approaches* to determine whether a particular strategy is more likely to enhance outcomes and to determine the best systems to implement those strategies effectively and reliably. For example, the introduction of surfactant during the 1980s and 1990s represented a novel drug for the neonate that required extensive research to establish its effectiveness and long-term effects, in addition to its dose and dosing schedule. CQI could then use large data from multiple institutions to better compare and understand different approaches to the use of surfactant in different systems and optimize protocols for surfactant use to specific contexts.

In attempting to assess the effectiveness of big data and neonatal quality improvement efforts, one needs to look at the respective roles of research versus CQI in the past several decades of neonatal medicine. How much of the improvement in neonatal outcomes can be attributed to research and how much to CQI?

If one accepts the concept that pure research involves the study of a novel therapy or approach to care, then it is helpful to examine when some of the game-changing therapies in newborn medicine were originally introduced:

- Surfactant (1967,[17] 1980[18])
- Neonatal Resuscitation Program (1987[19])
- Prenatal glucocorticoids (1972[20])

- Intravenous alimentation (1968[21])
- Continuous positive airway pressure and noninvasive ventilation (1970–1971[22])
- High-frequency ventilation (1980[23,24])
- Hypothermia and head-cooling for hypoxic-ischemic encephalopathy (1994–1998, more widespread 2005[25,26])
- Vitamin A for bronchopulmonary dysplasia (BPD) prevention (1985[27])
- Indomethacin for patent ductus arteriosus closure, intraventricular hemorrhage prevention (1978,[28] 1988[29])
- Steroid therapy for BPD (1985[30])
- Inhaled nitric oxide for persistent pulmonary hypertension of the newborn and respiratory failure (1993[31])
- Ultrasound, computed tomography, MRI for neurologic assessment (1970–80)
- Cryotherapy, laser surgery, bevacizumab for retinopathy of prematurity (ROP) (1985–2007[32,33])

Although this list is only partial, it highlights some of the most important *novel* therapies that have dramatically altered treatment and outcomes in the NICU. It should be noted that most of these advances became available well before the year 2005, which is around when systematic quality improvement efforts began to emerge as an important facet of practice in neonatal medicine (the American Academy of Pediatrics introduced Part IV CQI as part of Maintenance of Certification in 2008).

Progress toward reducing neonatal mortality, perhaps the most easily measured neonatal quality outcome, can then be examined in this context. If trends in neonatal mortality (**Fig. 2**) are closely examined, 3 phases can be identified:

1. 1990 to 1998: a period in which some of the novel therapies were still being introduced and mortality dropped significantly
2. 1998 to 2005: a plateau phase in which NICU change was modest and infant mortality improved only marginally
3. 2005 to present: the era in which CQI became a progressively widespread phenomenon and mortality again began to decrease significantly

Given the timing of the notable research advances listed earlier, this would suggest the recent improvement in mortality in the third phase of the graph is not likely to be attributable to the development of a novel new therapy or intervention.

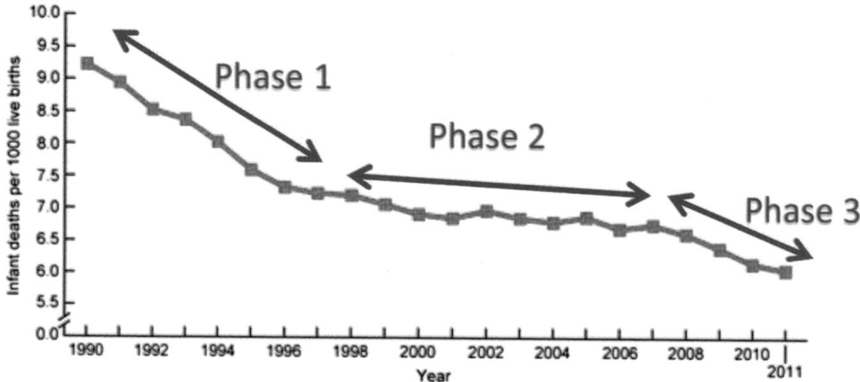

Fig. 2. The decline in neonatal mortality from 1990 to 2011 in the United States. (*Data from* National Vital Statistics Mortality Data.)

Similar to national trends, changes in mortality rates corresponding to the increase in CQI efforts can be seen in the MEDNAX, Inc CDW (**Fig. 3**). Before 2000, prior to systematic CQI initiatives, there was a steady mortality rate of about 2.6% to 2.8%. With the initial CQI efforts, the mortality began to decrease. Following the introduction of the 100,000 Babies CQI project in 2006, mortality declined significantly.[34] The VON recently reported outcomes for nearly 700 NICUs from 2005 to 2014, showing a decrease in in-hospital mortality rates for very-low-birth-weight infants in those NICUs from 14.0% in 2005 to 10.9% in 2014, with similar decreases in several important morbidities.[35] Therefore, if one accepts the concept that the focus on outcome measurement and organized quality improvement have been primary drivers for change in the NICU since 2005, then it does seem as if data-driven quality improvement has had an important impact in the current era.

Another way to examine the CQI effect, perhaps, is to review the work of the NICHD Neonatal Network. The Neonatal Network is composed of 17 of the finest academic centers in the United States. No group has been more persuasive in influencing neonatal care, not only in this country but around the world. Their controlled trials set the gold standard for the conduct of research, yet it is important to examine more precisely what the nature of their investigations has been. If one reviews the publications of the NICHD Neonatal Network, some very interesting aspects of their work can be discerned. Although the network is regarded as the paramount neonatal research group in the country, its publications reveal something slightly different. The network published 294 articles between 1991 and 2014.[36] In attempting to categorize these publications, the author examined whether the research findings fell into

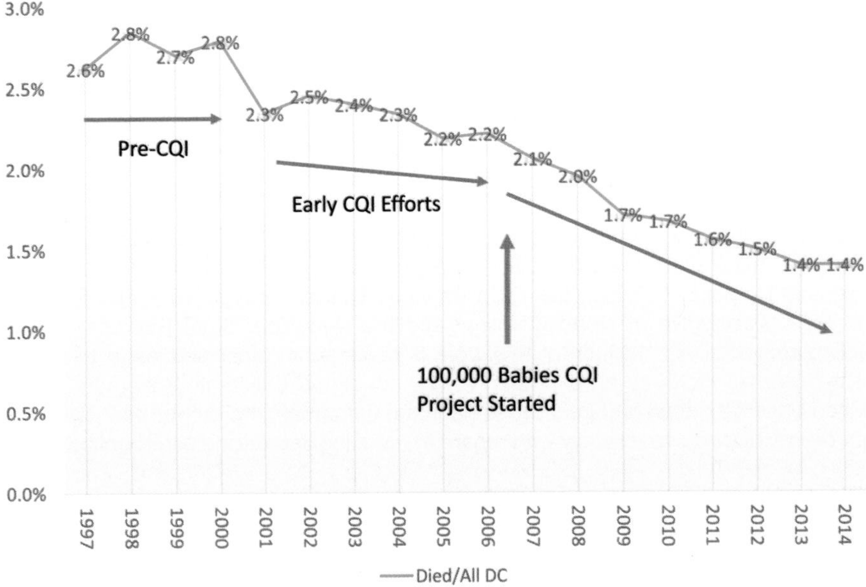

Fig. 3. Pediatrix Medical Group (MEDNAX, Inc) neonatal mortality data from 1997 to 2014. The *y* axis shows the mortality rate in Pediatrix NICUs during this period. The Pre-CQI era refers to a time when no organized CQI efforts were in place. Beginning in 2001, a director of quality improvement was appointed and CQI was initiated in the organization. From 2006 to 2007, a concerted effort in quality improvement called the 100,000 Babies Campaign was designed to focus on many aspects of modifiable neonatal outcomes. (*Data from* MEDNAX PSO, LLC.)

the following categories: (1) scientific assessment studies, which are essentially pilot trials to see if a therapy is reasonable and worth pursuing further; (2) prospective randomized trials, in which *novel* strategic approaches to care are being evaluated; (3) observational outcome studies, which examine the outcomes of some therapeutic approach in a relatively large population sample but do not necessarily have a comparison component; (4) quality outcomes or comparative outcomes research, which apply 2 established management efforts to determine whether one is more effective than the other; and (5) review articles. Although the author is certain that one might disagree with some of his categorizations for individual publications, he suspects that there would be reasonable agreement on most. What one finds is the following:

- Observational outcome studies: 64%
- Prospective randomized trials: 14%
- Scientific assessment studies: 11%
- Quality improvement/comparative outcome research studies: 9%
- Review articles: 2%

Thus, 73% of the network's publications could be classified as having a significant quality outcomes message. This observation in no way reduces the importance of the work of this outstanding collaborative group, whose value to neonatal practice cannot be overstated, but rather points out the fact that much of the improvement in neonatal care is not the result of emerging novel therapies but rather the thoughtful application, evaluation, and data collection to determine which approach results in *optimal* NICU care. The network has, therefore, performed high-quality research but primarily research in achieving quality outcomes as a primary part of its mission.

A CONCERTED APPROACH TO QUALITY IMPROVEMENT

In addition to being at least partly responsible for the reductions in neonatal mortality since 2000, a substantial and growing body of literature strongly suggests that a concerted approach to CQI throughout the field has resulted in significant improvements in a wide range of specific neonatal outcomes. Examples are documented in countless publications of focused quality improvement initiatives from single centers; in addition, large-scale improvements in outcomes from CQI initiatives have been shared in important publications from groups including VON, MEDNAX, the NICHD Neonatal Network, CPQCC, the Ohio Perinatal Quality Collaborative, the Perinatal Quality Collaborative of North Carolina, and the New York State Perinatal Quality Collaborative.[34,35,37–41] Much of this work is reviewed in other articles in this issue of this journal. Here, as an example of how concerted quality improvement efforts based on large datasets can improve neonatal outcomes, the author describes CQI efforts in MEDNAX, specifically with regard to reducing necrotizing enterocolitis (NEC).

Improvements in Necrotizing Enterocolitis in MEDNAX

MEDNAX neonatology began as a collaboration of private practice groups, focused on the clinical care of the NICU population; the outcome of patients was always of the highest priority. To best assess outcomes, a proprietary electronic medical record was developed by the organization to enter data and extract outcome information. The elimination of patient bias was achieved through *automated data extraction* from the daily medical record note entered by the clinicians. As the organization grew, the tabulated data collected provided a great deal of information on the changes in neonatal practice in this country and information on which approaches produced the best outcomes for babies. Starting in 2005, quality improvement initiatives became a mandatory part of neonatal practice in MEDNAX, with broad-scale improvement efforts complemented by focused initiatives targeting specific issues, such ROP, NEC, neonatal infection, and unnecessary medication administration.[34]

In 2007, clinicians in MEDNAX began a concerted effort to try to increase the rates of human milk use throughout the organization. An ongoing series of Quality Improvement Summits was organized to educate physicians on the values of human milk feeding, with many of the country's leading experts in neonatal nutrition as speakers. MEDNAX practices were invited to present their efforts in increasing human milk use in their NICUs as well as problems that they encountered and how they attempted to overcome barriers to human milk use. Most importantly, the MEDNAX CDW allowed them to see results of their efforts in real time by tracking outcomes, including: (1) use of human milk in the first week of life, (2) rates of human milk use in the NICU on a weekly basis, and (3) rates of human milk use at time of discharge from the NICU. **Fig. 4** demonstrates rates of human milk use in the first week of life from 2007 to 2015 during this CQI effort; the percentage of infants receiving human milk in the first week of life increased from 47% in 2007% to 78% in 2015, a 66% increase. This increase was accompanied by a reduction in the rates of NEC in the same NICU population during the same interval, shown in **Fig. 5**; the overall rate of NEC decreased from 6.8% in 2007 to 3.6% in 2015, a 47% decrease. In addition, the rate of surgical NEC decreased from 2.3% to 0.9%, a 61% decrease; sepsis rates decreased from 21% to 11%. Estimated costs of care for an infant with surgical NEC is approximately $198,000 per infant, approximately $50,000 more than the costs for a matched group of infants without NEC.[42] Thus, approximately $6.9 million was saved with the

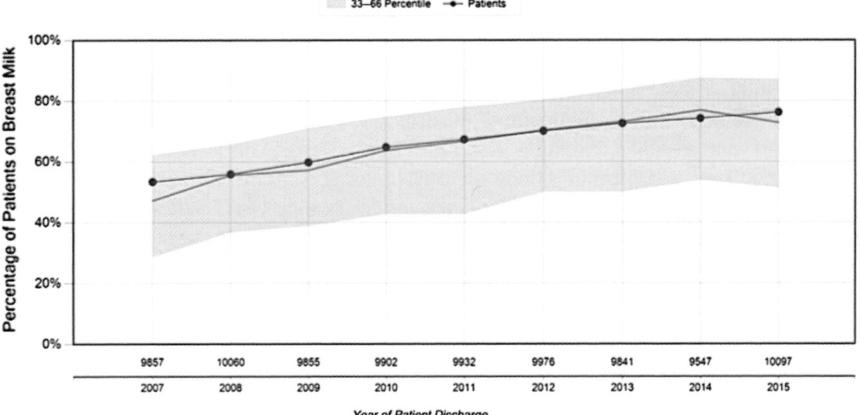

Fig. 4. Pediatrix Medical Group (MEDNAX, Inc) CDW illustration indicating the annual rate of human milk use in the first week of life for all Pediatrix neonatal sites between 2007 and 2015. This report, the information contained herein, and the underlying data from which the report is drawn are proprietary and constitute Patient Safety Work Product (PSWP) pursuant to the Patient Safety and Quality Improvement Act of 2005 and the regulations promulgated thereunder. Accordingly, this PSWP is both (1) privileged (not subject to any subpoena, order, or discovery request and not admissible as evidence in any kind of proceeding) and (2) confidential (not to be further disclosed for any purpose). (*Data from* MEDNAX PSO, LLC.)

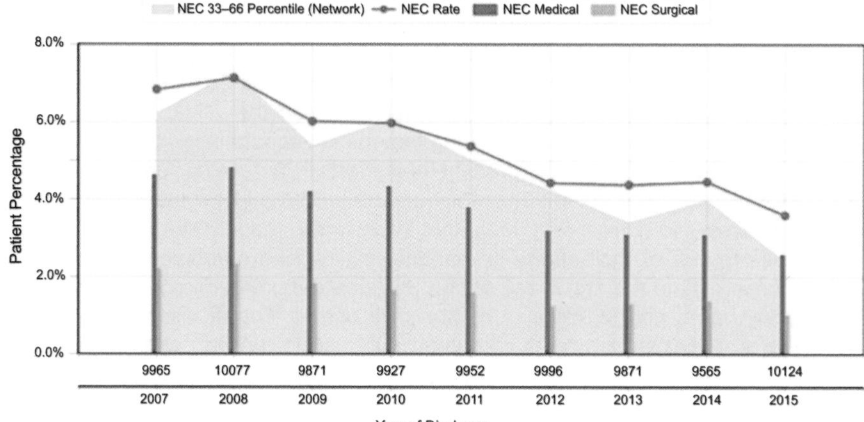

Fig. 5. Pediatrix Medical Group outcome data on NEC between 2007 and 2015. Rates of medical and surgical NEC are indicated as well as the overall rate of NEC, which declines substantially. This report, the information contained herein, and the underlying data from which the report is drawn are proprietary and constitute Patient Safety Work Product (PSWP) pursuant to the Patient Safety and Quality Improvement Act of 2005 and the regulations promulgated thereunder. Accordingly, this PSWP is both (1) privileged (not subject to any subpoena, order, or discovery request and not admissible as evidence in any kind of proceeding) and (2) confidential (not to be further disclosed for any purpose). (*Data from* MEDNAX PSO, LLC.)

improvements in human milk use and the reductions in NEC in our premature infant population.

Importantly, these improvements were not the result of some miraculous new medication or therapy that was suddenly introduced. Rather, the application of a well-researched and readily available product, human milk, applied consistently and thoughtfully, had a profound effect on outcomes for infants and the cost of care. Without question, the IHI Triple Aim objectives for quality were directly met: a better patient experience for the individual infant and family, enhancement of population outcomes, and provision of care at a substantially reduced cost.

SUMMARY

During the past decade, the emergence of outcome measurement and quality improvement in the NICU, far more than the introduction of new research approaches or novel therapies, has had a profound effect on improving outcomes for premature neonates. Collection of outcome data, review of those data, and strategies to identify and resolve problems using CQI methods can dramatically improve patient outcomes. It is likely that further initiatives in quality improvement will continue to have additional beneficial effects for the neonate.

REFERENCES

1. Berwick DM, Nolan TW, Whittington J. The triple aim: care, health, and cost. Health Aff 2008;27(3):759–69.

2. Fiore LD, Lavori PW. Integrating randomized comparative effectiveness research with patient care. N Engl J Med 2016;374(22):2152–8.
3. Schneeweiss S. Learning from big health care data. N Engl J Med 2014;370(23): 2161–3.
4. Obermeyer Z, Emanuel EJ. Predicting the future - big data, machine learning, and clinical medicine. N Engl J Med 2016;375(13):1216–9.
5. Aplenc R, Fisher BT, Huang YS, et al. Merging of the National Cancer Institute-funded Cooperative Oncology Group data with an administrative data source to develop a more effective platform for clinical trial analysis and comparative effectiveness research: a report from the Children's Oncology Group. Pharmacoepidemiol Drug Saf 2012;21(Suppl 2):37–43.
6. Quon BS, Goss CH. A story of success: continuous quality improvement in cystic fibrosis care in the USA. Thorax 2011;66(12):1106–8.
7. Horbar JD. The Vermont Oxford Network: evidence-based quality improvement for neonatology. Pediatrics 1999;103(1 Suppl E):350–9.
8. Spitzer AR, Ellsbury DL, Handler D, et al. The Pediatrix BabySteps Data Warehouse and the Pediatrix QualitySteps improvement project system–tools for "meaningful use" in continuous quality improvement. Clin Perinatol 2010;37(1): 49–70.
9. Institute of Medicine. Committee on Quality of Health Care in A. Crossing the quality chasm: a new health system for the 21st century. Washington, DC: 2001.
10. Batmangelich S, Adamowski S. Maintenance of certification in the United States: a progress report. J Contin Educ Health Prof 2004;24(3):134–8.
11. M.D BL. A Kennedy baby's life and death. 2013: Section D; Column 0; Science Desk; AFTER THE FACT. p. 3.
12. High-frequency oscillatory ventilation compared with conventional mechanical ventilation in the treatment of respiratory failure in preterm infants. The HIFI Study Group. N Engl J Med 1989;320(2):88–93.
13. Vermont Oxford Network. Available at: https://public.vtoxford.org/about-us/. Accessed November 16, 2016.
14. California Perinatal Quality Care Collaborative. Available at: https://www.cpqcc.org/about-us/mission-vision. Accessed November 16, 2016.
15. Eunice Kennedy Shriver Neonatal Research Network. Available at: https://neonatal.rti.org/about/network.cfm. Accessed September 18, 2016.
16. Centers for Disease Control and Prevention Perinatal Quality Collaborative Guide Working Group. Developing and sustaining perinatal quality collaboratives: a resource guide for states. 2016. Available at: https://www.cdc.gov/reproductivehealth/maternalinfanthealth/pdf/best-practices-for-developing-and-sustaining-perinatal-quality-collaboratives_tagged508.pdf. Accessed April 26, 2017.
17. Chu J, Clements JA, Cotton EK, et al. Neonatal pulmonary ischemia. I. Clinical and physiological studies. Pediatrics 1967;40(4:Suppl):709–82.
18. Fujiwara T, Maeta H, Chida S, et al. Artificial surfactant therapy in hyaline-membrane disease. Lancet 1980;1(8159):55–9.
19. American Academy of Pediatrics Neonatal Resuscitation Program. Available at: https://www.aap.org/en-us/continuing-medical-education/life-support/NRP/Pages/History.aspx. Accessed November 16, 2016.
20. Liggins GC, Howie RN. A controlled trial of antepartum glucocorticoid treatment for prevention of the respiratory distress syndrome in premature infants. Pediatrics 1972;50(4):515–25.
21. Wilmore DW, Dudrick SJ. Growth and development of an infant receiving all nutrients exclusively by vein. JAMA 1968;203(10):860–4.

22. Gregory GA, Kitterman JA, Phibbs RH, et al. Treatment of the idiopathic respiratory-distress syndrome with continuous positive airway pressure. N Engl J Med 1971;284(24):1333–40.
23. Bland RD, Kim MH, Light MJ, et al. High frequency mechanical ventilation in severe hyaline membrane disease an alternative treatment? Crit Care Med 1980; 8(5):275–80.
24. Boros SJ, Campbell K. A comparison of the effects of high frequency–low tidal volume and low frequency–high tidal volume mechanical ventilation. J Pediatr 1980;97(1):108–12.
25. Towfighi J, Housman C, Heitjan DF, et al. The effect of focal cerebral cooling on perinatal hypoxic-ischemic brain damage. Acta Neuropathol 1994;87(6): 598–604.
26. Gunn AJ, Gluckman PD, Gunn TR. Selective head cooling in newborn infants after perinatal asphyxia: a safety study. Pediatrics 1998;102(4 Pt 1):885–92.
27. Shenai JP, Chytil F, Stahlman MT. Vitamin A status of neonates with bronchopulmonary dysplasia. Pediatr Res 1985;19(2):185–8.
28. Merritt TA, DiSessa TG, Feldman BH, et al. Closure of the patent ductus arteriosus with ligation and indomethacin: a consecutive experience. J Pediatr 1978;93(4): 639–46.
29. Hanigan WC, Kennedy G, Roemisch F, et al. Administration of indomethacin for the prevention of periventricular-intraventricular hemorrhage in high-risk neonates. J Pediatr 1988;112(6):941–7.
30. Avery GB, Fletcher AB, Kaplan M, et al. Controlled trial of dexamethasone in respirator-dependent infants with bronchopulmonary dysplasia. Pediatrics 1985;75(1):106–11.
31. Kinsella JP, Abman SH. Inhalational nitric oxide therapy for persistent pulmonary hypertension of the newborn. Pediatrics 1993;91(5):997–8.
32. Tasman W. Management of retinopathy of prematurity. Ophthalmology 1985; 92(8):995–9.
33. Chung EJ, Kim JH, Ahn HS, et al. Combination of laser photocoagulation and intravitreal bevacizumab (Avastin) for aggressive zone I retinopathy of prematurity. Graefes Arch Clin Exp Ophthalmol 2007;245(11):1727–30.
34. Ellsbury DL, Clark RH, Ursprung R, et al. A multifaceted approach to improving outcomes in the NICU: the Pediatrix 100 000 Babies Campaign. Pediatrics 2016;137(4) [pii:e20150389].
35. Horbar JD, Edwards EM, Greenberg LT, et al. Variation in performance of neonatal intensive care units in the United States. JAMA Pediatr 2017;171(3): e164396.
36. Eunice Kennedy Shriver Neonatal Research Network. https://neonatal.rti.org/. Accessed November 15, 2015.
37. Wirtschafter DD, Powers RJ, Pettit JS, et al. Nosocomial infection reduction in VLBW infants with a statewide quality-improvement model. Pediatrics 2011; 127(3):419–26.
38. Walsh M, Laptook A, Kazzi SN, et al. A cluster-randomized trial of benchmarking and multimodal quality improvement to improve rates of survival free of bronchopulmonary dysplasia for infants with birth weights of less than 1250 grams. Pediatrics 2007;119(5):876–90.
39. Kaplan HC, Lannon C, Walsh MC, et al, Ohio Perinatal Quality Collaborative. Ohio statewide quality-improvement collaborative to reduce late-onset sepsis in preterm infants. Pediatrics 2011;127(3):427–35.

40. Fisher D, Cochran KM, Provost LP, et al. Reducing central line-associated bloodstream infections in North Carolina NICUs. Pediatrics 2013;132(6):e1664–71.
41. Schulman J, Stricof R, Stevens TP, et al. Statewide NICU central-line-associated bloodstream infection rates decline after bundles and checklists. Pediatrics 2011; 127(3):436–44.
42. Ganapathy V, Hay JW, Kim JH. Costs of necrotizing enterocolitis and cost-effectiveness of exclusively human milk-based products in feeding extremely premature infants. Breastfeed Med 2012;7(1):29–37.

National Quality Measures in Perinatal Medicine

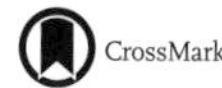

Scott A. Lorch, MD, MSCE[a,b,c,d,e,*]

KEYWORDS

• Quality measure • Perinatal care • Readmission • Mortality • Cesarean section

KEY POINTS

- There are a wide variety of quality measures that assess the quality of perinatal care at a hospital center.
- Ideal perinatal quality measures should be easy to classify and measure, show adequate reliability, and have adequate face and construct validity.
- Currently endorsed measures from the National Quality Foundation focus primarily on preventive care, mode and timing of delivery, and hospital infection rates.
- Future work should address what aspect of quality is assessed by current measures and research gaps including drivers of high quality care.

As health care costs continue to increase in both the developed and developing world, stakeholders and providers have placed an increased emphasis on providing improved outcomes at the lowest possible cost.[1] A key element to this goal is the development of quality measures to assess how well the system provides high-value care and best outcomes. National groups, such as the National Quality Forum (NQF), serve as a source for collating and endorsing measures of perinatal quality.[2] Although these measures may assess an individual hospital's care, these measures may also be used for other purposes, such as the public reporting of data[3,4] and payment strategies, such as pay-for-performance programs.[5–8]

Financial Disclosure: No financial relationships relevant to this article to disclose.
Conflict of Interest: No conflicts of interest to disclose.
Funding Source: Funded in part by AHRQ U18HS020508.

[a] Department of Pediatrics, Division of Neonatology, The Children's Hospital of Philadelphia, 2716 South Street, Room 10-251, Philadelphia, PA 19146, USA; [b] PolicyLab, The Children's Hospital of Philadelphia, 2716 South Street, Room 10-251, Philadelphia, PA 19146, USA; [c] Center for Perinatal and Pediatric Health Disparities Research, The Children's Hospital of Philadelphia, 2716 South Street, Room 10-251, Philadelphia, PA 19146, USA; [d] Department of Pediatrics, The University of Pennsylvania School of Medicine, 2716 South Street, Room 10-251, Philadelphia, PA 19146, USA; [e] Leonard Davis Institute of Health Economics, University of Pennsylvania, 3641 Locust Walk, Philadelphia, PA 19104, USA

* Corresponding author. The Children's Hospital of Philadelphia, 3535 Market Street, Suite 1029, Philadelphia, PA 19104.
E-mail address: lorch@email.chop.edu

Clin Perinatol 44 (2017) 485–509
http://dx.doi.org/10.1016/j.clp.2017.05.001
perinatology.theclinics.com
0095-5108/17/

The sheer number of endorsed metrics may lead to confusion about what these measures truly assess; how to interpret variation in these measures across hospitals, health care systems, and geographic regions; and how to use measures to drive performance improvement. This review presents the differences between *quality assessment* and *quality improvement*, as it pertains to assessing the validity and use of specific quality measures, a conceptual model for the endorsement of numerous measures of perinatal care, an overview of the types of measures endorsed for perinatal quality by NQF in 2016, and potential measures currently absent in recommendations from these national bodies. Unique challenges to the development of such measures for perinatal care, and ideal characteristics of quality metrics for quality assessment also are presented.

QUALITY ASSESSMENT VERSUS QUALITY IMPROVEMENT

Quality measures, as traditionally used by policy makers and insurers, are meant to assess quality of health care providers. Quality assessment identifies low-performing or high-performing health care providers for further intervention by a state or national public health agency; for the purposes of reimbursement, such as pay-for-performance plans in which some part of a facility's payment is tied to their outcomes on a specific set of quality measures; or for public reporting of information.[3,4] States often publicly report such statistics as the mortality rates of cardiothoracic surgeons in New York State[9] and hospital infection rates.[10] For a measure to be used for quality assessment, research needs to show (1) evidence of variation between sites, (2) adequate risk adjustment, (3) reliability and reproducibility of the measure, and (4) measure validity (**Box 1**).

Measures also may be used for quality improvement. As we see in several articles in this issue, quality improvement improves the performance of a specific health care organization, typically a single center or institution, on a measure using PDSA, or plan-do-study-act cycles. Improvement is typically assessed using run charts or other forms of evaluation at the level of the specific institution. Measures used for quality improvement need to be consistently measurable at the level of that institution, with interventions tailored to the specific issues that may be associated with a poor performance at that institution.

Thus, measures typically need to meet a different set of standards when applied across a number of centers for the purposes of quality assessment compared with

Box 1
Quality assessment versus quality improvement

Quality Assessment

- Measures the care of a specific health care entity, whether provider, facility, or region
- Used by public health agencies and insurers
- Recommended data and research include
  - Variation in measure across health care entities
  - Reproducibility and reliability of the measure
  - Validity of measure

Quality Improvement

- Measures improvement in process or outcome at a specific institution or set of institutions
- Used by individual hospitals, public health agencies, and insurers
- A facility's performance on the measure is assessed using run charts and other statistical processing tools

quality improvement at a single center. Despite the differences in quality assessment and quality improvement, measures may be used for both depending on their characteristics.

CONCEPTUAL MODEL FOR QUALITY MEASURES

A significant challenge faced by providers and stakeholders is the proliferation of measures either endorsed by a national group, such as NQF, or unendorsed but used by other stakeholders, such as the Vermont Oxford Network. This proliferation of measures is not confined to perinatal care; there is a similar landscape of quality measures for pediatric and adult care. Why is this? It helps to examine quality measures within the lens of a conceptual framework, such as a "flashlight" theory of quality (**Fig. 1**).[11]

First, we start with the idea that "quality" of care for a given health care provider or facility is a black box. Each quality measure is a flashlight that illuminates some aspect of this box. We can assess the measure based on 2 characteristics. First, we determine how much of the quality box the measure illuminates. It may illuminate a very small part of the box and thus assess a specific aspect of quality, or it may illuminate a much larger part of the box and thus capture many areas of quality that overlap with other quality measures. Second, we can assess how clearly the measure illuminates the box. Some measures may provide a very clear and accurate picture, with strong accuracy and reliability. Other measures provide a blurry assessment of the box, with less reliability and more noise.

Ideally, we would have a measure that illuminated the entire box, with perfect clarity. Because such a measure is not available for neonatal medicine, we see how there are numerous measures of "quality of care," which may have strong or poor correlations between them.

CHARACTERISTICS OF AN IDEAL PERINATAL QUALITY MEASURE

Stakeholders, such as NQF, use certain characteristics to assess perinatal measures (**Box 2**). These characteristics include the following:

1. *Easy to classify*: The definition of a measure should be clear to all stakeholders.
2. *Easy to measure*: Accurate data about a measure should be easy to collect. Data can come from a range of sources, including birth certificates or hospital administrative data, insurance data, or medical record/patient or provider report, ordered by the ease of obtaining such information.

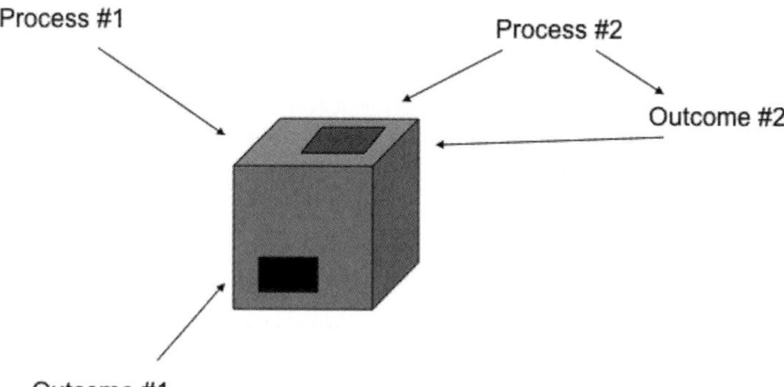

Fig. 1. Conceptual model for the use of multiple measures of perinatal quality. Different measures assess different aspects of the quality box, with different breadth and accuracy.

Box 2
Characteristics of an ideal quality measure

- Easy to classify
- Easy to measure
- High reliability and reproducibility
- Face and construct validity
- Present in sufficient numbers to minimize loss of statistical power to detect significant differences between health care providers or facilities
- Adequate risk adjustment

3. *Show adequate reliability*: Reliability of a measure assesses the consistency of the results. It is affected by the randomness of a measure. For example, measures that vary over time without any change in casemix or care delivery would have a lower reliability.
4. *Show adequate validity*: Validity of a measure assesses how well the measure assesses care quality. A measure should have face validity and construct validity. *Face validity* refers to the idea that stakeholders believe that the measure assesses quality of care. *Construct validity* refers to the idea that the measure is associated with some other measure of care quality. Construct validity may be easy or difficult to demonstrate depending on how broadly the measure illuminates the quality box and whether there are other measures that assess a similar aspect of quality to the measure of interest.

There are additional challenges specific to perinatal care. These include the following:

1. *Small number of patients and outcomes*: Although there are more than 4 million deliveries in the United States, fewer than 2% of these deliveries have a birth weight of less than 1500 g. These high-risk deliveries are not distributed equally across hospitals with obstetric services. Thus, the power to detect a difference in care between hospitals for this popular group of infants may be limited.
2. *Need for risk adjustment:* For some quality metrics, the baseline risk of developing the condition may be affected by factors outside the control of a provider, such as gestational age at birth or coexisting maternal medical conditions. The percentage of patients with these high-risk conditions measures the *casemix* of a health care provider or hospital. Any differences in casemix need to be adjusted to provide a valid assessment of a hospital's quality.
3. *Difficulty defining the measure accurately*: Clear definitions for a particular measure may be difficult. For example, bronchopulmonary dysplasia may use clinical judgment or the use of an oxygen reduction test to make a diagnosis. Similarly, measures such as neonatal death provide an incomplete assessment of a hospital's performance if fetal death, an alternative outcome of pregnancy, is not included in the assessment.

MEASURES ENDORSED BY THE NATIONAL QUALITY FORUM

NQF is a not-for-profit organization that convenes committees made up of multiple stakeholders to review and recommend submitted quality measures for endorsement along numerous topic areas, including perinatal health. There are currently 22 measures endorsed by NQF that apply to perinatal health as of 2016. These measures can be divided into 4 time periods (Appendix 1, **Box 3**):

Box 3
Endorsed measures by National Quality Forum, 2016

Time Period 1: Prenatal/Periconception
- Adult current smoking prevalence

Time Period 2: Intrapartum/Postpartum Care
- Appropriate deep venous thrombosis prophylaxis in women undergoing cesarean delivery
- Appropriate prophylactic antibiotic received within 1 hour before surgical incision: cesarean delivery
- Contraceptive care: postpartum
- Contraceptive care: most and moderately effective methods
- Contraceptive care: access to long-acting reversible method of contraception
- Incidence of episiotomy
- Intrapartum antibiotic prophylaxis for group B *Streptococcus*
- PC-01 elective delivery
- PC-02 cesarean birth
- PC-03 antenatal steroids
- Percentage of low birthweight births
- Rh immunoglobulin (Rhogam) for Rh-negative pregnant women at risk of fetal blood exposure.
- Unexpected complications in term newborns

Time Period 3: Newborn Care
- Gains in patient activation measure scores at 12 months
- Hepatitis B vaccine coverage among all live newborn infants before hospital or birthing facility discharge
- PC-05 exclusive breast milk feeding
- Pediatric all-condition readmission measure

Time Period 4: Care of the Very Low Birthweight (VLBW) Infant
- Late sepsis or meningitis in VLBW neonates (risk-adjusted)
- Neonatal blood stream infection rate (NQI 03)
- PC-04 health care–associated bloodstream infections in newborns
- Proportion of infants 22 to 29 weeks' gestation screened for retinopathy of prematurity.

Time period 1: Prenatal/Preconception: Measures in this time period focus on counseling and access to care.

Time period 2: Intrapartum/Postpartum care: Measures in this time period focus primarily on preventive therapies around delivery, mode and timing of delivery, and the outcomes of healthy term infants.

Time period 3A: Newborn care: Measures in this time period focus on general newborn care, all-condition readmission, and patient activation.

Time period 3B: Care of the very low birthweight (VLBW) infant: These measures assess hospital infection rates and screening for retinopathy of prematurity (ROP).

An overview of these measures as of 2016 follows, organized roughly by these areas. The endorsement status of these measures changes continually, so there could be the inclusion or exclusion of a specific measure. The reliability of most measures is difficult to assess given the lack of published information on this topic.

Prenatal/Preconception Time Period

Specific measures in this time period focus on processes of care including adequacy of prenatal care and counseling. A recent revision to the perinatal group of measures resulted in the unendorsement of the adequacy of prenatal care and counseling of women of childbearing age with epilepsy measures, leaving only the general smoking-cessation measure that applies to all adults as a quality measure reflective of care in this time period. As the prenatal care and counseling of women of childbearing age with epilepsy measures were only recently unendorsed, we include them in this review.

Ease of classification: Easy, as counseling and prenatal care visits either occur or do not.

Ease of measurement: Moderately difficult to difficult. Prenatal care visits are generally straightforward to measure by either self-report of the mother (as noted in birth certificates) or insurance data. On the other hand, counseling variables require specific information from patients or providers about the receipt of such counseling. This information is frequently only found in electronic health records or by self-report. Smoking prevalence can be obtained via birth certificate data[12]; but, despite the ability to easily measure and report smoking prevalence, information on cessation counseling is not easily obtained.

Validity: Moderate to strong. Counseling data are important to reduce the risk of associated congenital anomalies in women taking antiepileptic medications[13] and potential adverse neurocognitive outcomes particularly with valproate exposure.[14] Similarly, smoking cessation is important both for the health of the woman,[15] and to reduce the risk of fetal death,[16] preterm birth, and intrauterine growth retardation.[17] Adequate prenatal care has strong face validity as evidenced by publications such as *Healthy People 2020.*[18] However, there are limited data to support an association between receipt of prenatal care and improved pregnancy outcomes.[19,20] There are no studies to show variation in the rate of counseling of women taking antiepileptic drugs. In statewide studies of smoking counseling, there is variation between providers.[21]

Number of eligible patients: Generally large. These measures generally include all deliveries with the exception of some counseling measures specific to different exposures. For example, the recently retired measure of counseling of women with epilepsy applies to only 1% of the childbearing population,[22] or approximately 500,000 to 1 million women annually.[23]

Need for risk adjustment: None, as there are no known factors that should influence whether women receive recommended counseling or prenatal care.

Intrapartum/Postpartum Time Period

Mode and timing of deliveries

These measures focus on limiting early elective delivery (ie, delivery at a gestational age at 38 weeks or less without medical indications) and reducing cesarean delivery rates in nulliparous singleton pregnancies.

Ease of classification: Easy to moderately difficult. Cesarean deliveries are easy to classify based on mode of delivery. On the other hand, correctly classifying deliveries at a gestational age of less than 38 weeks is more challenging, depending on the accuracy of the data to determine the medical necessity of the early delivery.

Ease of measurement: Easy to moderately difficult. Claims datasets are typically used for these measures, with well-validated *International Classification of Diseases, Ninth Revision* (ICD-9) codes or delivery fields to identify cesarean deliveries in claims or birth certificate datasets respectively. One primary challenge is obtaining accurate gestational age data because most insurance and hospital discharge datasets do consistently not include this information through ICD-9 codes. Although gestational age is typically well coded in data that use birth certificates, data on maternal comorbidities used to help determine medical indication for an early delivery are less accurate on birth certificates than hospital administrative data.[24,25] Some endorsed measures recommend paper record collection to assess the medical necessity of early deliveries, which is more difficult to implement.

Validity: Moderate to strong. Early elective delivery at 37 to 38 weeks' gestation is associated with higher rates of respiratory distress, transient tachypnea of the newborn, and admission to the neonatal intensive care unit (NICU) compared with infants born at 39 weeks or later.[26–28] Hospital-level and provider-level variation in the rate of these deliveries exist.[29] One concerning aspect of this measure is the possible association between the passage of state and hospital policies that ban such early deliveries, the so-called "hard stop" rules and higher rate of fetal death, which would replace one set of adverse outcomes with another set.[30] Two other studies have not found such an association.[31,32]

There is more controversy related to the validity of higher cesarean delivery rates as a measure of poor care, even though national reductions in cesarean delivery rates have been the hallmark of public health campaigns for decades.[18] Hospital data from studies during the 1980s and 1990s show an association between higher hospital cesarean delivery rates and several adverse outcomes, including asphyxia and infection.[33,34] More recent multistate data from 1995 to 2005 found that hospitals with lower-than-expected rates of cesarean deliveries actually had higher rates of poorer maternal outcomes as measured by a maternal adverse composite measure, worse neonatal outcomes as measured by a neonatal adverse composite measure, and poorer patient safety as measured by 4 Agency for Healthcare Research and Quality patient safety indicators (PSIs 17–20).[35] Other studies have found an association between lower-than-expected rates of cesarean deliveries and higher rates of asphyxia.[36] Thus, although this measure has strong face validity, there are conflicting data on the construct validity of this measure.[37]

Numbers of eligible patients: Large, as all deliveries are included in the denominator and cesarean deliveries are performed at high rates in most developed countries.

Need for risk adjustment: No.

Therapies

Endorsed measures addressing therapies in the intrapartum and postpartum period are related to prophylaxis for Group B *Streptococcus* (GBS), deep vein thrombosis (DVT), or surgical infections; use of antenatal corticosteroids; provision of contraception after delivery; avoiding episiotomy; and offering of Rhogam for women whose blood type is Rh-negative.

Ease of classification: Easy, as each of these treatments are medications or therapies that are either given or not.

Ease of measurement: Difficult. None of these measures are available in standard administrative datasets except for episiotomy, and as a result, collection of these measures typically uses pharmacy claims or paper records. Some of this information, especially antenatal corticosteroid use, is now available on the most recent version of birth certificates, but the reliability of such data fields has not been published.

Validity: Strong. There is ample evidence for both the prevalence and importance of each condition that the therapies are preventing, including the following:

- High risk of neonatal infection in women not receiving antibiotic prophylaxis for GBS[38]
- High rates of DVT[39] or surgical site infections[40–42] in women receiving cesarean deliveries without appropriate prophylaxis
- High rate of mortality and neonatal morbidity in prematurely born infants who did not receive antenatal corticosteroids[43]
- Risk of iso-immunization and the development of hemolytic anemia, hydrops fetalis, and jaundice in future infants of iso-immunized Rh-negative women
- Higher risk of preterm birth and low birth weight in women with short interconception interval[44,45]

In addition, variations in each measure across facilities, states, and countries have been reported.[46]

Numbers of eligible patients: Large, as eligible women include all deliveries, those with GBS colonization, Rh-negative women, or cesarean deliveries.

Need for risk adjustment: No.

Pregnancy outcomes

Two endorsed measures focus on outcomes of pregnancy. First, the NQF-endorsed metric related to outcomes of healthy term deliveries[47] is the only outcome measure for low-risk term deliveries, identifying several potential adverse outcomes, including neonatal intensive care admission, respiratory distress, perinatal depression, and need to transfer for higher level of care.

Ease of classification: Moderately difficult, depending on the accuracy of the specified ICD-9 codes included in the measure.

Ease of measurement: Moderately difficult. The measure is designed for hospital administrative data, and thus it can be difficult to obtain the information needed to classify the infant as older than 37 weeks and heavier than 2500 g. Linking administrative data with birth certificates to obtain gestational age and birthweight information can solve this problem, but is difficult to implement.

Validity: Poor to moderate. A recent study from Florida found a 14-fold variation in hospital rates of this measure between 2004 and 2013. Hospital factors such as birth volume, level of care, and Medicaid volume were associated with higher rates.[48,49] Aside from this study, there is limited additional published information on the validity of this measure.

Numbers of eligible patients: Large. All term singleton deliveries without other serious fetal conditions are included in the denominator, although rates of these outcomes (numerator) are generally very low.

Need for risk adjustment: No, based on the measure guidelines, although the need for accurate coding to determine a low-risk delivery is essential for this measure.

Second, the measure of percentage of low birth weight deliveries is the only endorsed population health measure. Designed explicitly for state and larger population regions, it uses birth certificate data to quantify the percentage of infants born with a birth weight less than 2500 g in a region. This measure is not designed for insurers or health care providers within a given facility.

Newborn Measures

Measures for healthy newborns focus primarily on receipt of hepatitis B vaccine and exclusive breastfeeding rates. Although newborn infants fit into the pediatric all-condition readmission measure and the parents fit into the general patient activation measure, these groups per se are not a specific focus or subgroup of this metrics (see Appendix 1 for additional details), and these measures are not discussed further.

Ease of classification: Easy as receipt of the hepatitis B vaccine and formula to determine exclusive breastfeeding are either given or not.

Ease of measurement: Difficult. Both metrics require patient report or electronic health record data to obtain information.

Validity: Strong. Hepatitis B vaccine is associated with lower rates of seroconversion in newborns delivered to mothers with hepatitis B, as well as protection against contracting hepatitis B during adolescence and adulthood.[50] Similarly, exclusive breastfeeding has been associated with lower rates of asthma, allergic disease, mortality especially in developing countries, and improved growth.[51–54]

Numbers of eligible patients: Large, as all deliveries are included in the measure.

Need for risk adjustment: No.

Measures for Very Low Birthweight Infants

Measures for VLBW infants focus on infections and screening for ROP.

Infections

Infections are the most common assessment of quality of care for VLBW infants. NQF-endorsed measures include late sepsis or meningitis after 3 days of life, any neonatal bloodstream infection, and health care–associated bloodstream infections. The challenge comes in harmonizing across each of these measures of infection that are defined differently with different data sources and the absence of a measure of central-line associated bloodstream infections (CLABSI).

Ease of classification: Moderately difficult, primarily surrounding how to approach infections with coagulase-negative *Staphylococcus* rates, which are generally considered contaminants in other populations but may be a true pathogen in premature infants, and the phenomenon of "culture-negative" sepsis.

Ease of measurement: Moderately difficult to difficult. Measures that use administrative data rely on accurate coding of infections in their ICD-9 code list. However, this may be a challenge given the large number of diagnoses experienced by these infants and the limited number of ICD-9/10 code slots (12–24) included in a typical administrative dataset. Alternatively, studies may use pathology records or registry data through such organizations as the Vermont Oxford Network or the California Perinatal Quality Care Collaborative to identify eligible patients.

Validity: Moderate to strong, given that there is variation in infection rates across institutions, and that these rates vary by hospital characteristics, such as level of care.[55–58] Infants who experience 1 or more of these infections have worse outcomes, including mortality, prolonged length of stay, and chronic lung disease.[59–62] However, at the level of the facility, there are scant data to show a correlation between a facility's infection rate and rates of other adverse outcomes, such as bronchopulmonary dysplasia (BPD) or necrotizing enterocolitis (NEC).[56]

Numbers of eligible patients: Small. Overall VLBW infants account for only 1.4% to 2.0% of all deliveries in the United States. Therefore, measures that focus solely on VLBW infants suffer from the power issues around small numbers.

Need for risk adjustment: Yes, based on the measures currently endorsed that include a risk-adjustment tool that accounts for the association between infection risk and gestational age at birth. CLABSI rates have typically not been risk-adjusted.

Screening for retinopathy of prematurity
This measure assesses the percentage of infants born 22 0/7 weeks' gestation to 29 6/7 weeks' gestation who received at least 1 screening examination for ROP while hospitalized.

Ease of classification: Easy, because the screening examination was either completed or not.

Ease of measurement: Moderately difficult. Completion of this measure using the Vermont Oxford Network data requires manual data collection of the electronic or paper record. Insurance-based datasets may capture this information using CPT codes from an ophthalmologist.

Validity: Poor to moderate. Variation in screening rates has not been published, although a recent study did find variation in the method of screening between units.[63] Screening reduces the adverse visual outcomes of ROP.[64,65]

Numbers of eligible patients: Small. Measures that focus solely on VLBW infants suffer from the power issues around small numbers.

Need for risk adjustment: No.

Unendorsed Measures: Mortality and Hospital Readmission

There are a number of proposed quality measures that are not endorsed by national guidelines, but have been used either by national networks of NICUs (eg, the Vermont Oxford Network) or for other patient populations (readmission rates). The next section discusses the metrics of mortality and hospital readmission and describes potential challenges in using them as quality metrics.

Mortality as a quality measure
Neonatal death is a frequently proposed measure of quality of care because, in most medical situations, death is an easy-to-measure, easy-to-classify outcome that may reflect differences care practices after adjusting for a given patient's medical condition. However, perinatal medicine is more challenging, as pregnancies may end in a fetal death, a live birth with a neonatal death, or a live birth with a surviving infant. Also, the very low rates of neonatal and fetal death in the developed world limit the statistical power of mortality rates.

Ease of classification: Difficult. The division between a fetal death and neonatal death has been challenging, as these 2 measures are frequently assessed separately from each other. First, there is no universally accepted minimum gestational age needed to be considered a potential live birth: some states use a threshold as low as 16 weeks' gestation, whereas other states use a threshold as high as 24 weeks.[66] Differences in this definition may artificially increase or decrease a hospital's neonatal death rate by changing which infants are included in the measure.[56,67,68] Second, when assessing the care of a hospital, fetal deaths may be related to the quality of care provided by obstetricians, pediatricians, or neonatologists (preventable fetal deaths), or may be inevitable on presentation to medical care (nonpreventable fetal deaths). Because some proportion of fetal deaths may be preventable, ignoring these deaths in a neonatal death metric may again artificially increase the rates at hospitals that successfully resuscitate an infant (changing them from a fetal death to a live birth), but ultimately have the infant die.[56,67,69,70]

Ease of measurement: Moderately difficult. Mortality is easy to capture regardless of the data source. However, assigning deliveries and deaths to hospitals can be difficult depending on the percentage of infants transferred from their birth hospital. Also, sicker infants, with a younger gestational age at birth and/or greater illness severity, are more likely to be transferred, which biases against hospitals that receive large numbers of transfers. When care is split between centers for substantial periods of time at each hospital, it is difficult to assign the outcome to one or the other hospital. Most studies in this topic assign patients to the birth hospital regardless of where the death occurred, which may overestimate the impact of birth hospital on outcomes.

Validity: Strong. There is ample evidence of variation in mortality rates by the level and volume of care of the birth hospital.[56,67,69,70] Also, data from the Vermont Oxford Network shows wide variation in mortality rates from the 1990s,[71] although recently published data show a narrowing of this variation across hospitals.[55]

Number of eligible patients: Small, as typically these measures again include only VLBW infants. Even all-infant neonatal death measures are challenging given the relative rareness of neonatal death as an outcome.

Need for risk adjustment: Yes. Younger and sicker infants are more likely to die, but are not randomly distributed across perinatal hospitals in a given region.[56,67,71] Standard risk adjustment models include variables present at delivery, such as gestational age, birth weight, singleton or multiple birth, and gender. Although these models have relatively good reliability, one recent study found that mortality rates between these different levels of NICUs were only statistically significant using methods that accounted for unmeasured casemix differences, here an instrumental variables approach, and not with traditional risk-adjustment models.[56] Such findings are concerning given the need to adjust for casemix with this measure.

Although an intuitively appealing measure of quality, concerns about the small numbers, need for risk adjustment, and the need to include some but not all fetal deaths at a given hospital have raised concerns about the ability of neonatal mortality rates to assess care quality at a specific facility.

Readmissions from neonatal intensive care units as a quality measure

Readmissions are a common group of quality measures endorsed by NQF and other national bodies. As of 2016, there are 54 readmission measures endorsed by NQF for patients of all ages and health. Besides the added health care costs associated with hospital readmissions, readmissions may assess different areas of health care compared with other process or outcome measures. Many of the other measures we have discussed focus specifically on medical care, either the prevention and early identification of illness, or the provision of prophylactic treatment with strong benefit to patients. Unlike these measures, hospital readmission rates may assess the quality of discharge planning,[72,73] and the effective transition of care between the inpatient and outpatient care providers. But why have readmission rates not been endorsed for neonatal care?

Ease of classification: Moderately difficult to difficult. Most readmission metrics are all-condition measures; that is, any readmission that occurs within a specific time window postdischarge. For neonatal patients, this may include febrile illnesses or other infectious diseases that are unpreventable, and thus introduce random noise into the measure. Attempts to identify "preventable" readmissions have failed because of the lack of agreement about what constitutes a preventable readmission between study teams.[74–78]

Ease of measurement: Moderately difficult. Administrative data require linkages between hospitalizations to identify infants who were readmitted. Registry data typically cannot capture all readmissions, because many infants are readmitted to hospitals that did not discharge them from the NICU, based on data from California (**Fig. 2**).

Validity: Moderate. There is substantial variation in NICU readmission rates, with a sixfold to sevenfold difference in hospital readmission rates in California NICUs, and

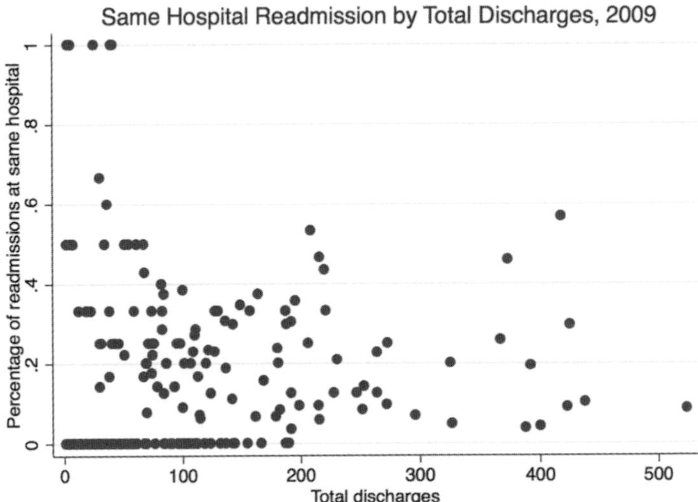

Fig. 2. Percentage of hospital readmissions readmitted to discharge hospital, California linked birth certificate–hospital discharge data, 2009.

a fivefold to sixfold difference in state readmission rates for Medicaid patients requiring NICU care.[79] This variation in readmission rates persists after controlling for differences in casemix. There are data from adults that show an association between readmissions and a hospital's performance in discharge planning[72,73] and transitions of care, but not other measures of poor care, such as hospital complication rates. Data in prematurely born infants find no correlation between a hospital's 30-day readmission rate and the hospital's rate of BPD, intraventricular hemorrhage (IVH), ROP, or NEC (**Fig. 3**), with no studies of the association between readmissions and either discharge planning or transitions of care.

Number of eligible patients: Moderate, although like most measures of perinatal care, readmission rates are relatively low with a hospital average of 2% to 5% by 7 days after discharge to 5% to 7% by 90 days after discharge. Medicaid patients showed higher readmission rates compared with privately insured patients.

Need for risk adjustment: Possibly. Younger infants and infants discharged with chronic conditions, such as BPD, are at higher risk of readmission.[80] As a result, most stakeholders expect to find readmission rates adjusted for these factors. Including these factors in a risk adjustment model, though, does not substantively change a hospital's performance on this measure. Readmission risk adjustment models in adults and children also have lower reliability than other measures, with c-statistics between 0.6 to 0.7, possibly because social and community factors are not included in the models.[75,81,82]

Although used for other patient populations, using readmissions as a quality measure for NICUs remains controversial, with limited validity at the current time. Also, this measure currently is limited to insurance-based datasets because most infants are admitted to a different hospital from where they were discharged (see **Fig. 2**). These datasets are lacking in other data elements, such as an accurate gestational age, which are necessary to calculate a valid readmission measure.[79] Collecting accurate data, and assessing the association of readmission rates with other measures of care such as the discharge process, will be important to validating the measure for neonatal care.

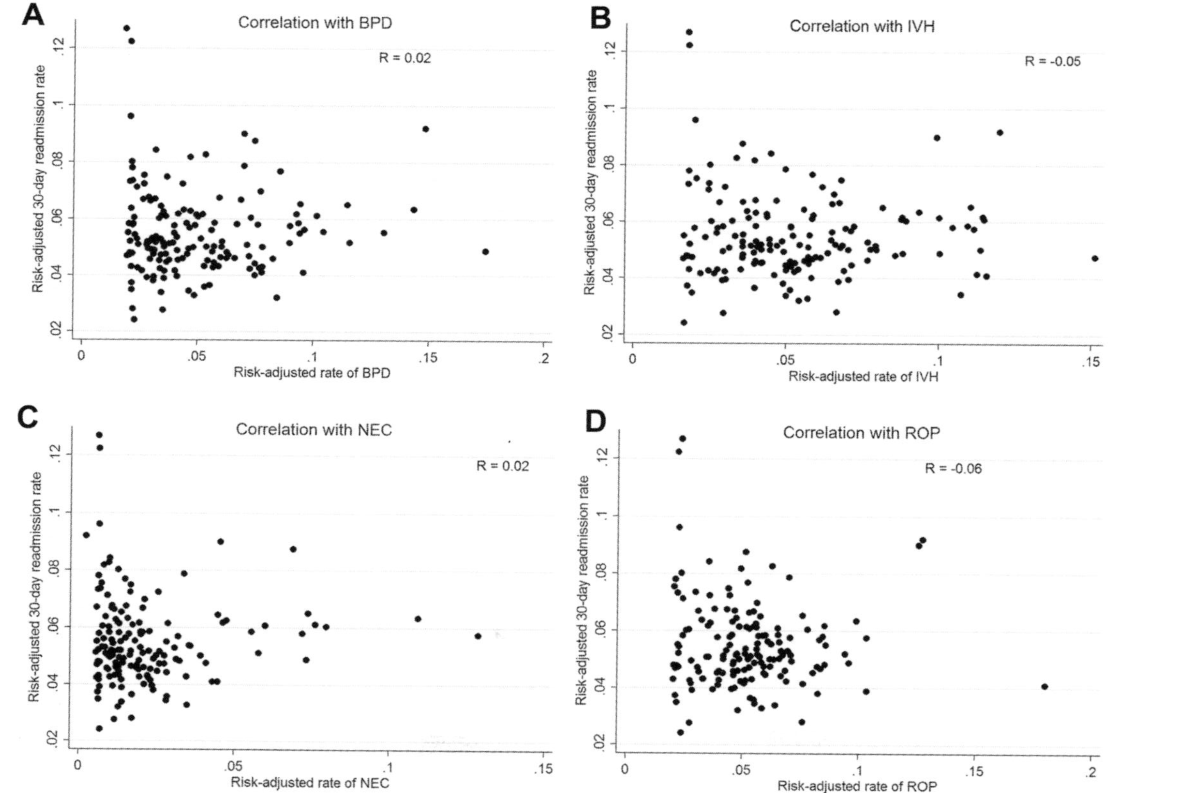

Fig. 3. Lack of correlation between 30-day all-cause hospital readmission rates and rates of BPD, IVH, NEC, and ROP, California linked birth certificate–hospital discharge data. All data risk-adjusted for gestational age, birth weight, maternal comorbid conditions, gender, and race/ethnicity. (*A*) Correlation with BPD. (*B*) Correlation with any IVH. (*C*) Correlation with NEC. (*D*) Correlation with any ROP.

SUMMARY

There are a plethora of quality measures, both endorsed and unendorsed, that assess different aspects of a hospital's "quality box." The process to obtain endorsement is rigorous and has resulted in a set of measures that focus primarily on preventive care, mode and timing of delivery, and hospital infection rates. Further work is needed to assess what these measures truly assess about care quality at the hospital level, and what is missing from our assessment of a hospital's quality of care. Such topics include parental education, transitions of care, and methods to address factors such as social determinants of health on pregnancy outcomes. With better understanding of what these measures truly say about the care provided at an individual NICU, we can identify metrics to optimize the outcomes of high-risk pregnancies.

REFERENCES

1. Institute of Medicine, Committee on the Learning Health Care System in America, Smith M, et al, editors. Best care at lower cost: the path to continuously learning health care in America. Washington, DC: The National Academies Press; 2013. Available at: https://www.nap.edu/catalog/13444/best-care-at-lower-cost-the-path-to-continuously-learning.
2. National Quality Forum. Measuring performance. Available at: http://www.qualityforum.org/Measuring_Performance/Measuring_Performance.aspx. Accessed January 23, 2017.
3. CMS.gov. Public reporting. Available at: https://www.cms.gov/Medicare/Quality-Initiatives-Patient-Assessment-Instruments/physician-compare-initiative/Public_Reporting.html. Accessed January 23, 2017.
4. County Health Rankings & Roadmaps. Health Policy Brief: Public Reporting on Quality and Costs, Health Affairs/RWJF Health Policy Briefs, March 8, 2012. Available at: http://www.countyhealthrankings.org/policies/public-reporting-health-care-quality-performance. Accessed January 23, 2017.
5. Das A, Gopalan SS, Chandramohan D. Effect of pay for performance to improve quality of maternal and child care in low- and middle-income countries: a systematic review. BMC Public Health 2016;16:321.
6. Gleeson S, Kelleher K, Gardner W. Evaluating a pay-for-performance program for Medicaid children in an accountable care organization. JAMA Pediatr 2016;170:259–66.
7. Spitzer AR. Pay for performance in neonatal-perinatal medicine–will the quality of health care improve in the neonatal intensive care unit? A business model for improving outcomes in the neonatal intensive care unit. Clin Perinatol 2010;37:167–77.
8. Profit J, Zupancic JA, Gould JB, et al. Implementing pay-for-performance in the neonatal intensive care unit. Pediatrics 2007;119:975–82.
9. New York State Department of Health. Cardiovascular Disease Data and Statistics. Available at: https://www.health.ny.gov/statistics/diseases/cardiovascular/. Accessed January 23, 2017.
10. Centers for Disease Control and Prevention. 2014 National and State Healthcare-Associated Infections Progress Report. Available at: https://www.cdc.gov/hai/pdfs/progress-report/hai-progress-report.pdf. Accessed January 23, 2017.
11. Lorch SA. Quality measurements in pediatrics: what do they assess? JAMA Pediatr 2013;167:89–90.
12. Curtin SC, Mathews TJ. Smoking prevalence and cessation before and during pregnancy: data from the birth certificate, 2014. National vital statistics reports;

vol. 65 no 1. Hyattsville (MD): National Center for Health Statistics. Available at: https://www.cdc.gov/nchs/data/nvsr/nvsr65/nvsr65_01.pdf. Accessed January 23, 2017.

13. Meador K, Reynolds MW, Crean S, et al. Pregnancy outcomes in women with epilepsy: a systematic review and meta-analysis of published pregnancy registries and cohorts. Epilepsy Res 2008;81:1–13.
14. Gedzelman E, Meador KJ. Antiepileptic drugs in women with epilepsy during pregnancy. Ther Adv Drug Saf 2012;3:71–87.
15. Phelan S. Smoking cessation in pregnancy. Obstet Gynecol Clin North Am 2014; 41:255–66.
16. Marufu TC, Ahankari A, Coleman T, et al. Maternal smoking and the risk of still birth: systematic review and meta-analysis. BMC Public Health 2015;15:239.
17. Kleinman JC, Madans JH. The effects of maternal smoking, physical stature, and educational attainment on the incidence of low birth weight. Am J Epidemiol 1985;121:843–55.
18. U.S. Department of Health and Human Services, Office of Disease Prevention and Health Promotion. Pregnancy health and behaviors. Washington, DC. Available at: https://www.healthypeople.gov/2020/topics-objectives/objective/mich-10. Accessed January 22, 2017.
19. Hillemeier MM, Domino ME, Wells R, et al. Effects of maternity care coordination on pregnancy outcomes: propensity-weighted analyses. Matern Child Health J 2015;19:121–7.
20. Fiscella K. Does prenatal care improve birth outcomes? A critical review. Obstet Gynecol 1995;85:468–79.
21. Tran ST, Rosenberg KD, Carlson NE. Racial/ethnic disparities in the receipt of smoking cessation interventions during prenatal care. Matern Child Health J 2010;14:901–9.
22. O'Connor SE, Zupanc ML. Women and epilepsy. J Paediatr Pharmacol Ther 2009;14:212–20.
23. Hirtz D, Thurman DJ, Gwinn-Hardy K, et al. How common are the "common" neurologic disorders? Neurology 2007;68:326–37.
24. Dietz P, Bombard J, Mulready-Ward C, et al. Validation of selected items on the 2003 U.S. standard certificate of live birth: New York City and Vermont. Public Health Rep 2015;130:60–70.
25. Lydon-Rochelle MT, Holt VL, Cardenas V, et al. The reporting of pre-existing maternal medical conditions and complications of pregnancy on birth certificates and in hospital discharge data. Am J Obstet Gynecol 2005;193:125–34.
26. Ganchimeg T, Nagata C, Vogel JP, et al. Optimal timing of delivery among low-risk women with prior caesarean section: a secondary analysis of the WHO Multi-country Survey on maternal and newborn health. PLoS One 2016;11:e0149091.
27. Tita AT, Eunice Kennedy Shriver National Institute of Child Health and Human Development Maternal–Fetal Medicine Units Network. What we have learned about scheduling elective repeat cesarean delivery at term. Semin Perinatol 2016;40:287–90.
28. Tita AT, Landon MB, Spong CY, et al. Timing of elective repeat cesarean delivery at term and neonatal outcomes. N Engl J Med 2009;360:111–20.
29. Kozhimannil K, Macheras M, Lorch SA. Trends in childbirth before 39 weeks' gestation without medical indication. Med Care 2014;52:649–57.
30. Nicholson JM, Kellar LC, Ahmad S, et al. US term stillbirth rates and the 39-week rule: a cause for concern? Am J Obstet Gynecol 2016;214:621.e1-9.

31. Little SE, Zera CA, Clapp MA, et al. A multi-state analysis of early-term delivery trends and the association with term stillbirth. Obstet Gynecol 2015;126:1138–45.
32. Snowden JM, Muoto I, Darney BG, et al. Oregon's hard-stop policy limiting elective early-term deliveries: association with obstetric procedure use and health outcomes. Obstet Gynecol 2016;128:1389–96.
33. Gould JB, Danielsen B, Korst LM, et al. Cesarean delivery rates and neonatal morbidity in a low-risk population. Obstet Gynecol 2004;104:11–9.
34. Bailit JL, Garrett JM, Miller WC, et al. Hospital primary cesarean delivery rates and the risk of poor neonatal outcomes. Am J Obstet Gynecol 2002;187:721–7.
35. Srinivas SK, Fager C, Lorch SA. Evaluating risk-adjusted cesarean section rates as a measure of obstetric quality. Obstet Gynecol 2010;115:1007–13.
36. Bailit JL, Love TE, Dawson NV. Quality of obstetric care and risk-adjusted primary cesarean delivery rates. Am J Obstet Gynecol 2006;194:402–7.
37. Gibson K, Bailit JL. Cesarean delivery as a marker for obstetric quality. Clin Obstet Gynecol 2015;58:211–6.
38. Verani JR, McGee L, Schrag SJ, Division of Bacterial Diseases, National Center for Immunization and Respiratory Diseases, Centers for Disease Control and Prevention (CDC). Prevention of perinatal group B streptococcal disease–revised guidelines from CDC, 2010. MMWR Recomm Rep 2010;59:1–36.
39. Bain E, Wilson A, Tooher R, et al. Prophylaxis for venous thromboembolic disease in pregnancy and the early postnatal period. Cochrane Database Syst Rev 2014;(2):CD001689.
40. Tita AT, Szychowski JM, Boggess K, et al. Adjunctive azithromycin prophylaxis for cesarean delivery. N Engl J Med 2016;375:1231–41.
41. Mackeen AD, Packard RE, Ota E, et al. Timing of intravenous prophylactic antibiotics for preventing postpartum infectious morbidity in women undergoing cesarean delivery. Cochrane Database Syst Rev 2014;(12):CD009516.
42. Smaill FM, Grivell RM. Antibiotic prophylaxis versus no prophylaxis for preventing infection after cesarean section. Cochrane Database Syst Rev 2014;(10):CD007482.
43. Roberts D, Dalziel S. Antenatal corticosteroids for accelerating fetal lung maturation for women at risk of preterm birth. Cochrane Database Syst Rev 2006;(3):CD004454.
44. Cofer FG, Fridman M, Lawton E, et al. Interpregnancy interval and childbirth outcomes in California, 2007-2009. Matern Child Health J 2016;20:43–51.
45. Wendt A, Gibbs CM, Peters S, et al. Impact of increasing inter-pregnancy interval on maternal and infant health. Paediatr Perinat Epidemiol 2012;26(Suppl 1): 239–58.
46. Vogel JP, Souza JP, Gulmezoglu AM, et al. Use of antenatal corticosteroids and tocolytic drugs in preterm births in 29 countries: an analysis of the WHO Multi-country Survey on Maternal and Newborn Health. Lancet 2014;384:1869–77.
47. California Maternal Quality Care Collaborative. Unexpected complications in term newborns. Available at: https://www.cmqcc.org/focus-areas/quality-metrics/unexpected-complications-term-newborns. Accessed January 24, 2017.
48. Sebastião YV, Womack LS, Castillo HL, et al. Hospital variations in unexpected complications among term newborns. Pediatrics 2017;139(3) [pii:e20162364].
49. Lorch SA. Challenges to measuring the quality of low-risk newborns. Pediatrics 2017;139(3) [pii:e20164025].
50. Kar P, Mishra S. Management of hepatitis B during pregnancy. Expert Opin Pharmacother 2016;17:301–10.
51. Gdalevich M, Mimouni D, Mimouni M. Breast-feeding and the risk of bronchial asthma in childhood: a systematic review with meta-analysis of prospective studies. J Pediatr 2001;139:261–6.

52. Patnode CD, Henninger ML, Senger CA, et al. Primary care interventions to support breastfeeding: updated evidence report and systematic review for the US Preventive Services Task Force. JAMA 2016;316:1694–705.
53. Huang P, Zhou J, Yin Y, et al. Effects of breast-feeding compared with formula-feeding on preterm infant body composition: a systematic review and meta-analysis. Br J Nutr 2016;116:132–41.
54. Sankar MJ, Sinha B, Chowdhury R, et al. Optimal breastfeeding practices and infant and child mortality: a systematic review and meta-analysis. Acta Paediatr 2015;104:3–13.
55. Horbar JD, Edwards EM, Greenberg LT, et al. Variation in performance of neonatal intensive care units in the United States. JAMA Pediatr 2017;171:e164396.
56. Lorch SA, Baiocchi M, Ahlberg CE, et al. The differential impact of delivery hospital on the outcomes of premature infants. Pediatrics 2012;130:270–8.
57. Profit J, Gould JB, Bennett M, et al. The association of level of care with NICU quality. Pediatrics 2016;137:e20144210.
58. Aziz K, McMillan DD, Andrews W, et al. Variations in rates of nosocomial infection among Canadian neonatal intensive care units may be practice-related. BMC Pediatr 2005;5:22.
59. Ting JY, Synnes A, Roberts A, et al. Association between antibiotic use and neonatal mortality and morbidities in very low-birth-weight infants without culture-proven sepsis or necrotizing enterocolitis. JAMA Pediatr 2016;170:1181–7.
60. Adams-Chapman I, Bann CM, Das A, et al. Neurodevelopmental outcome of extremely low birth weight infants with *Candida* infection. J Pediatr 2013;163:961–7.e3.
61. Schlapbach LJ, Aebischer M, Adams M, et al. Impact of sepsis on neurodevelopmental outcome in a Swiss National Cohort of extremely premature infants. Pediatrics 2011;128:e348–57.
62. Stoll BJ, Hansen NI, Adams-Chapman I, et al. Neurodevelopmental and growth impairment among extremely low-birth-weight infants with neonatal infection. JAMA 2004;292:2357–65.
63. Vartanian RJ, Besirli CG, Barks JD, et al. Trends in the screening and treatment of retinopathy of prematurity. Pediatrics 2017;139 [pii:e20161978].
64. Kennedy KA, Wrage LA, Higgins RD, et al. Evaluating retinopathy of prematurity screening guidelines for 24- to 27-week gestational age infants. J Perinatol 2014;34:311–8.
65. Fierson WM, American Academy of Pediatrics Section on Ophthalmology, American Academy of Ophthalmology, American Association for Pediatric Ophthalmology and Strabismus, American Association of Certified Orthoptists. Screening examination of premature infants for retinopathy of prematurity. Pediatrics 2013;131:189–95.
66. MacDorman MF, Kirmeyer S. Fetal and perinatal mortality, United States, 2005. National Vital Statistics Reports; vol. 57 no 8. Hyattsville (MD): National Center for Health Statistics. Available at: https://www.cdc.gov/nchs/data/misc/itop97.pdf. Accessed January 23, 2017.
67. Phibbs CS, Baker LC, Caughey AB, et al. Level and volume of neonatal intensive care and mortality in very-low-birth-weight infants. N Engl J Med 2007;356:2165–75.
68. Gibson E, Culhane J, Saunders T, et al. Effect of nonviable infants on the infant mortality rate in Philadelphia, 1992. Am J Public Health 2000;90:1303–6.

69. Chung JH, Phibbs CS, Boscardin WJ, et al. Examining the effect of hospital-level factors on mortality of very low birth weight infants using multilevel modeling. J Perinatol 2011;31:770–5.
70. Chung JH, Phibbs CS, Boscardin WJ, et al. The effect of neonatal intensive care level and hospital volume on mortality of very low birth weight infants. Med Care 2010;48:635–44.
71. Rogowski JA, Horbar JD, Staiger DO, et al. Indirect vs direct hospital quality indicators for very low-birth-weight infants. JAMA 2004;291:202–9.
72. Kociol RD, Peterson ED, Hammill BG, et al. National survey of hospital strategies to reduce heart failure readmissions: findings from the Get with the Guidelines-Heart Failure registry. Circ Heart Fail 2012;5:680–7.
73. Henke RM, Karaca Z, Jackson P, et al. Discharge planning and hospital readmissions. Med Care Res Rev 2016. [Epub ahead of print].
74. Toomey SL, Peltz A, Loren S, et al. Potentially preventable 30-day hospital readmissions at a children's hospital. Pediatrics 2016;138 [pii:e20154182].
75. Sills MR, Hall M, Colvin JD, et al. Association of social determinants with children's hospitals' preventable readmissions performance. JAMA Pediatr 2016; 170:350–8.
76. Jonas JA, Devon EP, Ronan JC, et al. Determining preventability of pediatric readmissions using fault tree analysis. J Hosp Med 2016;11:329–35.
77. Amin D, Ford R, Ghazarian SR, et al. Parent and physician perceptions regarding preventability of pediatric readmissions. Hosp Pediatr 2016;6:80–7.
78. Hain PD, Gay JC, Berutti TW, et al. Preventability of early readmissions at a children's hospital. Pediatrics 2013;131:e171–81.
79. Lorch SA, Passarella M, Zeigler A. Challenges to measuring variation in readmission rates of neonatal intensive care patients. Acta Paediatr 2014;14:S47–53.
80. Ray KN, Lorch SA. Hospitalization of early preterm, late preterm, and term infants during the first year of life by gestational age. Hosp Pediatr 2013;3:194–203.
81. Lorch SA, Enlow E. The role of social determinants in explaining racial/ethnic disparities in perinatal outcomes. Pediatr Res 2016;79:141–7.
82. Ray KN, Lorch SA. Hospitalization of rural and urban infants during the first year of life. Pediatrics 2012;130:1084–93.

APPENDIX 1: PERINATAL QUALITY MEASURES ENDORSED BY NATIONAL QUALITY FORUM, 2017

Measure	Numerator	Denominator	Risk Adjustment	Data Sources[a]
Time period 1: prenatal/periconception				
Adult current smoking prevalence	The numerator is current adult smokers (age 18 and older) in the United States who live in households.	The adult (age 18 and older) population of the United States who live in households. One adult per household is interviewed.	No	Other
Time period 2: intrapartum/postpartum care				
Appropriate DVT prophylaxis in women undergoing cesarean delivery	Number of women undergoing cesarean delivery who receive either fractionated or unfractionated heparin or heparinoid, or pneumatic compression devices before surgery.	All women undergoing cesarean delivery.	No	Other, paper records, pharmacy
Appropriate prophylactic antibiotic received within 1 hour before surgical incision – cesarean delivery	Percentage of women who receive recommended antibiotics within 1 hour before the start of cesarean delivery. This requires that (1) the antibiotic selection is consistent with current evidence and practice guidelines, and (2) that the antibiotics are given within an hour before delivery.	All patients undergoing cesarean delivery without evidence of prior infection or already receiving prophylactic antibiotics for other reasons. Patients with significant allergies to penicillin and/or cephalosporins AND allergies to gentamicin and/or clindamycin are also excluded.	No	Claims, electronic health record, other, paper records
Contraceptive care postpartum	Women ages 15 through 44 who had a live birth and were provided the most (sterilization, intrauterine device, implant) or a moderately (pill, patch, ring, injectable, diaphragm) effective method of contraception within 3 and 60 d of delivery.	Women ages 15 through 44 who had a live birth in a 12-mo measurement year.	No	Claims
Contraceptive care: most and moderately effective methods	Women aged 15–44 y of age at risk of unintended pregnancy who are provided a most (sterilization, intrauterine device, implant) or moderately (pill, patch, ring, injectable, diaphragm) effective method of contraception.	Women aged 15–44 y of age who are at risk of unintended pregnancy.	No	Claims

(continued on next page)

(continued)

Measure	Numerator	Denominator	Risk Adjustment	Data Sources[a]
Contraceptive care: access to LARC	Women aged 15–44 y of age at risk of unintended pregnancy who were provided an LARC, that is, intrauterine device or implant.	All women aged 15–44 y of age who are at risk of unintended pregnancy.	No	Claims
Incidence of episiotomy	Number of episiotomy procedures (ICD-9 code 72.1, 72.21, 72.31, 72.71, 73.6; ICD-10 PCS:0W8NXZZ) performed on women undergoing a vaginal delivery (excluding those with shoulder dystocia ICD-10; O66.0).	All vaginal deliveries during the analytical period (ie, monthly, quarterly, yearly), excluding those coded with a shoulder dystocia ICD-1: O66.0).	No	Claims, paper records
Intrapartum antibiotic prophylaxis for GBS	All eligible patients who receive intrapartum antibiotic prophylaxis for GBS.	All women delivering live infants, except certain classes who are specifically deemed not to be at risk of vertical transmission of GBS.	No	Claims, electronic health record, other, paper records
PC-01 elective delivery	Patients with elective deliveries with ICD-10-PCS Principal Procedure Code or ICD-10-PCS Other Procedure Codes for 1 or more of the following: • Medical induction of labor as defined in Appendix A, Table 11.05 available at: http://manual.jointcommission.org/releases/TJC2016A/ while not in labor before the procedure • Cesarean birth as defined in Appendix A, Table 11.06 available at: http://manual.jointcommission.org/releases/TJC2016A/ and all of the following: ○ Not in labor ○ No history of a prior uterine surgery	Patients delivering newborns with $\geq$37 and <39 wk of gestation completed with ICD-10-PCS Principal or Other Procedure Codes for delivery and with ICD-10-CM Principal Diagnosis Code or ICD-10-CM Other Diagnosis Codes for planned cesarean birth in labor.	No	Electronic health record, paper records

PC-02 cesarean birth	Patients with cesarean births with ICD-10-PCS Principal Procedure Code or ICD-10-PCS Other Procedure Codes for cesarean birth.	Nulliparous patients delivered of a live term singleton newborn in vertex presentation ICD-10-PCS Principal or Other Diagnosis Codes for delivery.	No	Paper records
PC-03 antenatal steroids	Patients with antenatal steroids initiated before delivering preterm newborns.	Patients delivering live preterm newborns with $\geq$24 and <34 wk gestation completed with ICD-10-PCS Principal or Other Procedure Codes for delivery.	No	Paper records
Percentage of low birthweight births	The number of babies born weighing <2500 g at birth in the study population.	All births in the study population.	No	Claims
Rh immunoglobulin (Rhogam) for Rh-negative pregnant women at risk of fetal blood exposure	Number of appropriate patients who receive Rhogam.	All women, confirmed pregnant, who are at significant risk of fetal blood exposure.	No	Claims, electronic health record, other, paper records
Unexpected complications in term newborns	The numerator is divided into 2 categories: severe complications and moderate complications. Severe complications include neonatal death, transfer to another hospital for higher level of care, extremely low Apgar scores (=3 at either 5 or 10 min of life), severe birth injuries such as intracranial hemorrhage or nerve injury, neurologic damage, severe respiratory and infectious complications, such as sepsis. Moderate complications include diagnoses or procedures that raise concern but at a lower level than the list for severe (eg, use of continuous positive airway pressure or bone fracture).	Singleton, liveborn infants who are at least 37.0 wk of gestation, and more than 2500 g in birth weight. The denominator excludes most serious fetal conditions that are "preexisting" (present before labor), including prematurity, multiple gestations, poor fetal growth, congenital malformations, genetic disorders, other specified fetal and maternal conditions and infants exposed to maternal drug use in utero.	No	Claims

(*continued on next page*)

(continued)

Measure	Numerator	Denominator	Risk Adjustment	Data Sources[a]
Time period 3: newborn care				
Hepatitis B vaccine coverage among all live newborn infants before hospital or birthing facility discharge	The number of live newborn infants administered hepatitis B vaccine before discharge (or within 1 mo of life, if the infant had an extended hospital stay) from the hospital/birthing facility.	The number of live newborn infants born at the hospital/birthing facility during the reporting window (1 calendar year).	No	Electronic health record, other, paper records, pharmacy, registry
PC-05 exclusive breast milk feeding	Newborns that were fed breast milk only since birth.	Single term liveborn newborns discharged alive from the hospital with ICD-10-CM Principal Diagnosis Code for single liveborn newborn.	No	Electronic health record, paper records
Pediatric all-condition readmission measure	The numerator consists of hospitalizations at general acute care hospitals for patients <18 years old who are followed by 1 or more readmissions to general acute care hospitals within 30 d. Readmissions are excluded from the numerator if the readmission was for a planned procedure or for chemotherapy.	Hospitalizations at general acute care hospitals for patients <18 years old.	Yes	Claims
Time period 4: care of the VLBW infant				
Late sepsis or meningitis in VLBW neonates (risk-adjusted)	Eligible infants with 1 or more of the following criteria: Criterion 1: Bacterial pathogen. A bacterial pathogen is recovered from a blood and/or cerebral spinal fluid culture obtained after day 3 of life. OR	Eligible infants who are in the reporting hospital after day 3 of life.	Yes	Registry

	Criterion 2: Coagulase-negative *Staphylococcus*. The infant has all 3 of the following: 1. Coagulase-negative *Staphylococcus* is recovered from a blood culture obtained from either a central line, or peripheral blood sample, and/or is recovered from cerebrospinal fluid obtained by lumbar puncture, ventricular tap, or ventricular drain. 2. One or more signs of generalized infection (such as apnea, temperature instability, feeding intolerance, worsening respiratory distress, or hemodynamic instability). 3. Treatment with 5 or more days of intravenous antibiotics after the previously mentioned cultures were obtained.			
Neonatal blood stream infection rate (National Quality Indicator [NQI] 03)	Discharges, among cases meeting the inclusion and exclusion rules for the denominator, with any of the following: • Any secondary ICD-9-CM or ICD-10-CM diagnosis codes for other septicemia; or • Any secondary ICD-9-CM or ICD-10-CM diagnosis codes for newborn septicemia or bacteremia; and • Any secondary ICD-9-CM or ICD-10-CM diagnosis codes for staphylococcal or gram-negative bacterial infection.	All newborns and outborns with any of the following: • A birth weight of 500–1499 g (birth weight categories 2, 3, 4 and 5); or • Any-listed ICD-9-CM or ICD-10-CM diagnosis codes for gestational age between 24 and 30 wk; or • A birth weight $\geq$ 1500 g (birth weight category 6, 7, 8, or 9) and death (DISP = 20); or • A birth weight $\geq$ to 1500 g (birth weight category 6, 7, 8, or 9) and any-listed ICD-9-CM or ICD-10-PCS procedure codes for operating room procedure; or	Yes	Claims

(*continued on next page*)

(continued)

Measure	Numerator	Denominator	Risk Adjustment	Data Sources[a]
		• A birth weight $\geq$ to 1500 g (birth weight category 6, 7, 8, or 9) and any-listed ICD-9-CM or ICD-10-PCS procedure codes for mechanical ventilation; or • A birth weight $\geq$ to 1500 g (birth weight category 6, 7, 8, or 9) and transferring from another health care facility within 2 days of birth.		
PC-04 health care–associated bloodstream infections in newborns	Newborns with septicemia or bacteremia with ICD-10-CM other diagnosis codes for newborn septicemia or bacteremia with a bloodstream infection confirmed OR ICD-10-CM other diagnosis codes for sepsis as defined in Appendix A, Table 11.10.1 available at: http://manual.jointcommission.org/releases/TJC2016A/ with a bloodstream infection confirmed.	The outcome target population being measured is as follows: liveborn newborns with ICD-10-CM other diagnosis codes for birth weight between 500 and 1499 g as defined in Appendix A, Table 11.12, 11.13 or 11.14 OR birth weight between 500 and 1499 g OR ICD-10-CM other diagnosis codes for birth weight $\geq$1500 g as defined in Appendix A, Table 11.15 or 11.16 OR Birth Weight $\geq$1500 g who experienced 1 or more of the following: • Experienced death • ICD-10-PCS Principal Procedure Code or ICD-10-PCS Other Procedure Codes for major surgery • ICD-10-PCS Principal Procedure Code or ICD-10-PCS Other Procedure Codes for mechanical ventilation • Transferred in from another acute care hospital or health care setting within 2 d of birth.	Yes	Paper records

Proportion of infants 22–29 wk gestation screened for ROP	Number of infants born from 22 wk, 0 d to 29 wk, 6 d gestational age who were in the reporting hospital at the postnatal age recommended for ROP screening by the AAP and who received a retinal examination for ROP before discharge.	All eligible infants born from 22 wk, 0 d to 29 wk, 6 d gestational age who were in the reporting hospital at the postnatal age recommended for ROP screening by the AAP.	No	Registry

Data taken directly from the National Quality Forum Web site, endorsed measures for perinatal health. http://www.qualityforum.org/QPS/.

Abbreviations: AAP, American Academy of Pediatrics; DISP, DISP variable, reflecting discharge status of infant in hospital claims database; DVT, deep venous thrombosis; GBS, Group B Streptococcus; ICD-9-CM, International Classification of Diseases, Ninth Revision, Clinical Modification; ICD-10-CM, International Classification of Diseases, 10th Revision, Clinical Modification; ICD-10-PCS, ICD-10 Procedure Coding System; LARC, long-acting reversible method of contraception; ROP, retinopathy of prematurity; VLBW, very low birthweight.

[a] Data source definitions, as classified by the measure developers: claims: administrative records, including vital statistics and hospital administrative data; electronic health records: data from electronic health record sources; registry: data specifically collected for submission to a cohort, which may come from review of any health record; paper records: data from chart review of a nonelectronic record; pharmacy: data from pharmacy records, typically within a hospital; other: other sources of data including patient or provider report.

The Hard Work of Improving Outcomes for Mothers and Babies

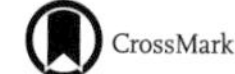

Obstetric and Perinatal Quality Improvement Initiatives Make a Difference at the Hospital, State, and National Levels

Patrick D. Schneider, MD[a], Bethany A. Sabol, MD[b], Patricia Ann Lee King, PhD, MSW[c], Aaron B. Caughey, MD, PhD[b], Ann E.B. Borders, MD, MSc, MPH[d,*]

KEYWORDS

• Quality • Improvement • Obstetrics • Perinatal

KEY POINTS

- Quality improvement and patient safety efforts are a growing focus for perinatal care providers.
- The maternal-focused and perinatal-focused quality improvement initiative results offer strong examples of the impact that perinatal quality improvement and safety work have in improving the delivery of care.
- Expanded work at the hospital, state, and national levels is essential to drive sustainable quality improvement and patient safety efforts that will make every hospital a safer and better place to give birth and be born.

[a] Maternal-Fetal Medicine, NorthShore University HealthSystem, University of Chicago, 2650 Ridge Avenue, Walgreen Building Suite 1506, Evanston, IL 60201, USA; [b] Department of Obstetrics and Gynecology, Oregon Health & Science University, 3181 Southwest Sam Jackson Park Road, Portland, OR 97239-3098, USA; [c] Feinberg School of Medicine, Northwestern University, 633 North St. Clair Street, Chicago, IL 60611, USA; [d] Department of Obstetrics and Gynecology, NorthShore University HealthSystem Evanston Hospital, Pritzker School of Medicine, University of Chicago, Walgreen Building, Suite 1507, Evanston, IL 60201, USA

* Corresponding author. Department of Obstetrics and Gynecology, NorthShore University HealthSystem Evanston Hospital, Pritzker School of Medicine, University of Chicago, Walgreen Building, Suite 1507, Evanston, IL 60201

E-mail address: aborders@northshore.org

Clin Perinatol 44 (2017) 511–528
http://dx.doi.org/10.1016/j.clp.2017.05.007

INTRODUCTION

Quality improvement and patient safety efforts are a growing focus for perinatal care providers. This work has developed in response to major public health goals to reduce maternal and neonatal morbidity and mortality while balancing pressures from consumers and payers to ensure that care is safe, reliable, and effective.[1] Although quality improvement work has been present in medicine for more than 3 decades, it is only recently that a focus on quality improvement and patient safety has become an integral part of perinatal care.[2–8]

In obstetrics, quality improvement efforts have gradually expanded from local initiatives at single institutions to statewide efforts through state-based perinatal quality collaboratives (PQCs), and recently to national initiatives incorporating multiple state PQCs. Hospital-level work continues to expand as hospitals and health care networks realize the benefits of standardized data measures, quality improvement science, and team-based training and communication strategies to drive improvements in outcomes for mothers and babies.[9–13] At the state level, PQCs are networks of perinatal care providers and public health professionals working to improve pregnancy outcomes for women and newborns by advancing evidence-based clinical practices and processes through continuous quality improvement. At the national level, numerous initiatives now seek large-scale improvements in obstetric outcomes. The Centers for Disease Control and Prevention (CDC) have taken a leadership role in supporting state PQCs, recognizing PQCs in 39 of 50 states, and supporting 6 (California, New York, Ohio, Illinois, Massachusetts, North Carolina) with Division of Reproductive Health funding for further project development.[14]

In addition, the CDC has developed a guide, *Developing and Sustaining Perinatal Quality Collaboratives*, outlining how to initiate and support state-based perinatal quality improvement collaboratives with a goal of achieving a PQC in every state.[1] A launch meeting for the National Network of Perinatal Quality Collaboratives (NNPQC) in 2016, sponsored by the March of Dimes/CDC, was attended by teams representing PQCs in different stages of development from 49 of 50 states.[15] Other national organizations designed to help state collaboratives and hospital perinatal quality improvement teams have also launched major initiatives. These groups include The Alliance for Innovation on Maternal Health (AIM) program with the American Congress of Obstetricians and Gynecologists (ACOG) and the Council for Patient Safety in Women's Health Care; the Collaborative Improvement and Innovation Network (COIN) to Reduce Infant Mortality; Hospital Engagement Networks; March of Dimes Big 5 State Prematurity Collaborative (including California, New York, Texas, Illinois, Florida); and National Institute for Children's Health Quality.[16–19] Most of these national initiatives have developed since the mid-2000s and have progressed rapidly. At all of these levels, the need for better obstetric data and appropriate performance measures has been clear.

This article highlights key perinatal-focused and obstetric-focused quality improvement initiatives at the local, state, and national levels that have shown improved patient outcomes and clinical care. Quality improvement work with published data is divided into initiatives focused on birth and neonatal outcomes (perinatal quality improvement), reducing maternal morbidity and mortality (obstetric quality improvement), and team-based training. Birth and neonatal outcome–focused quality initiatives include reducing early elective delivery before 39 weeks' gestation, increasing antenatal corticosteroid administration for eligible women, increasing risk-appropriate perinatal care, optimizing prenatal care and access, and optimizing breastfeeding at discharge. Maternal-focused topics include cesarean section rates, surgical site infection, and postpartum hemorrhage. Reports on team-based training initiatives that may include communication, simulation, or other skills used to help teams improve quality and safety outcomes are included. The article also reviews emerging topics in perinatal quality and safety that are the current work of state and national efforts.

Quality Improvement Terminology

Quality improvement efforts use a unique set of terms to describe quality improvement methodology. Although these terms share similarities with existing concepts and paradigms that physicians, nurses, public health professionals, and other researchers use in existing evidence-based research practices, it is important to understand their subtle differences. **Box 1** includes a selection of these terms for further reference.[14,20–22]

Box 1
Definitions for perinatal quality improvement collaboratives

Outcome measures

- Evaluate the impact of system changes on maternal or infant health outcomes.
- Example: a project to reduce severe maternal morbidity associated with severe-range blood pressure would have an outcome measure of percentage of cases with new-onset severe hypertension with any adverse maternal outcomes.

Process measures

- Evaluate the impact of system change on steps or parts of the system that have been shown to lead to improved maternal or infant health outcomes.
- Example: a process measure for a perinatal quality improvement project to reduce severe maternal morbidity associated with severe-range blood pressure would be percentage of cases with new-onset severe hypertension treated within 60 minutes.

Balancing measures

- Evaluate the impact of system change in one part of the system on other parts of the system.
- Help hospital teams and perinatal quality monitor for unintended consequences of system change that are causing problems in other parts of the system.
- Example: a balancing measure for a perinatal quality improvement project to reduce severe maternal morbidity associated with severe-range blood pressure would be percentage of cases with new-onset severe hypertension with diastolic pressure decreasing to less than 80 mm Hg within 1 hour of medication administration.

Collaborative learning

- Core quality improvement tool used by perinatal quality collaboratives in which hospital quality improvement teams learn quality improvement strategies from each other through interaction on webinars, conference calls, LISTSERV discussions, Web-based discussion boards, hospital site visits, and exchange of quality improvement data reports.

Plan-Do-Study-Act cycles

- Method to test system changes by creating a plan to test a change (Plan), conducting the test of change (Do), learning from the change (Study), and modifying the test based on the results (Act).

Rapid-response data

- Core quality improvement tool used by perinatal quality collaboratives in which data are submitted by hospital quality improvement teams at least monthly and immediately returned in graphic report format for review of progress toward process and outcome measure goals over time and compared with other hospitals.

Perinatal Quality Improvement

Morbidity and mortality associated with preterm birth, maternal complications of pregnancy, fetal anomalies, and sudden infant death syndrome are the primary causes of infant deaths in the United States. The preterm birth rate in the United States is approximately 1 in 10 and African American women are twice as likely to deliver preterm compared with white women.[23] Local and state quality initiatives have focused on birth and neonatal outcomes work to affect morbidity and mortality across the country, some of which is highlighted later.

Reducing elective delivery before 39 weeks

Reduction of non–medically indicated deliveries before 39 weeks (early elective delivery [EED]) has been one of the most successful perinatal quality improvement initiatives. Recognition of adverse neonatal outcomes associated with early term delivery before 39 weeks, including neonatal intensive care unit (NICU) admission, respiratory distress syndrome, and long-term neonatal morbidity, prompted a nationwide reexamination of elective delivery policies.[24–27] Initiatives to reduce the rate of EED have ranged from single-center to multistate collaborative efforts, with initial elective delivery rates ranging from 9.6% to 33.1% and postinitiative rates decreasing to as low as less than 2.5% to 16.2%.[24–29] NICU admissions, which are another outcome measure, were either unchanged[26,29] or significantly decreased.[30,31] Stillbirth rates, which are a balancing measure, have overall not increased following initiative implementation.[29–32]

Most of these efforts incorporated hospital policy changes and provider education, dissemination, and feedback.[12,28–35] The Ohio Perinatal Quality Collaborative initiative worked with 20 Ohio hospitals to reduce the rate of EED. Hospital improvement teams implemented interventions and identified key drivers for success, such as optimal determination of gestational age with ultrasonography and implementation of hard-stop polices for scheduling delivery. These efforts reduced EED from 25% to less than 5% ($P<.05$).[36,37]

The March of Dimes Big 5 State Prematurity Initiative was a multistate collaborative effort between California, Florida, Illinois, New York, and Texas to decrease EED. The collaborative selected 26 hospitals without previous EED initiatives to participate. Each hospital used the Elimination of Non-medically Indicated (Elective) Deliveries before 39 Weeks Gestational Age toolkit as an implementation guide along with associated training, policy development, and patient education. The initiative saw a decrease in scheduled EED from 2010 to 2011 by 83%, from 27.8% to 4.8% ($P<.001$).[38] This multistate quality improvement program was able to engage diverse national stakeholders and was effective across a diverse population of patients, hospitals, and health care systems, and provides an important example of what broader collaboration can achieve.[31,33]

Increasing antenatal corticosteroid administration for eligible women

Antenatal corticosteroid (ACS) administration before preterm delivery results in decreased rates of respiratory distress syndrome, intraventricular hemorrhage, necrotizing enterocolitis, and other morbidities associated with prematurity.[39,40] Current guidelines recommend that all preterm deliveries before 34 weeks and certain preterm deliveries before 36 (6/7) weeks receive ACS.[41] However, baseline data from 1998 suggested that only 76% to 85% of eligible women receive ACS before a preterm delivery, and administration rates may be lower for fetuses of less than 28 weeks' gestation.[42–45]

The California Perinatal Quality Care Collaborative (CPQCC) implemented a state-based quality improvement initiative to increase ACS rates in women at risk for preterm delivery between 24 and 34 weeks' gestation. Maternal-fetal medicine specialists served as champions to support and facilitate local quality improvement work through an ACS quality improvement toolkit. The toolkit included quality improvement methodologies and sample documents for policies, procedures, staff education, and competency testing. Toolkit resources were also disseminated through workshops and presentations throughout the state. ACS rates increased for eligible infants from 76% in 1998 to 86% in 2001. Participating hospitals continued to have higher rates of administration approximately 5 years later (85% versus 69%; $P<.001$). However, there is still significant variation of reported rates of ACS administration across California, ranging from 68.4% to 92.9%, with hospitals with lower-level NICUs having lower rates.[43]

Additional work in other states has suggested that a component of the variability in ACS rates may be related to poor documentation and under-reporting of ACS use. The Ohio Perinatal Quality Collaborative incorporated improved documentation and birth certificate reporting as a component of their ACS initiative.[46] In addition, they reported elements identified during the Ohio ACS initiative that were needed for high-reliability use of ACS.[47] The March of Dimes Big 5 State Collaborative launched its second multistate quality initiative in 2015 through 2017, to continue to support hospital work toward increased ACS administration among eligible women.

Increasing risk-appropriate perinatal care

The initial regionalization of perinatal health services in the 1970s was a collaborative effort that led to reduced perinatal mortality and improved outcomes for preterm infants.[3,48–50] Current guidelines for regionalized perinatal care recommend that neonates less than 32 weeks and less than 1500 g (ie, those that represent the most critically ill neonates and account for significant neonatal morbidity and mortality) deliver at a hospital with a level III NICU because of the improved morbidity and survival rates seen at these centers.[50] With changing health care environments some areas have seen increased numbers of high-risk deliveries occurring outside level III centers.[51,52]

Numerous organizations and states have undertaken initiatives to improve the regionalization of perinatal care, focusing primarily on risk-appropriate care for very low birth weight (VLBW) infants.[53] One example, the maternal-fetal medicine (MFM) division at the University of Arkansas with the support of the state's Medicaid agency, Department of Health, and medical society launched a statewide program, Antenatal & Neonatal Guidelines, Education, and Learning System (ANGELS) in 2003 to provide an enhanced level of care to the more rural parts of the state and increase referral to higher perinatal levels of care.[13,54] Using telemedicine support for select high-volume birth centers without neonatal intensive care support services in Arkansas, maternal-fetal medicine specialists collaborated with local providers to develop and adopt best-practice guidelines. These telemedicine-supported hospitals without neonatal intensive care support services were able to decrease their deliveries of VLBW infants from 13.1% in 2009 to 7.0% in 2010 ($P = .01$). Similar hospitals without neonatal intensive care support services in Arkansas that did not receive telemedicine support saw no change in the percentage of deliveries of VLBW infants (23.5% in 2009 vs 23.7% in 2010). There was also a reduction in neonatal mortality for VLBW infants (12% to 6.7% before and after the program, respectively) at the targeted hospitals.[55]

Risk-appropriate perinatal care is a Healthy People 2020 goal, a National Quality Forum process measure, and a major driver in the national Collaborative Improvement and Innovation Network to Reduce Infant Mortality (IM CoIIN). To achieve these goals and increase the percentage of mothers and newborns delivered and cared for at appropriate-level facilities, national standard hospital classifications and improved reliability of hospital discharge data for accurate data collection and interpretation are needed.[51] In addition, although not all indicated transfers to level III hospitals occur before delivery, improving the neonatal transport process warrants further evaluation.[49,51,56] Implementation and adoption of the CDC Levels of Care Assessment Tool (LOCATe), based on American Academy of Pediatrics, ACOG, and Society for Maternal-Fetal Medicine guidelines, should help states and hospitals assess levels of care in birthing hospitals, and is another important step in this process.[57] Achieving these improvements in risk-appropriate perinatal care at the hospital and state levels has become an important quality measure and goal given the potential for improved maternal and neonatal outcomes.

Prenatal care optimization and improved access

Access to care and preventive medicine is paramount to long-term improved health outcomes. In pregnancy, this includes early access to prenatal care and expanded coverage to include preconception, postpartum care, mental health, and ancillary social services. In 2010, the Centers for Medicare and Medicaid Services (CMS) implemented the Strong Start for Mothers and Newborns initiative involving selected hospitals and birth centers across the United States. Participating sites tested 3 models for enhanced prenatal care: (1) centering or group prenatal care to foster peer interaction and psychosocial support; (2) comprehensive prenatal care at birth centers with access to health professionals, social work, and case management; and (3) maternity care homes, combining traditional prenatal care with education, health promotion, and additional health services in a single care facility. The goals of the project include testing ways to encourage best practices for reducing the number of early elective deliveries that lack medical indication for all payer types and to reduce preterm birth and adverse outcomes among women enrolled in Medicaid and other public-payer services. Preliminary results have shown significant improvements in outcomes over the course of the project for participating hospitals, including a 64% reduction in early elective deliveries, 58% to 94% increases in breastfeeding rates, 23% reduction in cesarean delivery rates, and 12% reduction in preterm birth rates compared with national averages. In addition, participating hospitals enjoyed high patient satisfaction scores.[58,59]

In 2014, the CMS Maternal and Infant Health initiative launched the Postpartum Care Action Learning Series in 11 states, designed to strengthen the postpartum visit through quality improvement strategies. One year after its launch, there were 18 active initiatives at hospital, local, and state collaborative levels, including home visits, texting programs, modifications to the electronic medical record for postpartum visit tracking and billing, and reducing language barriers to care.[60] One promising preliminary result is the effort of a single hospital to reduce its language barrier through bilingual, bicultural prenatal partners, resulting in an improvement in postpartum visits in the intervention group (73% vs 51%).[61]

The Geisinger Health System is an integrated health service organization in multiple states that implemented its ProvenCare model to decrease the variability and improve the utility of prenatal care. Twenty-two outpatient sites established 103 unique best-practice measures that were incorporated into a single standardized prenatal care pathway. This pathway was then implemented and tracked, with improvement seen on all clinical measures, including decreased rates of primary cesarean deliveries and NICU admissions.[62]

The medical home model is designed to improve the quality of prenatal care, improve maternal and perinatal outcomes, and reduce cost. In North Carolina, 90%

of providers caring for the pregnant Medicaid population are part of a pregnancy medical home program. This program requires practitioners to have no elective delivery before 39 weeks; offer and provide 17alpha-hydroxyprogesterone (17-OHP) to patients with a prior spontaneous preterm birth; maintain a cesarean delivery rate less than 16% for term, nulliparous, vertex pregnancies; have a postpartum visit within 60 days of delivery; and coordinate with pregnancy care managers.[63] Although the results of this effort are still pending, they represent a substantive effort to address access to care and expanded services to improve maternal and perinatal outcomes.

Optimizing breastfeeding at hospital discharge

Quality improvement efforts to optimize breastfeeding at the time of hospital discharge have been linked to improved perinatal outcomes. The benefits of breast milk for infants include decreased infections, sudden infant death syndrome, asthma and atopy, childhood leukemia, obesity, and diabetes.[64,65] A team of global experts developed an evidence-based guide called *Ten Steps to Successful Breastfeeding* to increase breastfeeding initiation and duration in the hospital setting.[66] Using this guide, San Francisco General Hospital saw an increase in rates of breastfeeding initiation from 81% in 2002 to 98% in 2010.[65]

In 2010, the New York State Department of Health in collaboration with the Obesity Prevention Program and National Initiative for Children's Healthcare Quality engaged 12 hospitals in the New York State Breastfeeding Quality Improvement in Hospitals Learning Collaborative. The goal was to increase rates of exclusive breastfeeding and improve hospital practice and policies. Using a multistep Plan-Do-Study-Act improvement cycle, policies and process changes were implemented to comply with the recommendations of *The Ten Steps to Successful Breastfeeding* by the World Health Organization and the United Nations Children's Fund (UNICEF). Seven process measures were identified, including establishment of skin-to-skin contact after birth, efforts to room in (keep mother and baby together), and variations in work flow. The results showed increased rates of skin-to-skin (up to 90%), rooming in (from 0% to 70%), and exclusive breastfeeding (6% to 44%) by 24 months following implementation.[67]

Recognizing that successful breastfeeding on hospital discharge is just 1 milestone on the way to exclusive breastfeeding for the first 6 months of life, the Washington State Department of Health piloted an adapted version of the *Ten Steps to Successful Breastfeeding* to the outpatient community setting to boost rates of continued breastfeeding postpartum in 8 health centers. Using provider-based assessment tools, adjustments to clinic process flow, and reference documents, participating centers implemented, on average, 7 of the 10 steps within the first 6 months.[68] The program's efficacy once fully operational is yet to be determined.

Maternal-Focused Quality Improvement

The care of mothers at the time of delivery has been a primary focus of obstetric quality improvement efforts. Leaders in maternal-fetal medicine have issued calls for improved efforts to address increasing maternal morbidity and mortality and to put the "M back into maternal-fetal medicine".[69,70] This article highlights outcome data from quality improvement initiatives focused on reducing maternal morbidity and mortality, including reductions in primary cesarean section rates, surgical site infection, postpartum hemorrhage, and team-based training.

Safe reduction of primary cesarean section

One of the early focuses of obstetric quality improvement has been reduction of cesarean section rates. However, obstetricians have long recognized that cesarean section rates alone are not an ideal measure of quality care. Although cesarean delivery is associated with adverse maternal health, rates can be affected by provider and hospital practice patterns as well as the baseline health of patient populations, making meaningful comparisons between hospitals and health systems potentially challenging.[71] As such, there has been a transition in quality improvement work from simple reduction of cesarean section rates to promoting vaginal birth, reducing the first cesarean, and appropriate use of the cesarean procedure.

Two San Francisco–based hospitals starting in the late 1980s showed the impact of large-scale data collection, review, and provision to hospitals and providers to inform them of process measures and balancing measures relative to each other regarding cesarean section rates. Focusing on individual and coded group comparison statistics, the Perinatal Data Center (and outcomes and report-generating software) was used to implement policies and guidelines such as checklists and indications for cesarean section that made identification of appropriate process and balancing measures easier. The results of this work showed decreases in overall cesarean section rates from 25% to 18.5% collectively at both centers.[72] Similar declines were also seen with hospital-level quality improvement work at Cedars-Sinai in Los Angeles, California, and state-level work in Michigan through the Michigan Patient Outcome Measures Project. These two quality improvement projects also showed the importance of data collection using process, balancing, and outcome measures and dissemination to compare measures across sites. They showed reductions of overall cesarean rates of between 3% and 6.5% by evaluating provider variation and using oxytocin protocols and vaginal birth after cesarean section (VBAC).[73,74]

Since 2000, attention has focused on reducing the cesarean section rate of vertex, nulliparous women at term and the safe prevention of the first cesarean section. Originally developed as a potential process measure for affecting cesarean section rates, health system–level quality improvement work at Sutter Health System in northern California in 2000 sought to look for approaches to improve the outcomes of vertex, term, nulliparous mothers while using appropriate clinical tools to effect provider delivery of care through effective measures and data collection systems. Labor practices, including early labor admission and elective induction of labor with an unfavorable Bishop score, were strongly correlated with higher rates of cesarean section in nulliparous, term, singleton, vertex patients. Five-minute Apgar scores less than 7 at term were not correlated with cesarean section rates.[75,76] These findings provided a unique consideration that balanced the need for cesarean sections in certain cases, but taking appropriate and safe evidence-based actions to avoid excessive use.

Since that time there have been ongoing efforts to better promote safe reduction of cesarean delivery. Published in 2014, "Obstetric Care Consensus No. 1: Safe Prevention of the Primary Cesarean Delivery" outlined practices that could be incorporated into labor and delivery care to safely prevent primary cesarean section.[77] Penn State University between 2013 and 2014 showed an overall cesarean section rate reduction of 26.9% to 18.8% with significant gains through reduced cesarean rates following induction or augmentation (35.%–24.5%).[11]

Finding differences in neonatal outcomes, as a balancing measure for initiatives reducing cesarean rates, has proved particularly vexing for these single-institutional studies. It is possible that state-based PQCs may be able to better characterize the neonatal impact by aggregating larger numbers. The California Maternal Quality Care Collaborative in 2016 initiated a project entitled Support Vaginal Birth and Reduce Primary Cesarean Sections, designed to further address this issue.[78]

Reduction of surgical site infection

Another effort that arose from optimizing cesarean section has been the reduction in surgical site infections for cesarean deliveries. Taking the existing literature that has showed the effectiveness of antibiotic prophylaxis and surgical site preparation with chlorhexidine, multiple groups have been able to show a reduction in infection rates through hospital-level quality improvement initiatives. At the University of California, Los Angeles Medical Center, a quality improvement initiative reduced infection rates following cesarean delivery from 10.8% to 2.3% from 2005 to 2008.[79] Components of the initiative included efforts to observe operating room functioning, surveys to assess knowledge gaps and attitudes about infection control, development of process measures such as handwashing compliance and antibiotic administration, and interventions to affect the delivery of care. Similar findings were noted at University of Minnesota and Johns Hopkins University.[9,80]

Management of postpartum hemorrhage

Postpartum hemorrhage is the primary driver of maternal morbidity and mortality both in the United States and worldwide and generated substantive quality improvement work. New York Hospital Medical Center highlighted their response to maternal deaths related to hemorrhage that occurred from 2000 to 2005. Process changes were implemented following recommendations from a multidisciplinary patient safety team including a rapid-response model. Protocols that led to early diagnosis, assessment, and management of patients at high risk for hemorrhage were associated with a reduction in cases of maternal mortality and no increase in rate of cesarean hysterectomy despite increasing their cases of major obstetric hemorrhage 4-fold from 2000 to 2005 (defined as estimated blood loss >1500 mL, need for blood transfusion, need for operative procedure to control bleeding, and hysterectomy).[81]

Similar hospital-level work has confirmed the impact of protocols for hemorrhage management to improve patient care. Marian Medical Center in Santa Barbara, California between 2008 and 2010 showed that implementation of hemorrhage protocols led to improved outcome measures such as fewer blood products for transfusion (16.7 vs 6.3 units/mo, $P<.01$, before and after the protocol, respectively) and a 64% reduction in the incidence of disseminated intravascular coagulation.[82] Moreover, these protocols were perceived by providers as improving patient safety. The introduction of a hemorrhage protocol at Northwestern University between 2007 and 2011 saw improvement in process measures related to management of postpartum hemorrhage with increased use of proven interventions including uterotonic medications (47% before vs 64.8% after, $P<.001$), intrauterine balloon tamponade (2.9% before vs 6.2% after, $P = .002$), B-Lynch suture placement (3.9% before vs 6.0% after, $P = .042$), uterine artery embolization (0.7% before vs 1.8% after, $P = .05$), and cryoprecipitate (1.9% before vs 3.8% after, $P = .022$), which led to a decreased frequency of intensive care unit (ICU) admission over the same time period.[83]

State-level PQCs have been essential to education and dissemination efforts within their respective states as well as nationally. New York and California and their associated maternal quality collaboratives have published online safety bundles and toolkits that show how to operate, develop, and execute statewide hemorrhage quality improvement work.[84–86] The Association of Women's Health, Obstetric, and Neonatal Nurses has also created useful resources and data collection strategies to support hemorrhage initiatives with participating hospitals and states.[87]

Team-Based Training

Hospitals and practitioners may have difficulty adopting new protocols and multiple efforts simultaneously.[88,89] Team-based training seeks to address these difficulties through the use of safety programs, expert review, protocols and guidelines, simulation and drills, alterations in nursing and provider staffing, event reporting, and safety committees to affect how medical team members approach clinical care. Although initial efforts did not seem to suggest substantive effects when used across multiple hospital centers in New England,[86] later results from other multiple hospital efforts showed that team-based efforts could be effectively used to enhance patient safety and quality improvement and improve outcomes.[88,90]

The use of composite measures of adverse maternal and neonatal outcomes (such as ICU admission and traumatic birth injury, in addition to traditional maternal and neonatal mortality) has been particularly helpful toward team-based training efforts. Beth Israel Deaconess Hospital showed the impact of changing the teamwork practices. They found that using communication, situation monitoring, mutual support, and leadership led to a reduced composite measure of adverse maternal and neonatal outcomes.[91] Similar findings were seen at several other hospital-level initiatives.[89,92–94]

Team-based training initiatives have shown economic impact, particularly with regard to liability claims. Working with the 120 hospitals that comprise the Hospital Corporation of America between 1996 and 2006, an emphasis on uniform processes and procedures, development of unambiguous practice guidelines, and effective peer review showed a decrease in malpractice claims from a high of 13 per 10,000 deliveries (1998) to 6 per 10,000 deliveries (2006).[88] Similar decreases in claims and payments at Yale New Haven Hospital occurred between 1998 to 2002 and 2003 to 2007 following the implementation of a comprehensive safety program. Claims decreased from 30 to 14 and payments from $50.7 million versus $2.9 million over each time period, whereas overall claims across the state of Connecticut were stable with increased costs per claim.[95]

Team-based training has also begun to transition to the state-level PQCs. California and New York have both been actively developing methods to train and educate providers with patient safety bundles for the reduction of morbidity. California's focus has been on hemorrhage and hypertension in pregnancy through the California Partnership for Maternal Safety with conclusion of their work in 2016.[96] Through its Safe Motherhood Initiative, New York has focused on hypertension, hemorrhage, and thromboembolism with protocols addressing diagnosis, prevention, and management and is in the midst of an ongoing effort that commenced in 2011.[97] When this work is published it will provide additional understanding of the challenges and benefits of hospital team-based training supported by a state-level collaborative.

Emerging Topics

The immediate future for obstetric quality collaboratives and PQCs is exciting. At the hospital and state levels, work in hypertension in pregnancy, hemorrhage, neonatal abstinence syndrome, reduction of primary cesarean section, provision of 17-OHP for preterm birth prevention, long-acting reversible contraception placement immediately postpartum, and birth certificate accuracy projects are all currently in process. These major projects will shed light on timely and important considerations for perinatal care in the United States.[14]

Multiple states are working on reducing maternal morbidity associated with preeclampsia and severe hypertension in pregnancy and the postpartum period.

California and New York have led the way with initiatives directed at improving care for maternal hypertension. Their toolkits and resources are available on their Web sites and have contributed to the development of the AIM Hypertension Bundle. California is showing preliminary reduction in population-level maternal mortality, whereas other states, including Michigan, Oklahoma, Illinois, Florida, and North Carolina, have embarked on similar work reducing time to treatment of severe hypertension, appropriate preeclampsia management, patient education and follow-up, and decrease in incidence of associated maternal morbidity.[14,98,99] Incorporating work with hypertension, the development of maternal early warning triggers (MEWTs) and similar tools designed to use maternal vital signs to identify patients at risk of clinical deterioration and subsequent morbidity have emerged.[100,101] Work from California using MEWTs has shown substantive reductions in maternal morbidity and provides a model for implementation and further testing by other hospital-level and PQC efforts.[100] Neonatal abstinence syndrome has the attention of numerous states (Ohio, Illinois, Massachusetts, New York, West Virginia, Kentucky, Michigan, Tennessee, Utah, Vermont, New Hampshire) across the country with projects reflecting the national opioid epidemic. Initiatives to increase use of 17-OHP for recurrent preterm birth prevention with hospital-level initiatives in Massachusetts and the state PQC in Ohio expand PQC work into the prenatal care setting to identify at-risk women and increase rates of timely and sustained 17-OHP use.[14] Placement of long-acting reversible contraception (LARC), including an intrauterine device or implantable contraceptive such as etonorgestrel implant, immediately after delivery has been recognized for its potential to increase usage rates for effective, reliable postpartum birth control. State PQC work in South Carolina has made that state a prominent leader in quality improvement work to increase the use of LARC with Medicaid backing.[102] Ohio and Illinois have performed substantive work in optimization of birth certificate accuracy, making a notoriously inaccurate data source increasingly accurate and reliable.[14]

The state-based nature of these efforts has the potential to affect outcomes, cost, and resource allocation within states and nationally. The foundation of state PQCs occurs through hospital-level improvement teams. Improved patient outcomes occur through individual hospitals' efforts to use collaborative resources, collaborative learning, and shared data to drive quality improvement strategies that create sustainable systems-level and team culture change driven by providers and nurses.

Future Considerations

To achieve expanded and sustained quality improvement, hospital, state, and national level quality improvement efforts need perinatal provider champions. Physicians, midwives and nurses, and other staff need quality improvement training to contribute their clinical and systems expertise to the quality improvement process. With education comes improved understanding by staff and providers of the importance of quality improvement work to improve patient care and outcomes. Hospital teams need institutional support for their quality improvement work. Patient and family engagement in hospital-level quality improvement teams helps initiatives to better understand the patient perspective and is associated with faster improvement and improved outcomes overall. State PQCs support hospital-level initiatives with rapid-response data, opportunities for collaborative learning, and quality improvement strategies and support. National initiatives and organizations provide resources, bundles, and toolkits to support state PQCs and their initiatives, assist development, expansion and sustainability of PQCs nationwide, and opportunities for sharing and support across initiatives and collaboratives.

State PQCs require resources, particularly reliable and responsive data collection and reporting processes and funding. Low-burden data collection processes and easily interpreted reports help hospitals direct their quality improvement efforts and allow state PQCs to track progress and provide resources to support hospital teams' work toward improvement goals.[1] Government funding sources of state PQCs include CDC and Division of Reproductive Health, IM CoIIN, Agency for Healthcare Research and Quality (AHRQ), Centers for Medicare Services (CMS), Title V Maternal and Child Health Block Grant Program, state departments of public health, and Medicaid. Private funding sources of state PQCs include insurers, March of Dimes, ACOG, and pharmaceutical company foundations such as Merck for Mothers. The March of Dimes supports the NNPQC.[14–18,97] A mix of public and private funding is essential to foster, develop, and sustain perinatal quality collaborative work into the future.

Despite the significant advances by perinatal and obstetric quality initiatives over the years and their increasing prominence and recognition, there is still much work to be done. There are resources available at the state and national levels to support this work by providing evidence-based toolkits, bundles, and standardized measures to assist the start-up of quality initiatives. At present, many quality collaboratives have comprehensive and detailed resources, including safety bundles and toolkits for implementation of quality improvement work, available on their Web sites.[14–18,97] In addition, the Council on Patient Safety in Women's Healthcare with the AIM in collaboration with ACOG and other partners has laid out comprehensive safety bundles and tools. Available bundles include reduction of primary cesarean birth, obstetric hemorrhage, prevention of preterm birth, severe hypertension in pregnancy, prevention of neonatal abstinence syndrome, venous thromboembolism, mental health, reduction of peripartum racial/ethnic disparities, and support after a severe maternal event.[18] Further publication and dissemination of the findings and work of these organizations should help to highlight these resources and familiarize providers and staff with quality improvement methodology. The expansion of PQCs will need to continue to be sustained and supported. Physician leaders should use organizations at the state (departments of health and Medicaid) as well as national levels (NNPQC, Medicaid, Title V, ACOG, and CDC) to determine available resources and support for their work. Such support includes, but is not limited to, effective data systems, collaborative teams, and advisory groups to allow for effective engagement in ongoing quality initiatives.[1,15]

The work that quality improvement initiatives have achieved is significant. The maternal-focused and perinatal-focused quality improvement initiative results reviewed earlier offer strong examples of the impact that perinatal quality improvement and safety work has in improving the delivery of care. Expanded work at the hospital, state, and national levels is essential to drive sustainable quality improvement and patient safety efforts that will make every hospital a safer and better place to give birth and be born.

REFERENCES

1. Centers for Disease Control and Prevention's Division of Reproductive Health Perinatal Quality Collaborative Guide Working Group. Developing and sustaining perinatal quality collaboratives. Available at: https://www.cdc.gov/reproductivehealth/maternalinfanthealth/pqc.htm. Accessed November 30, 2016.
2. Pettker CM, Grobman WA. Obstetric safety and quality. Obstet Gynecol 2015; 126(1):196–206.

3. Hein HA. Regionalized perinatal care in North America. Semin Neonatol 2004; 9(2):111–6.
4. American College of Obstetricians Gynecologists. Society for maternal-fetal medicine. Levels of maternal care. Am J Obstet Gynecol 2015;212(3):259–71.
5. Myers SA, Gleicher N. The Mount Sinai Cesarean Section Reduction Program: an update after 6 years. Soc Sci Med 1993;37(10):3.
6. Caron A, Neuhauser D. The effect of public accountability on hospital performance: trends in rates for cesarean sections and vaginal births after cesarean section in Cleveland, OH. Qual Manag Health Care 1999;7(2):1–10.
7. Studnicki J, Remmel R, Campbell R, et al. The impact of legislatively imposed practice guidelines on cesarean section rates: the Florida experience. Am J Med Qual 1997;12(1):62–8.
8. Ransom SB, McNeely SG, Yono A, et al. The development and implementation of a normal vaginal delivery clinical pathways in a large multihospital system. Am J Manag Care 1998;4(5):723–7.
9. Witter FR, Lawson P, Ferrell J. Decreasing cesarean section surgical site infection: an ongoing comprehensive quality improvement program. Am J Infect Control 2014;42(4):429–31.
10. Pettker CM, Thung SF, Raab CA, et al. A comprehensive obstetrics patient safety program improves safety climate and culture. Am J Obstet Gynecol 2011;204(3):216.e1-6.
11. Wilson-Leedy JG, DiSilvestro AJ, Repke JT, et al. Reduction in the cesarean delivery rate after obstetric care consensus guideline implementation. Obstet Gynecol 2016;128(1):145–52.
12. Reisner DP, Wallin TK, Zingheim RW, et al. Reduction of elective inductions in a large community hospital. Am J Obstet Gynecol 2009;200(6):674.e1-7.
13. Lowery C, Bronstein J, McGhee J, et al. ANGELS and University of Arkansas for Medical Sciences paradigm for distant obstetrical care delivery. Am J Obstet Gynecol 2007;196(6):534.e1-9.
14. Centers for Disease Control and Prevention's Division of Reproductive Health Perinatal Quality Collaborative Guide Working Group. State Perinatal Quality Collaboratives. Available at: https://www.cdc.gov/reproductivehealth/maternalinfanthealth/pqc-states.html. Accessed November 30, 2016.
15. March of Dimes. National Network of Perinatal Quality Collaboratives Launch. Available at: http://www.marchofdimes.org/professionals/national-network-of-perinatal-quality-collaboratives-launch.aspx. Accessed December 3, 2016.
16. Lee V. The Collaborative Improvement & Innovation Network (CoIIN) to Reduce Infant Mortality: update on regions IV, V and VI. 2014. Available at: https://www.hrsa.gov/advisorycommittees/mchbadvisory/InfantMortality/Meetings/20140709/lee.pdf. Accessed December 3, 2016.
17. Berns SD. March of Dimes Prematurity Collaborative: March of Dimes Big 5 State Prematurity Collaborative. 2009. Available at: http://www.amchp.org/AboutAMCHP/Newsletters/Pulse/Archive/2009/November%202009/Pages/Feature1.aspx. Accessed December 3, 2016.
18. Council on Patient Safety in Women's Health Care. Alliance for Innovation on Maternal Health. Available at: http://safehealthcareforeverywoman.org/aim-program/. Accessed December 3, 2016.
19. National Institute for Children's Health Quality. About NICHQ. Available at: http://www.nichq.org/about. Accessed December 3, 2016.
20. Institute for Healthcare Improvement. Science of improvement: establishing measures. Available at: http://www.ihi.org/resources/Pages/HowtoImprove/

ScienceofImprovementEstablishingMeasures.aspx. Accessed December 11, 2016.
21. Nembhard IM. Learning and improving in quality improvement collaboratives: which collaborative features do participants value most? Health Serv Res 2009;44(2 Pt 1):359–78.
22. Institute for Healthcare Improvement. Plan-Do-Study-Act (PDSA) Worksheet. Available at: http://www.ihi.org/resources/pages/tools/plandostudyactworksheet.aspx. Accessed December 11, 2016.
23. Centers for Disease Control and Prevention Chronic Disease Prevention and Health Promotion. Infant Health. Available at: https://www.cdc.gov/chronicdisease/resources/publications/aag/infant-health.htm. Accessed December 3, 2016.
24. Sengupta S, Carrion V, Shelton J, et al. Adverse neonatal outcomes associated with early-term birth. JAMA Pediatr 2013;167(11):1053–9.
25. Zhang X, Kramer MS. Variations in mortality and morbidity by gestational age among infants born at term. J Pediatr 2009;154(3):358–62, 362.e1.
26. Reddy UM, Bettegowda VR, Dias T, et al. Term pregnancy: a period of heterogeneous risk for infant mortality. Obstet Gynecol 2011;117(6):1279–87.
27. Seikku L, Gissler M, Andersson S, et al. Asphyxia, neurologic morbidity, and perinatal mortality in early-term and postterm birth. Pediatrics 2016;137(6):e20153334.
28. Clark SL, Frye DR, Meyers JA, et al. Reduction in elective delivery at <39 weeks of gestation: comparative effectiveness of 3 approaches to change and the impact on neonatal intensive care admission and stillbirth. Am J Obstet Gynecol 2010;203(5):449.e1-6.
29. Ehrenthal DB, Hoffman MK, Jiang X, et al. Neonatal outcomes after implementation of guidelines limiting elective delivery before 39 weeks of gestation. Obstet Gynecol 2011;118(5):1047–55.
30. Fisch JM, English D, Pedaline S, et al. Labor induction process improvement: a patient quality-of-care initiative. Obstet Gynecol 2009;113(4):797–803.
31. Oshiro BT, Kowalewski L, Sappenfield W, et al. A multistate quality improvement program to decrease elective deliveries before 39 weeks of gestation. Obstet Gynecol 2013;121(5):1025–31.
32. El Haj Ibrahim S, Gregory KD, Kilpatrick SJ, et al. A quality improvement intervention to reduce the rate of elective deliveries < 39 weeks. Jt Comm J Qual Patient Saf 2013;39(6):274–8.
33. Yamasato K, Bartholomew M, Durbin M, et al. Induction rates and delivery outcomes after a policy limiting elective inductions. Matern Child Health J 2015;19(5):1115–20.
34. Berrien K, Devente J, French A, et al. The perinatal quality collaborative of North Carolina's 39 Weeks Project: a quality improvement program to decrease elective deliveries before 39 weeks of gestation. N C Med J 2014;75(3):169–76.
35. Snowden JM, Muoto I, Darney BG, et al. Oregon's hard-stop policy limiting elective early-term deliveries: association with obstetric procedure use and health outcomes. Obstet Gynecol 2016;128(6):1389–96.
36. Donovan EF, Lannon C, Bailit J, et al. A statewide initiative to reduce inappropriate scheduled births at 36(0/7)-38(6/7) weeks' gestation. Am J Obstet Gynecol 2010;202(3):243 e1-8.
37. Bailit JL, Iams J, Silber A, et al. Changes in the indications for scheduled births to reduce nonmedically indicated deliveries occurring before 39 weeks of gestation. Obstet Gynecol 2012;120(2 Pt 1):241–5.

38. Main E, Oshiro B, Chagolla B, et al. Elimination of non-medically indicated (elective) deliveries before 39 weeks gestational age (California Maternal Quality Care Collaborative Toolkit to Transform Maternal Care). 2010; Available at: www.marchofdimes.com/professionals/medicalresources_39weeks.html. Accessed November 11, 2016.
39. Liggins GC, Howie RN. A controlled trial of antepartum glucocorticoid treatment for prevention of the respiratory distress syndrome in premature infants. Pediatrics 1972;50(4):515–25.
40. Crowley P. Prophylactic corticosteroids for preterm birth. Cochrane Database Syst Rev 2000;(2):CD000065.
41. American College of Obstetricians Gynecologists. Committee opinion no.677: antenatal corticosteroid therapy for fetal maturation. Obstet Gynecol 2016; 128(4):e187–94.
42. Wirtschafter DD, Danielsen BH, Main EK, et al. Promoting antenatal steroid use for fetal maturation: results from the California Perinatal Quality Care Collaborative. J Pediatr 2006;148(5):606–12.
43. Lee HC, Lyndon A, Blumenfeld YJ, et al. Antenatal steroid administration for premature neonates in California. Obstet Gynecol 2011;117(3):603–9.
44. Bronstein JM, Cliver SP, Goldenberg RL. Practice variation in the use of interventions in high-risk obstetrics. Health Serv Res 1998;32(6):825–39.
45. Bronstein JM, Goldenberg RL. Practice variation in the use of corticosteroids: a comparison of eight data sets. Am J Obstet Gynecol 1995;173(1):296–8.
46. Ohio Perinatal Quality Collaborative Writing Committee. Abstract 521: a statewide project to promote optimal use of antenatal corticosteroids (ANCS). Am J Obstet Gynecol 2013;208(1):S224.
47. Kaplan HC, Sherman SN, Cleveland C, et al. Reliable implementation of evidence: a qualitative study of antenatal corticosteroid administration in Ohio hospitals. BMJ Qual Saf 2016;25(3):173–81.
48. Staebler S. Regionalized systems of perinatal care: health policy considerations. Adv Neonatal Care 2011;11(1):37–42.
49. Brantley MD, Davis NL, Goodman DA, et al. Perinatal regionalization: a geospatial view of perinatal critical care, United States, 2010-2013. Am J Obstet Gynecol 2017;216(2):185.e1-10.
50. Phibbs CS, Baker LC, Caughey AB, et al. Level and volume of neonatal intensive care and mortality in very-low-birth-weight infants. N Engl J Med 2007;356(21): 2165–75.
51. Nowakowski L, Barfield WD, Kroelinger CD, et al. Assessment of state measures of risk-appropriate care for very low birth weight infants and recommendations for enhancing regionalized state systems. Matern child Health J 2012;16(1): 217–27.
52. Howell EM, Richardson D, Ginsburg P, et al. Deregionalization of neonatal intensive care in urban areas. Am J Public Health 2002;92(1):417–23.
53. Laswell SM, Barfield WD, Rochat RW, et al. Perinatal regionalization for very low-birth-weight and very preterm infants. JAMA 2010;304(9):992–1000.
54. Bronstein JM, Ounpraseuth S, Jonkman J, et al. Improving perinatal regionalization for preterm deliveries in a Medicaid covered population: initial impact of the Arkansas ANGELS intervention. Health Serv Res 2011;46(4):1082–103.
55. Kim EW, Teague-Ross TJ, Greenfield WW, et al. Telemedicine collaboration improves perinatal regionalization and lowers statewide infant mortality. J Perinatol 2013;33(9):725–30.

56. Akula VP, Gould JB, Kan P, et al. Characteristics of neonatal transports in California. J Perinatol 2016;36(12):1122–7.
57. Grant J. The journey to LOCATe levels of neonatal & maternal care. 2016. Available at: http://www.nichq.org/blog/2016/august/locate_perinatal_care_levels. Accessed December 3, 2016.
58. Daniel-Robinson L, Cha S, Lillie-Blanton M. Efforts to improve perinatal outcomes for women enrolled in Medicaid. Obstet Gynecol 2015;126(2):435–41.
59. Hill I, Benatar S, Courtot B, et al. Strong Start Mothers Newborns Eval Year 1 Annu Rep. 2014. Available at: https://innovation.cms.gov/Files/reports/strongstart-enhancedprenatal-yr1evalrpt.pdf. Accessed December 3, 2016.
60. Centers for Medicare and Medicaid Services Maternal & Infant Health Initiative. Resources on strategies to improve postpartum care among Medicaid and CHIP populations. 2015. Available at: https://www.medicaid.gov/medicaid/quality-of-care/downloads/strategies-to-improve-postpartum-care.pdf. Accessed December 3, 2016.
61. Marsiglia FF, Bermudez-Parsai M, Coonrod D. Familias Sanas: an intervention designed to increase rates of postpartum visits among Latinas. J Health Care Poor Underserved 2010;21(3):119–31.
62. Berry SA, Laam LA, Wary AA, et al. ProvenCare perinatal: a model for delivering evidence/guideline-based care for perinatal populations. Jt Comm J Qual Patient Saf 2011;37(5):229–39.
63. Berrien K, Ollendorff A, Menard K. Pregnancy medical home care pathways improve quality of perinatal care and birth outcomes. N C Med J 2015;76(4):263–6.
64. Vasquez MJ, Berg OR. The baby-friendly journey in a US public hospital. J Perinat Neonatal Nurs 2012;26(1):37–46.
65. Magri EP, Hylton-McGuire K. Transforming a care delivery model to increase breastfeeding. MCN Am J Matern Child Nurs 2013;38(3):177–82.
66. Baby-Friendly USA. The ten steps to successful breastfeeding. 2012. Available at: http://www.babyfriendlyusa.org/about-us/baby-friendly-hospital-initiative/the-ten-steps. Accessed December 3, 2016.
67. Grummer-Strawn LM, Shealy KR, Perrine CG, et al. Maternity care practices that support breastfeeding: CDC efforts to encourage quality improvement. J Womens Health (Larchmt) 2013;22(2):107–12.
68. Schwartz R, Ellings A, Baisden A, et al. Washington 'Steps' up: a 10-step quality improvement initiative to optimize breastfeeding support in community health centers. J Hum Lact 2015;31(4):651–9.
69. D'Alton ME, Bonanno CA, Berkowitz RL, et al. Putting the "M" back in maternal-fetal medicine. Am J Obstet Gynecol 2013;208(6):442–8.
70. Creanga AA, Berg CJ, Syverson C, et al. Pregnancy-related mortality in the United States, 2006-2010. Obstet Gynecol 2015;125(1):5–12.
71. Gibson K, Bailit JL. Cesarean delivery as a marker for OB quality. Clin Obstet Gynecol 2015;58(2):211–6.
72. Main EK. Reducing cesarean birth rates with data-driven quality improvement activities. Pediatrics 1999;103(1):374–83.
73. Rosen LS, Schroeder K, Hagan M, et al. Adapting a statewide patient database for comparative analysis and quality improvement. Jt Comm J Qual Improv 1996;22(7):468–81.
74. Gregory KD, Hackmeyer P, Gold L, et al. Using the continuous quality improvement process to safely lower the cesarean section rate. Jt Comm J Qual Improv 1999;25(12):619–29.

75. Main EK, Bloomfield L, Hunt G, Sutter Health, First Pregnancy and Delivery Clinical Initiative Committee. Development of a large-scale obstetric quality-improvement program that focused on the nulliparous patient at term. Am J Obstet Gynecol 2004;190(6):1747–56 [discussion: 1756–8].
76. Main EK, Moore D, Farrell B, et al. Is there a useful cesarean birth measure? Assessment of the nulliparous term singleton vertex cesarean birth rate as a tool for obstetric quality improvement. Am J Obstet Gynecol 2006;194(6): 1644–51 [discussion 1651–2].
77. American College of Obstetricians and Gynecologists. Society for Maternal-Fetal Medicine. Obstetric care consensus no. 1: safe prevention of the primary cesarean delivery. Obstet Gynecol 2014;123(3):693–711.
78. California Maternal Quality Care Collaborative. Support vaginal birth and reduce primary cesareans: collaborative and toolkit. Available at: https://www.cmqcc.org/projects/support-vaginal-birth-and-reduce-primary-cesareans-collaborative-and-toolkit. Accessed November 11, 2016.
79. Riley MM, Suda D, Tabsh K, et al. Reduction of surgical site infections in low transverse cesarean section at a university hospital. Am J Infect Control 2012; 40(9):820–5.
80. Rauk PN. Educational intervention, revised instrument sterilization methods, and comprehensive preoperative skin preparation protocol reduce cesarean section surgical site infections. Am J Infect Control 2010;38(4):319–23.
81. Skupski DW, Lowenwirt IP, Weinbaum FI, et al. Improving hospital systems for the care of women with major obstetric hemorrhage. Obstet Gynecol 2006; 107(5):977–83.
82. Shields LE, Smalarz K, Reffigee L, et al. Comprehensive maternal hemorrhage protocols improve patient safety and reduce utilization of blood products. Am J Obstet Gynecol 2011;205(4):368.e1-8.
83. Einerson BD, Miller ES, Grobman WA. Does a postpartum hemorrhage patient safety program result in sustained changes in management and outcomes? Am J Obstet Gynecol 2015;212(2):140–4.e1.
84. Burgansky A, Montalto D, Siddiqui NA. The safe motherhood initiative: the development and implementation of standardized obstetric care bundles in New York. Semin Perinatol 2016;40(2):124–31.
85. Bingham D, Lyndon A, Lagrew D, et al. A state-wide obstetric hemorrhage quality improvement initiative. MCN Am J Matern Child Nurs 2011;36(5):297–304.
86. California Maternal Quality Care Collaborative. Improving health care response to obstetric hemorrhage, Version 2.0: a California toolkit to transform maternity care. Available at: https://www.cmqcc.org/resources-tool-kits/toolkits/ob-hemorrhage-toolkit. Accessed November 11, 2016.
87. Association of Women's Health Obstetric and Neonatal Nurses. Postpartum hemorrhage (PPH). Available at: https://www.awhonn.org/?page=PPH.
88. Clark SL, Belfort MA, Byrum SL, et al. Improved outcomes, fewer cesarean deliveries, and reduced litigation: results of a new paradigm in patient safety. Am J Obstet Gynecol 2008;199(2):105.e1-7.
89. Gilbert WM, Bliss MC, Johnson A, et al. Improving recording accuracy, transparency, and performance for obstetric quality measures in a community hospital-based obstetrics department. Jt Comm J Qual Patient Saf 2013;39(6):258–66.
90. Nielsen PE, Goldman MB, Mann S, et al. Effects of teamwork training on adverse outcomes and process of care in labor and delivery: a randomized control trial. Obstet Gynecol 2007;109(1):48–55.

91. Pratt SD, Mann S, Salisbury M, et al. Impact of CRM-based team training on obstetric outcomes and clinicians' patient safety attitudes. Jt Comm J Qual Patient Saf 2007;33(12):720–5.
92. Iverson RE Jr, Heffner LJ. Patient safety series: obstetric safety improvement and its reflection in reserved claims. Am J Obstet Gynecol 2011;205(5): 398–401.
93. Tolcher MC, Torbenson VE, Weaver AL, et al. Impact of a labor and delivery safety bundle on a modified adverse outcomes index. Am J Obstet Gynecol 2016;214(3):401.e1-9.
94. Pettker CM, Thung SF, Norwitz ER, et al. Impact of a comprehensive patient safety strategy on obstetric adverse events. Am J Obstet Gynecol 2009; 200(5):492.e1-8.
95. Pettker CM, Thung SF, Lipkind HS, et al. A comprehensive obstetric patient safety program reduces liability claims and payments. Am J Obstet Gynecol 2014;211(4):319–25.
96. California Maternal Quality Care Collaborative. California Partnership for Maternal Safety. Available at: https://www.cmqcc.org/projects/california-partnership-maternal-safety.
97. American College of Obstetricians District II. ACOG district II Safe Motherhood Initiative (SMI). Available at: http://www.acog.org/About-ACOG/ACOG-Districts/District-II/Safe-Motherhood-Initiative.
98. Kilpatrick SJ, Abreo A, Greene N, et al. Severe maternal morbidity in a large cohort of women with acute severe intrapartum hypertension. Am J Obstet Gynecol 2016;215(1):91.e1-7.
99. Kilpatrick SJ, Berg C, Bernstein P, et al. Standardized severe maternal morbidity review: rationale and process. Obstet Gynecol 2014;124(2 Pt 1):361–6.
100. Shields LE, Wiesner S, Klein C, et al. Use of maternal early warning trigger tool reduces maternal morbidity. Am J Obstet Gynecol 2016;214(4):527.e1-6.
101. Mhyre JM, D'Oria R, Hameed AB, et al. The maternal early warning criteria: a proposal from the National Partnership for Maternal Safety. Obstet Gynecol 2014;124(4):782–6.
102. Crockett AH, Pickell LB, Heberlein EC, et al. Six- and twelve-month documented removal rates among women electing postpartum inpatient compared to delayed or interval contraceptive implant insertions after Medicaid payment reform. Contraception 2017;95(1):71–6.

Eliminating Undesirable Variation in Neonatal Practice

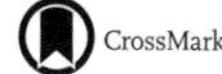

Balancing Standardization and Customization

Maya Balakrishnan, MD, CSSBB[a], Aarti Raghavan, MD[b], Gautham K. Suresh, MD, DM, MS[c,*]

KEYWORDS

• Quality improvement • Variation in health care • Standardization • Customization

KEY POINTS

- Variation in health care occurs at multiple levels, including geographic, institutional, and individual provider.
- Efforts to improve care quality should attempt to balance customization and standardization of care, to decrease unwanted variation and still promote favorable variation in practice.
- Finding the correct balance involves understanding what needs to be standardized as well as how it can be incorporated into practice.

INTRODUCTION

In its influential report, *Crossing the Quality Chasm*, the Institute of Medicine[1] described 6 domains of quality in health care: safety, timeliness, effectiveness, efficiency, equity, and patient-centeredness. These are important areas of focus for any effort to measure and improve health care quality. However, 2 additional aspects of health care quality require attention and improvement, but have generally been underemphasized: consistency of care, and the elimination of unnecessary and harmful variation. This article describes the prevalence and patterns of practice variation in both health care and neonatology; discusses the potential role of standardization as a

Disclosure: The authors have nothing to disclose.

[a] Division of Neonatology, Department of Pediatrics, University of South Florida Morsani College of Medicine, 2 Tampa General Circle, Tampa, FL 33606, USA; [b] Division of Neonatology, Department of Pediatrics, UIC Hospital, University of Illinois College of Medicine at Chicago, 1740 West Taylor Street, Chicago, IL 60612, USA; [c] Division of Neonatology, Department of Pediatrics, Texas Children's Hospital, Baylor College of Medicine, 6621 Fannin Street, W6104, Houston, TX 77030, USA

* Corresponding author.

E-mail address: gksuresh@bcm.edu

Clin Perinatol 44 (2017) 529–540

http://dx.doi.org/10.1016/j.clp.2017.04.002

solution to eliminating wasteful and harmful practice variation, particularly when it is founded on principles of evidence-based medicine[2,3]; and proposes ways to balance standardization with customization of practice to ultimately improve the quality of neonatal care.

VARIATION IN HEALTH CARE

Variation in care exists when patients with the same or reasonably similar conditions receive different care based on the geographic location or institution where the care is provided, or on the health professionals providing the care.

An abundance of literature has shown that variation in care is widespread, at both a geographic and institutional level. Differences in practice patterns from one country to another are well known, and the United States is no exception. Within the United States, numerous publications have described these variations in practice patterns for adult patients, including both medical (eg, screening for breast cancer or diabetes) and surgical care (eg, hip replacement). The Dartmouth Atlas of Healthcare, published annually, provides cartographic descriptions of such variations based on Medicare data.[4] Similar methodology has been applied to pediatric patients and has uncovered variations in perioperative care,[5] treatment of bronchiolitis,[6] treatment of sepsis,[7] among others. Interinstitutional variation is also well described with both neonatal practices and outcomes in reports from large networks of neonatal intensive care units, as well as in multicenter studies.[8–16] This variation occurs among different neonatal intensive care units (NICUs) and within a single NICU, as well as among providers.[17] The databases of the Vermont Oxford Network,[12] Neonatal Research Network,[13,14] Canadian Neonatal Network,[15] and Pediatrix[16] highlight NICU to NICU differences in neonatal practices and outcomes for very-low-birth-weight infants. Similar differences are described in early-onset sepsis risk management strategies,[18] as well as in the incidence of neonatal outcomes such as chronic lung disease, retinopathy of prematurity, and necrotizing enterocolitis.[12] Another example, variation in mortality and neurodevelopmental outcomes in extremely preterm infants based on practice approach (initiating active treatment vs comfort care at birth) is also reported.[19] Institutional variation in outcomes for term infants has also been described. One study noted that the geographic region in which a hospital is located, along with other hospital characteristics (level of care, birth volume, and percentage of Medicaid births), was associated with unexpected complications among term newborns.[20] Although the health care industry is decades behind other high-reliability organizations in standardization of practices, evidence in health care suggests that divergence of practice and lack of standardization are linked to poor outcomes.[21]

One type of variation that is not yet well studied is intrainstitutional variation or variation occurring within a single institution or NICU. When modifications in a management plan are based solely on changes in a patient's condition or on family preferences, it is likely both justified and desirable. The structure of NICU work schedules (ie, shift work, service rotations, or off-hour coverage) causes the same NICU patients to be cared for by different health professionals every shift or every service block. Anecdotally, there is general agreement that there are major differences in the philosophy, attitudes, decision-making style, and practice style among NICU physicians, nurse practitioners, nurses, respiratory therapists, and other health professionals. When care of an NICU patient transitions from one physician or nurse to another, these differences can lead to changes in patient care that are predominantly or solely based on a provider's preferences or decision-making style. Such undesirable variation breeds frustration among the patient's family, bedside staff, and colleagues. It also represents a form of poor-quality care that increases health care cost and waste, and potentially causes poor outcomes. Because inter-neonatologist or inter-practitioner differences in management style are common, trainees, nurses, and nurse practitioners often adapt by learning each neonatologist's preferences and styles, which develops a unit lore. Staff learn the preferred practice style of each specific physician and change patient care practices according to the physician in charge at any given time. Another common form of undesirable variation occurs when the primary neonatology team's management plan and goals differ from that of consulted subspecialists.

ADDRESSING VARIATION IN PRACTICE

Minimizing undesirable geographic, interinstitutional, and intrainstitutional variations in care practice requires an understanding of the underlying reasons for such variation. This variation can result from characteristics of the health professionals, of the patient (or family), and of the intervention (ie, the diagnostic test or treatment), as shown in **Box 1**. Clinicians' practice preferences can be affected by their knowledge bases and training, personal and professional experience, inherent biases, priorities (eg, fear of litigation, medicolegal or financial incentives, mandates), and personality (ie,

Box 1
Potential factors associated with health care variation

Factors related to health care provider:

- Place of training
- Experience
- Last patient seen
- Knowledge of evidence (ie, sources of knowledge, system of keeping informed, study habits)
- Willingness to change (ie, physicians' openness to questioning their own practices)
- Biases (eg, special interest in a disease or condition)
- Priorities
- Fear of litigation
- Incentives
- Specialty or discipline
- Personality (eg, risk averse)

Factors related to the health care intervention:

- Quality of evidence
- Uncertainty
- Diffusion of innovations[22]: perceived benefit, relative advantage, compatibility, simplicity, suitability for trials, observability

Factors related to the patient or family:

- Information and perceptions
- Health literacy and awareness
- Cultural factors
- Influences from peer pressure (eg, from friends or relatives), the Internet, or social media

willingness to change, degree of risk aversion). Factors related to an intervention that may contribute to practice variation include quality of evidence, as well as adaptability of a practice. Patient and family characteristics include their personal beliefs and values, degree of health literacy, and the influence attributed to the patient's culture, family, friends, and social media. Rogers and colleagues[22] identified major elements that affect the acceptance of a practice, including the perceived relative advantage, compatibility with existing norms or experience, complexity (ie, in understanding and application into practice), suitability for trials (ie, exposure allowing observation and testing of the intervention), and observability of an intervention's outcomes.

After analyzing the underlying sources of practice variation, the next step is to identify which types of variation should be encouraged and which types should be minimized or eliminated. Not all variation is bad and patient care sometimes improves with other perspectives, fresh insights, and different experiences that new health professionals bring when they take over the care of a patient. A simple principle that is helpful in distinguishing beneficial from harmful variation is that beneficial variation is based on a patient's condition; family preference; new insights; or previously overlooked diagnostic possibilities or therapeutic options. In contrast, variation that is based solely on a health professional's practice style or preferences (ie, it is arbitrary) is harmful, and should be minimized to promote consistency of care. Care of the patient and family therefore should be customized where appropriate, and standardized when appropriate.

Balancing customization with standardization in this manner requires an understanding of the evolution, principles, and application of standardization. Because many tools and techniques currently used for quality improvement (QI) in health care were imported from other industries, first understanding the evolution of QI and standardization in industry is important.

STANDARDIZATION IN OTHER INDUSTRIES

Standardization is successfully used in manufacturing of products, industrial processes, service industries, car manufacturing, commercial aviation, nuclear energy, accounting, and the military. Here, the underlying goal of standardization is generally to consistently produce a good service or product that meets agreed-upon requirements. Standardization is evident in many aspects of daily life. Examples are the design of electrical plugs and sockets, computer connections, diesel nozzles not fitting the opening of fuel tanks of gasoline-fueled cars, the use of standard operating procedures in aviation, computer coding, and manufacturing. Standardization makes it easier to do the right thing, and at times has the added benefit of conferring safety to the operation. For example, it reduces the likelihood of a driver incorrectly refueling a gasoline-powered car with diesel, and allows any pilot to competently fly a particular type of plane regardless of the airline.[23]

Frederick Taylor transformed standardization and the understanding of work flow by decreasing work complexity and increasing its efficiency. He did this by thoroughly understanding tasks involved in a process and outlining them, allowing people unfamiliar with a complex process to be successfully trained to perform simpler subprocesses. Working together using a standardized process, this team of people accomplishing multiple subprocesses could then more efficiently complete a task.[24,25] Henry Ford took standardization a step further with the mass production of automobiles. He understood the value of standardizing vehicle parts, which both simplified work and allowed both parts and workers to be interchangeable.[24,25] Ford found that standardization increased productivity, resulting in decreased cost of automobiles, which could then be purchased by more of the public, as well as increased wages for workers, which increased retention at the automobile plant. The Toyota Production Systems applied these lessons to develop a lean system of customized mass production, with the focus on eliminating non–value-added activities and waste (eg, overproduction, long setup times, rework), and on flexibility in job assignment. The gains realized were many, particularly that the increased efficiencies brought about increased production with fewer resources.[24,25] To standardize and control variation in their product line, Motorola successfully used QI methodology, such as the Shewhart statistical quality control principles, to decrease the number of defects.[24,25] Underlying industry's progress with QI (total quality management) and standardization are the contributions of QI leaders such as Shewhart, Deming, and Juran.

There are drawbacks to the types of standardization and scientific management listed earlier, including pressure to achieve results, which can induce workers to exaggerate the level of success and falsify data. Such approaches can also lead to demoralization of front-line workers who may believe themselves undervalued and depersonalized. A downstream effect of an inflated sense of efficiency might be unrealistic work expectations. It also does not account for the psychology of management, and can engender fears that workers are made to perform on "autopilot," mandated to do their tasks in the perceived single, most efficient way.[26]

The origins of the QI movement in health care were in industry and manufacturing. Early pioneers of QI in health care used principles developed by leaders such as Deming, Juran, and Shewhart. They successfully applied and widely used these principles from industries outside of health care. Therefore, it is not surprising that standardization was proposed very early on as a potential solution to minimize variation and improve quality in health care as well.

STANDARDIZATION IN HEALTH CARE

Understanding the Role of Standardization in Health Care

Standardization in health care has the potential to decrease practice variation in the industry, improve patient safety and care quality, increase efficiency, and make care more cost-effective.[27,28] Thus standardization is an important change concept in QI initiatives.[29] There is no single, agreed-on definition of standardization in health care. One definition is that it is a "process by which healthcare products or services are chosen by a committee of key stakeholders, taking into account evidence-based results, to ensure quality patient care while adhering to fiscal responsibility."[2] Furthermore, the lens with which standardization is viewed colors its meaning. For example, suppliers (eg, pharmaceutical or insurance companies) may focus primarily on the benefits of standardization on financial impact,[2,30,31] whereas hospital management may concentrate on efficiency balanced with quality patient care.[2]

There are many instances of standardization being successful in health care. A classic example is the Neonatal Resuscitation Program (NRP), introduced in the 1980s and now widely accepted as the standard way to assess and resuscitate newborn infants. NRP's international acceptance involved expert consensus opinion regarding resuscitation practices based on best available evidence with routine revisions; providing a standardized method to approach resuscitation that is adaptable to differing provider skill sets; and a dissemination and implementation plan that supports education, training, and sustainability.[32] Another example, and perhaps one of the greatest successes of standardization in health care, has been the implementation of the Directly Observed Therapy, Short-Course by the World Health Organization

(WHO) to reduce the global burden of tuberculosis (TB). Since 1990, this program has resulted in worldwide reduction of TB prevalence by standardizing the dispensation and monitoring consumption of anti-TB chemotherapy in endemic areas.[33] Similar achievements have been made in neonatology, including decreased rates of neonatal group B *Streptococcus* through the standardization of testing and intrapartum antibiotic prophylaxis in pregnant women[28] and reduced necrotizing enterocolitis rates and length of NICU stay with the use of standardized feeding protocols.[34] In health care, attempts at standardization using guidelines or policies may add layers of defense to prevent errors from occurring.[35] Having 100% of providers execute appropriate tasks on 100% of their patients, 100% of the time, may reduce inevitable human error and enhance reliability of care. An important benefit of standardizing practice is that it allows both patients and providers to seamlessly transition from one health care facility to another without compromising quality or safety. The WHO High 5s project is an example of international collaboration between more than 11 countries across 4 continents. The goals of this project were to identify the feasibility of establishing standardized protocols and practices across hospitals in different countries and the impact of this standardization on patient safety. The High 5s project focused on standardization of management for concentrated injectable medicines, ensuring medication accuracy at transitions of care, correct site procedure, communication during handoffs, and improved hand hygiene.[36] Standardized newborn screening in the United States has facilitated early identification of hearing loss, critical congenital heart disease, and various metabolic disorders. Administering antiretroviral treatment in neonates exposed to human immunodeficiency virus (HIV) within hours of birth has reduced the incidence of neonatal HIV infection.[37] Central line–associated bloodstream infections have decreased when facilities used targeted bundles of care that consistently applied evidence-based practices.[38]

Standardization is not intended to be, nor should it be, a panacea for every health care process. There are aspects in the diagnosis and management of individual patients that can and should be standardized to improve safety or quality of care. However, it would be nearly impossible to remove all sources of variation in health care; for example, the variations in neonatal management with regard to the choice of inotrope for hypotension, treatment of retinopathy of prematurity (ROP; eg, bevacizumab vs laser therapy), or use of high-frequency ventilation.[37]

Understanding How to Use Evidence-Based Medicine to Promote Standardization

Practicing evidence-based medicine means integrating the highest available quality of evidence and clinical expertise with patient values.[39] Batalden and Davidoff[40] describe how generalizable scientific evidence customized for a given context and executed through planned changes, with close performance monitoring, is necessary to achieve performance improvement. Recognizing that some degree of variation always remains, providers should, when appropriate, attempt to integrate standardization into everyday practice. This process starts with recognition of a suitable process or method of management to standardize. Processes that are suitable for standardization are ideally those involving issues supported by high-quality evidence (eg, exclusive human milk diet for neonates), or being repeatedly done in the same way every time (eg, medication administration), affecting a homogenous population of patients (eg, very-low-birth-weight infants and oxygen saturation targeting related to ROP), or engaging a large population of practitioners performing high-stakes tasks (eg, those performing neonatal resuscitation). For neonatal medical or nursing teams, this means reaching some internal consensus regarding how to identify an appropriate topic to standardize and reviewing the evidence supporting the suggested practices.

Although standardization of health care delivery using clinical practice guidelines and pathways is advocated as a potential method to decrease practice variation, it can also be problematic. A guideline is not enough to change behavior. Examples of guideline limitations include poor understanding of the local environment, using low-quality evidence to develop guidelines, lack of guideline consensus or compliance, overlooking needed customization of care, and medicolegal considerations. Health care systems, particularly NICUs, are unique, complex multisystems in which individual providers interface with their environments in intricate ways. A critical element of successful standardization efforts is having deep knowledge of the local environment and the ability to adapt systems to work in the settings for which they were created. It is incumbent on local teams to specify how to implement recommendations into their local environments. For example, studies encourage early continuous positive airway pressure (CPAP) use for treatment of respiratory distress syndrome. A NICU may have guidelines that support this practice, including criteria for how and when to provide surfactant. Executing this in the NICU is not so straightforward. For example, a team would need to consider who is responsible for having CPAP readily available in the delivery room and whether they have CPAP available as a resource in their NICU. Solutions to this may consist of delivery room role assignments and use of an equipment checklist. Another limitation of guidelines is developing practice recommendations if there are low levels of evidence by using expert consensus opinion, which may produce consistent, low-quality care.[41] A guideline's recommendations must be based on scientific evidence and have on-going evaluation.[42] Perhaps one of the greatest limitations is the adoption of, and adherence to, guidelines by practicing clinicians. Interinstitutional differences in operating procedures and protocols encourage lack of consensus. Beyond that, the belief that too much standardization results in automated behavior may limit provider compliance.[43] Other reported physician barriers include the shortcomings in knowledge (eg, awareness of or familiarity with the guideline), attitudes (eg, agreement with recommendations, self-efficacy, outcome expectancy, motivation to change from previous practices), and behavior (eg, external barriers, such as lack of time, ease of use, clarity, insufficient ancillary support, or patient resistance).[44] Widespread adoption of guidelines without consideration for individual patient characteristics that support customization of care poses risk of harm and may not reflect the preferences of the patient or family. There are also medicolegal implications related to lack of guideline compliance and risks to insurance reimbursement when specified criteria from guidelines are not met.[42]

There is risk in not accounting for a patient's unique characteristics or understanding the nuances of complex diseases or treatments. For example, overusing standardization in health care can prompt providers to make incorrect correlations between patients and diagnoses, and lead to inappropriate treatments. Physicians may view enforced standardization as so-called cookbook medicine and only be persuaded to accept it if provided with rationales based on strong evidence to support the standardization. In some studies, physicians have reported viewing standardization as a means of control, arguing for a greater need for transparency of assumed benefit.[45] Nurses may think standardization improves efficiency of care through time saving (ie, less time searching for equipment, allowing more time for patient interaction), whereas patients may consider it important only if it does not adversely affect their own care.[2,3] A study of patient attitudes toward standardization of their care reported that, although many are not aware of how standardization affects their care quality, approximately 90% believe it is driven by hospital administration and roughly 70% think that clinicians are directly affected by it.[3] These differing opinions highlight the need for all stakeholders to be involved in the standardization process in order to improve outcomes. Furthermore, there is some value to the art or customization of care, particularly when there is unavoidable variability (eg, type of respiratory support required for a newborn infant with rapidly evolving respiratory disease) or a complicated or unique diagnosis (eg, conjoined twins or other unique combination of birth defects).[46] In these types of situations, standardizing the management plan may not be advantageous. Harmonizing this pull between standardizing and customizing care is key to providing good patient care.

CUSTOMIZATION IN HEALTH CARE

Customization of care means treating a particular patient, at a particular time or place, in a particular way. Although customization cannot be completely avoided, it contributes to significant practice variation. However, much of the supposedly high-quality evidence that is reported from trials is developed with the intention of capturing homogenous populations of patients to test an intervention or treatment. Standardization does not explicitly account for necessary changes in treatment based on the heterogeneity of patients who are treat each day and who may have several coexisting morbidities and complex treatment regimens. Underlying themes of QI in health care are to understand variation, control the degree of variation, and minimize its impact so that, as much as possible, care can be delivered in a predictable manner to produce a predictable and reliable outcome. This approach is often perceived as advocating for standardization of care practices. However, this perception implies that all variation is harmful, wasteful, or inequitable, whereas customization may be warranted in order to tailor or target treatment of particular patients.[47]

Although standardization is designed to help care providers use evidence-based medicine in a systematic way that guarantees that patients receive high-quality care, consideration should be given to individual factors such as patient belief systems, treatment preferences, comorbidities, genomics, and the local environment. In addition, there exists the complex interaction of patients with their health care providers, who have the moral and ethical responsibility to adhere to the best-interest standard.[48] Patient-centered care and personalized medicine are representations of customized care.[49] Providers' beliefs regarding the individual nature of a problem[48] and the patients' beliefs that customized care is better quality care[49] are barriers to standardization. Patient-centered care incorporates the individual preferences of patients and providers, and fosters mutual trust between the two. It has shown clear improvement in patient satisfaction, increased employee satisfaction, and reduced burnout.[48] An example of customization in neonatology relating to an infant's human milk diet occurs when supplemental calories, protein, or fat are administered based on nutrition information provided by a breast milk analyzer. Genomics studies reveal the value of personalized medicine, in which care can be tailored to individuals based on genetic characteristics, as in breast cancer–screening protocols based on individual genome and risk stratification. Although applications of genomics are underexplored in neonatology, it offers potential for future therapeutic developments.

FINDING THE RIGHT BALANCE

Ultimately, both standardization and customization of care have value. Efforts to improve the quality of care should both attempt to decrease unwanted variation and promote favorable variation in practice. Therefore, leaders and QI teams should attempt to find the correct balance, which can support standardization while still allowing flexibility to customize care, ultimately leading to improved effectiveness, efficiency, and equity of care, as well as consistency of care and elimination of waste.[47]

To find this balance, there are useful principles that can be applied to the "what," as well as to the "how," of the practice. These principles outline how evidence can be transformed by QI to improve performance. The "what" is the medical intervention, such as a diagnostic test, therapy, or the medical decision or communication regarding risks or prognosis. The "how" refers to the process, which includes the implementation of the decision and execution of actions. Frameworks for integrating the concepts of the "what" and the "how" of a practice are described in the Batalden and Davidoff[40] formula and by Bohmer.[50]

Batalden and Davidoff[40] describe 5 knowledge systems that should be integrated for successful improvement of patient outcomes: generalizable scientific evidence, particular context awareness, performance measurement, plans for change, and execution of planned changes. A deficiency in any of these may cause an improvement initiative to be unsuccessful. The "what" is determined by the quality of evidence for a specific intervention, and the benefit/risk ratio. Highly standardized practices should have high-quality evidence in which benefits clearly outweigh risks. For example, removal of unnecessary central lines is important in decreasing central line–associated bloodstream infections. In neonatology, randomized controlled trials to guide management are often lacking and there may be an equivocal benefit/risk ratio. In these cases, lower quality evidence, expert consensus opinion, or benchmarking can be used to develop unit-specific guidelines. The goals would be to develop general agreement to promote consistency of care, to measure and monitor the developed process, and to make appropriate revisions based on data analysis.[40]

Bohmer[50] describes a framework for the "how" of implementing a practice. His structure can help providers consider a balanced approach by understanding patient situations using the following options: separate and select; separate and accommodate; integrate; and modularize. When a standardized process and a mechanism for recognizing patient patterns exist, the separate-and-select or separate-and-accommodate path makes sense. In essence, the separate-and-select model identifies a homogenous group of patients who can receive treatment following a standardized algorithm and separates them from those who require customized or other specialized care. This strategy can be changed into a separate-and-accommodate approach to address patients who, although initially classified to the homogenous group, may later be reallocated to receive customized care, or vice versa. For example, all infants born at 24 weeks' gestation require intravenous (IV) access for fluid management (separate and select), whereas infants born at 39 weeks' gestation may need only enteral feeds. However, if the 39-week infant develops severe hypoglycemia, IV fluids may be required (separate and accommodate). Clearly designating patients into a pathway or providing comprehensive care for complex patients is not always straightforward, and, as such, a combination of customization and standardization may be prudent. Incorporating standardized elements of care into a customized treatment course is called integration. For instance, all infants admitted into a NICU may require cardiopulmonary monitoring, but the remainder of their care may be customized. Customized care can be delivered from multiple independent standardized subprocesses that can combine to produce a desired result, which is modularization. For example, one NICU's delivery process may include separate standardized processes for predelivery preparation (eg, role assignment, equipment check, antenatal consult), delivery room care (eg, following NRP algorithm), and post-delivery care (eg, determine the infant's admitting service, debriefing).[50] Although an established process for one NICU may successfully achieve desired outcomes, it may not be applicable to all NICUs. Resource availability or hospital layout may affect how a process is performed (eg, a standard process for resuscitation in a stand-alone resuscitation room will not work in an institution where neonatal resuscitation is performed in the mother's hospital room). This concept of understanding a patient situation and clinical environment can be used in combination with quality of evidence to determine whether practice variation is justified. In situations in which there is low-quality or insufficient evidence to support a practice, providers may choose consistent arbitrariness. In this approach, a practice group develops a consensus about patient care practices, and agrees to use this consensus-based practice consistently to minimize variation in practice.

The challenge in neonatal care lies in the dichotomy between ensuring that neonates in all parts of the world are equally likely to receive the best evidence-based care, while allowing for individualization. The art of practicing medicine lies in navigating these types of decisions, and wisely judging when to standardize based on science or customize based on the patient's (and family's) needs and the clinician's intuition.

SUMMARY

Although standardization and individualization are often seen as opposing approaches in health care, when taken as a layered approach, they may together ensure outstanding quality of care, offering the patient the benefits of a wide range of knowledge and experience, while retaining individual preferences and suitability of care.

REFERENCES

1. Institute of Medicine. Crossing the quality chasm: a new health system for the 21st century. Washington, DC: National Academy Press; 2001.
2. Soll RF. Evaluating the medical evidence for quality improvement. Clin Perinatol 2010;37(1):11–28.
3. Zarzuela S, Ruttan-Sims N, Nagatakiya L, et al. Defining standardization within the healthcare industry: an in-depth analysis of standardization from the perspective of key stakeholders. Standardization - Mohawk Shared Services. Mohawk Shared Services; 2016. Available at: http://www.mohawkssi.com/en/resourcesSection/resources/DefiningstandardizationwithinhealthcareindustryPoster.pdf. Accessed June 15, 2017.
4. The Dartmouth Atlas of Health Care. 2017. Available at: http://www.dartmouthatlas.org. Accessed August 1, 2016.
5. Ramprasad VH, Ryan MA, Farjat AE, et al. Practice patterns in supraglottoplasty and perioperative care. Int J Pediatr Otorhinolaryngol 2016;86:118–23.
6. Carroll CL, Faustino EV, Pinto MG, et al. A regional cohort study of the treatment of critically ill children with bronchiolitis. J Asthma 2016;53(10):1006–11.
7. Giuliano JS, Markovitz BP, Brierley J, et al. Comparison of pediatric severe sepsis managed in U.S. and European ICUs. Pediatr Crit Care Med 2016;17(6):522–30.
8. Laughon M, Bose C, Allred E, et al. Factors associated with treatment for hypotension in extremely low gestational age newborns during the first postnatal week. Pediatrics 2007;119(2):273–80.
9. Christakis DA, Cowan CA, Garrison MM, et al. Variation in inpatient diagnostic testing and management of bronchiolitis. Pediatrics 2005;115(4):878–84.
10. Florin TA, French B, Zorc JJ, et al. Variation in emergency department diagnostic testing and disposition outcomes in pneumonia. Pediatrics 2013;132(2):237–44.
11. Slaughter JL, Stenger MR, Reagan PB. Variation in the use of diuretic therapy for infants with bronchopulmonary dysplasia. Pediatrics 2013;131(4):716–23.

12. Horbar JD, Edwards EM, Greenberg LT, et al. Variation in performance of neonatal intensive care units in the United States. JAMA Pediatr 2017;171(3): e164396.
13. Truog WE, Nelin LD, Das A, et al. Inhaled nitric oxide usage in preterm infants in the NICHD Neonatal Research Network: inter-site variation and propensity evaluation. J Perinatol 2014;34(11):842–6.
14. Alleman BW, Bell EF, Li L, et al. Individual and center-level factors affecting mortality among extremely low birth weight infants. Pediatrics 2013;132(1):e175–84.
15. Lee SK, McMillan DD, Ohlsson A, et al. Variations in practice and outcomes in the Canadian NICU network: 1996-1997. Pediatrics 2000;106(5):1070–9.
16. Spitzer AR, Kirkby S, Kornhauser M. Practice variation in suspected neonatal sepsis: a costly problem in neonatal intensive care. J Perinatol 2005;25(4):265–9.
17. Lagatta J, Uhing M, Panepinto J. Comparative effectiveness and practice variation in neonatal care. Clin Perinatol 2014;41(4):833–45.
18. Mukhopadhyay S, Taylor JA, Von Kohorn I, et al. Variation in sepsis evaluation across a national network of nurseries. Pediatrics 2017;139(3) [pii:e20162845].
19. Rysavy MA, Li L, Bell EF, et al. Between-hospital variation in treatment and outcomes in extremely preterm infants. N Engl J Med 2015;372(19):1801–11.
20. Sebastião YV, Womack LS, López Castillo H, et al. Hospital variations in unexpected complications among term newborns. Pediatrics 2017;139(3) [pii: e20162364].
21. Rozich JD, Howard RJ, Justeson JM, et al. Standardization as a mechanism to improve safety in health care. Jt Comm J Qual Saf 2004;30(1):5–14.
22. Rogers EM. Diffusion of innovations. 5th edition. New York: Free Press; 2003.
23. Lehmann CU, Miller MR. Standardization and the practice of medicine. J Perinatol 2004;24(3):135–6.
24. Sheingold BH, Hahn JA. The history of healthcare quality: the first 100 years 1860-1960. International Journal of Africa Nursing Sciences 2014;1:18–22.
25. Pyzdek T, Keller PA. The six sigma handbook. 4th edition. New York: McGraw-Hill Education; 2014.
26. Lepore J. Not so fast: scientific management started as a way to work. How did it become a way of life? New York: The New Yorker; 2009.
27. Spitzer AR. Pay for performance in neonatal-perinatal medicine–will the quality of health care improve in the neonatal intensive care unit? A business model for improving outcomes in the neonatal intensive care unit. Clin Perinatol 2010; 37(1):167–77.
28. Davies MA, Tales H. Enhancing patient safety through a standardized model of physiologic monitoring. Healthc Q 2005;8(Spec No):49–52.
29. Provost LP, Langley GJ. The importance of change concepts in creativity and improvement. Qual Prog 1998;31(3):31–8.
30. Neil R. Taking control of supply spending. Hosp Health Netw 2005;79(6):44–6, 48–50, 52.
31. Mckone-Sweet K, Hamilton P, Willis S. The ailing healthcare supply chain: a prescription for change. J Supply Chain Manag 2005;41(1):4–17.
32. Halamek LP. Educational perspectives: the genesis, adaptation, and evolution of the neonatal resuscitation program. Neoreviews 2008;9(4):e142–9.
33. Profit J, Goldstein BA, Tamaresis J, et al. Regional variation in antenatal corticosteroid use: a network-level quality improvement study. Pediatrics 2015;135(2): e397–404.

34. Viswanathan S, McNelis K, Super D, et al. Standardized slow enteral feeding protocol and the incidence of necrotizing enterocolitis in extremely low birth weight infants. JPEN J Parenter Enteral Nutr 2015;39(6):644–54.
35. Trembath AN, Iams JD, Walsh M. Quality initiatives related to moderately preterm, late preterm, and early term births. Clin Perinatol 2013;40(4):777–89.
36. Leotsakos A, Zheng H, Croteau R, et al. Standardization in patient safety: the WHO High 5s project. Int J Qual Health Care 2014;26(2):109–16.
37. Pfaff H, Driller E, Ernstmann N, et al. Standardization and individualization in care for the elderly: proactive behavior through individualized standardization. Open Longevity Sci 2010;4:51–7.
38. Schulman J, Stricof RL, Stevens TP, et al. Development of a statewide collaborative to decrease NICU central line-associated bloodstream infections. J Perinatol 2009;29(9):591–9.
39. Isaac CA, Franceschi A. EBM: evidence to practice and practice to evidence. J Eval Clin Pract 2008;14(5):656–9.
40. Batalden PB, Davidoff F. What is "quality improvement" and how can it transform healthcare? Qual Saf Health Care 2007;16(1):2–3.
41. Isaac A, Saginur M, Hartling L, et al. Quality of reporting and evidence in American Academy of pediatrics guidelines. Pediatrics 2013;131(4):732–8.
42. Merritt TA, Gold M, Holland J. A critical evaluation of clinical practice guidelines in neonatal medicine: does their use improve quality and lower costs? J Eval Clin Pract 1999;5(2):169–77.
43. Toft B, Mascie-Taylor H. Involuntary automaticity: a work-system induced risk to safe health care. Health Serv Manage Res 2005;18(4):211–6.
44. Cabana MD, Rand CS, Powe NR, et al. Why don't physicians follow clinical practice guidelines? A framework for improvement. JAMA 1999;282(15):1458–65.
45. Ellingsen G. Tightrope walking: standardization meets local work practice in a hospital. Int J IT Stand Stand Res 2004;2(1):1–22.
46. Hall J, Johnson M. When should a process be art, not science? Boston: Harvard Business Review; 2009. p. 58–65.
47. Crawford AG. The need for customized and standardized health care quality measures. Am J Med Qual 2012;27(2):94–5.
48. Rodkin S. Purchasing for safety: standardization in intravenous equipment. Br J Nurs 2007;16(19):1186, 1188–90.
49. Minvielle E, Waelli M, Sicotte C, et al. Managing customization in health care: a framework derived from the services sector literature. Health Policy 2014; 117(2):216–27.
50. Bohmer RM. Medicine's service challenge: blending custom and standard care. Health Care Manage Rev 2005;30(4):322–30.

Context in Quality of Care

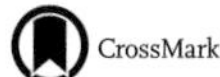

Improving Teamwork and Resilience

Daniel S. Tawfik, MD[a,b,*], John Bryan Sexton, PhD[c,d], Kathryn C. Adair, PhD[c,d], Heather C. Kaplan, MD, MSCE[e], Jochen Profit, MD, MPH[b,f,g]

KEYWORDS

• Safety climate • Teamwork • Quality • Burnout • Resilience

KEY POINTS

- Wide variation in neonatal intensive care unit quality of care exists, with differences in part attributable to variation in care context.
- Teamwork is an important driver of health care quality, and can be improved with established team-training tools.
- Individual resilience is a key contextual factor that may affect health care quality directly and indirectly via teamwork, and it can be coached.
- Improvements in teamwork and resilience are expected to enhance health care quality improvement initiatives.

INTRODUCTION

Improving the quality of health care is a substantial and widespread effort throughout the United States and the world, but patients continue to experience preventable harm on a daily basis.[1] Despite the variability in estimates of preventable deaths (ranging

---

Disclosures: The authors have no relevant financial relationships to disclose.
Funding: This work was supported by the Eunice Kennedy Shriver National Institute of Child Health and Human Development [R01 HD084679-01, principal investigators: Sexton and Profit] and the Jackson Vaughan Critical Care Research Fund.
[a] Division of Pediatric Critical Care Medicine, Department of Pediatrics, Stanford University School of Medicine, 770 Welch Road, Suite 435, Stanford, CA 94304, USA; [b] Lucile Packard Children's Hospital, 725 Welch Road, Palo Alto, CA 94304, USA; [c] Department of Psychiatry, Duke University School of Medicine, Duke University Health System, 2213 Elba Street, Durham, NC 27705, USA; [d] Duke Patient Safety Center, Duke University Health System, 2213 Elba Street, Durham, NC 27705, USA; [e] Department of Pediatrics, Perinatal Institute, James M. Anderson Centre for Health Systems Excellence, Cincinnati Children's Hospital Medical Center, 3333 Burnet Avenue, MLC 7009, Cincinnati, OH 45229, USA; [f] Perinatal Epidemiology and Health Outcomes Research Unit, Neonatology, Division of Neonatal and Developmental Medicine, Department of Pediatrics, Stanford University School of Medicine, Stanford University, 1265 Welch Road, MSOB, MC: 5415, Stanford, CA 94305, USA; [g] California Perinatal Quality Care Collaborative, 1265 Welch Road, MSOB, MC: 5415, Stanford, CA 94305, USA
* Corresponding author. Division of Pediatric Critical Care Medicine, Department of Pediatrics, Stanford University School of Medicine, 770 Welch Road, Suite 435, Stanford, CA 94304.
E-mail address: dtawfik@stanford.edu

Clin Perinatol 44 (2017) 541–552
http://dx.doi.org/10.1016/j.clp.2017.04.004 perinatology.theclinics.com
0095-5108/17/

from 25,000–250,000 per year in the United States alone), it is clear that mortality from medical error remains a serious problem.[2–4] Furthermore, nonfatal medical errors have been found to occur millions of times yearly.[1] Adults and children receive recommended care only about half the time,[5,6] with premature infants cared for in neonatal intensive care units (NICUs) experiencing similar variations in use, quality of health care, and in clinical outcomes.[7–10] For example, health care–associated infection rates,[11,12] growth velocity,[13] and treatment of persistent pulmonary hypertension[14] vary considerably. Up to 3-fold differences in mortality[9] and up to 44-fold variation in antibiotic use have been observed among NICUs.[15]

This observed variation in care is not merely a function of discrete differences in patient risk factors and care process guidelines but is an expression of differences in care contexts, which includes the contribution of each individual as well as the team. High-quality health care delivery is inherently reliant on providers maintaining individual excellence and working together effectively as a team. Poor teamwork and communication have been implicated in up to 72% of perinatal deaths and injuries and up to 30% of voluntary error reports.[16]

CONTEXT-SENSITIVE QUALITY OF CARE

The current challenges inherent in health care need not serve as discouragement for achieving marked improvement in quality and safety, but emphasize the importance of thinking broadly about creating a context, or environment, that supports quality and safety at the sociopolitical, organizational, mesosystem, microsystem, and team levels as opposed to tackling 1 problem at a time.[1,17,18] Numerous models and frameworks have been proposed to help policy makers, organizational leaders, and frontline staff create a context that supports quality and safety.

One framework designed to address the role of context in quality and safety is the Model for Understanding Success in Quality (MUSIQ), which describes 25 contextual factors across all levels of the health care system that are likely to influence the success of quality improvement (QI) endeavors, as shown in **Fig. 1**.[19] Although they are interconnected, most of the factors described are in the realm of microsystem (team members), macrosystem (organizational), or environment (community and society). MUSIQ suggests that the ability to achieve improvements in quality and safety is a result of the supporting context, including such factors as organizational and microsystem leadership, data infrastructure, QI culture, resource availability, workforce development, staff capability for QI, and team composition and effectiveness (both the QI team and microsystem team).

Another framework that highlights the important role of context in safety is the idea of the high-reliability organization (HRO) developed by Weick and Sutcliffe.[18] The HRO concept was originally applied to highly complex and high-risk industries, including aviation and nuclear power, but the principles are insensitive to the specific field in which they are applied, including in health care. HROs share 5 core characteristics: sensitivity to operations, reluctance to simplify, preoccupation with failure, deference to expertise, and resilience, as shown in **Fig. 2**.[20] Key contextual factors must be in place for an organization to develop as an HRO, including strong organizational leadership, a culture of safety and teamwork, and resilience.

Both of these models identify engagement of team members as a key aspect of context supporting quality and safety and the engagement of team members has been described as one of the significant factors predicting success in QI endeavors.[21] Common to both models is an emphasis on seemingly intangible features of organizational life: the relentless pursuit of better care undergirded by a culture that prizes

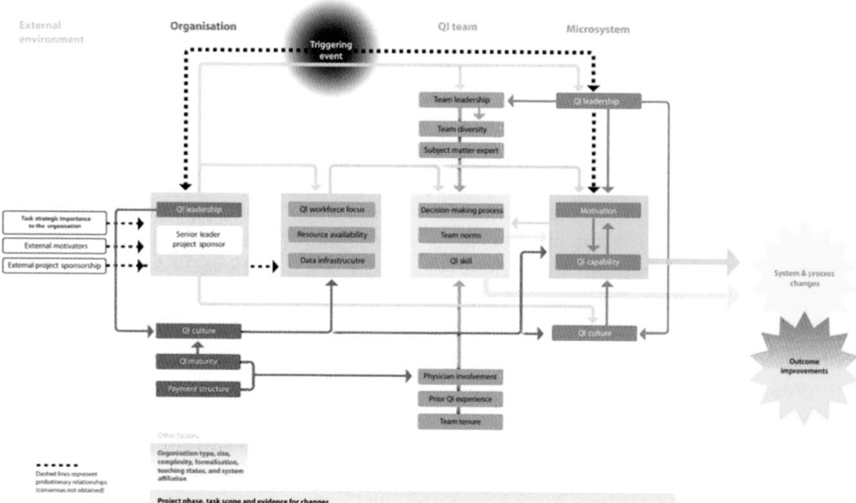

Fig. 1. MUSIQ, showing the contributions of organizational (*red*), macrosystem (*orange*), and microsystem (*green*) factors. (*From* Kaplan HC, Provost LP, Froehle CM, et al. The model for understanding success in quality (MUSIQ): building a theory of context in healthcare quality improvement. BMJ Qual Saf 2012;21(1):17; with permission.)

patient safety. The shared perceptions of leadership and the organizational attitudes toward patient safety and QI reflect the prevailing culture. The culture of safety construct is primarily measured based on health worker perceptions via surveys. The measured domains are called climates (ie, teamwork climate or safety climate). Climate reflects that perceptions are shared among health workers, meaning that they cluster more strongly within a work unit (eg, the NICU) than between work units

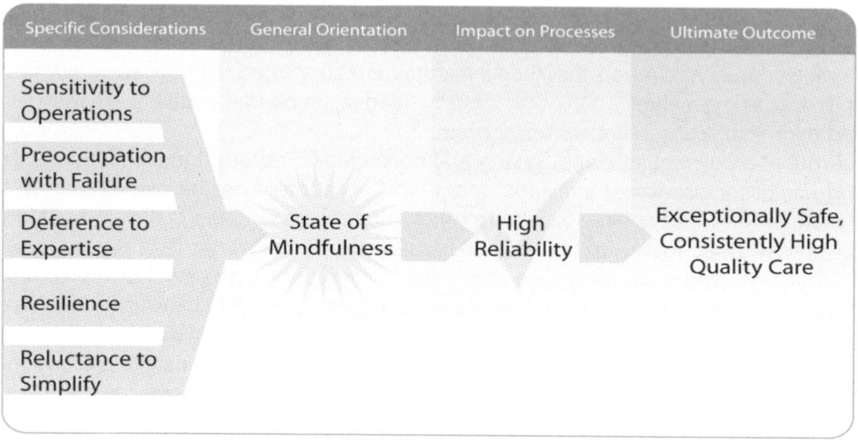

Specific Considerations
General Orientation
Impact on Processes
Ultimate Outcome
Sensitivity to Operations
Preoccupation with Failure
Deference to Expertise
Resilience
Reluctance to Simplify
State of Mindfulness
High Reliability
Exceptionally Safe, Consistently High Quality Care

Fig. 2. The 5 specific concepts that help create the state of mindfulness needed for a high-reliability organization. (*From* AHRQ Publication No. 08-0022. Agency for Healthcare Research and Quality. 2008. Available at: https://archive.ahrq.gov/professionals/quality-patient-safety/quality-resources/tools/hroadvice/hroadvice.pdf. Accessed December 27, 2016.)

either in the same institution (NICU vs PICU) or work units in other institutions (NICU in hospital A vs NICU in hospital B).[22] Two key subfactors of safety culture that affect health worker and patient well-being are teamwork and resilience, which are reviewed in detail here.

TEAMWORK IN THE NEONATAL INTENSIVE CARE UNIT

Across health care, improving teamwork has been recognized as an ongoing challenge. Moving from a team of experts to expert teams requires skills and training not often provided through traditional education. Paul Schyve,[23] MD, Senior Vice President of the Joint Commission stated, "Our challenge ... is not *whether* we will deliver care in teams but rather *how well* we will deliver care in teams." Although continually under development and refinement, teamwork measurement and intervention tools have been growing in concert with an increased emphasis on teamwork's role in health care delivery.

Salas and colleagues[25] identified 7 principal components relevant to teamwork: (1) cooperation, which depends on mutual trust and team-oriented mindset; (2) coordination, which requires shared performance monitoring, adaptability, and support; (3) communication, which must be clear, precise, and timely; (4) cognition, which refers to a shared understanding of roles and abilities of teammates; (5) coaching, which refers to team leadership, recognizing the importance of clear expectations; (6) conflict, the resolution of which is highly dependent on interpersonal skills and a climate of psychological safety; (7) conditions, which refers to the requisite supportive context for teams, because teamwork must be perceived as important to the leadership, and with positive reinforcement for good performance.[24,25]

Within a health care delivery unit, these factors interplay to create a composite climate of teamwork, which can vary widely across settings. Several tools exist to estimate the teamwork climate of a unit, including the Safety Attitudes Questionnaire (SAQ), Team Emergency Assessment Measure, Fundamental Interpersonal Relations Orientation–Behavior, Hospital Survey on Patient Safety Culture, and Team Climate Inventory.[26,27] Common to each of these measurement tools is an emphasis on the interpersonal interactions and adaptability of the team members. For example, the teamwork climate scale of the SAQ represents a composite measure of the extent to which caregivers report that they think they are supported, can speak up comfortably, can ask questions, think that input is heeded, think that conflicts are resolved, and think that team members collaborate.[28]

Profit and colleagues[29] and Sexton and colleagues[30] reported the SAQ to be valid and useful for assessing individual team work in addition to the overall teamwork climate in the NICU setting. Similar to other critical care settings,[31] physicians in the NICU have been found to have higher perceptions of teamwork than nurses, nurse practitioners, and respiratory care providers.[32] Physicians may be in leadership roles more frequently, resulting in the potential to elevate the physician's own perspective of adequate teamwork, even though the teamwork climate is weak in a given setting. It is unclear whether this difference is secondary to personal characteristics, professional responsibilities, or other unmeasured factors, but it has implications for the overall functioning of the NICU. Personal attributes, reputation, expertise, and seniority have been found to affect the ability of critical care providers to work together effectively.[31]

However, neither individual teamwork perception nor teamwork climate are static. Interventions focused on improving the teamwork of a health care unit include generalized training courses, such as crew resource management[33,34]; task-specific training[35,36]; or the implementation of process checklists.[37] A meta-analysis of 93 team training interventions showed consistent moderate improvements in teamwork measures, with more pronounced benefits seen following training programs combining generalized and task-specific approaches.[38] Within pediatric residency training, Thomas and colleagues[35] reported that randomization to a teamwork-based neonatal resuscitation curriculum results in up to 3-fold higher use of teamwork behaviors among interns compared with standard training, and that benefits can persist for at least 6 months.[36]

Across NICUs, teamwork climate has been found to vary widely.[32] Providing excellent care consistently throughout the clinical spectrum, from routine rounds to high-intensity resuscitations, relies on the adaptability of team members. NICUs with low teamwork climate may struggle to anticipate or adapt to changing clinical needs. However, teamwork is a malleable construct and interventions to improve teamwork are available. Although many of the teamwork interventions with measurable benefits reported in the published literature have focused on task-specific training for particular situations, such as surgical procedures or neonatal resuscitation, the same teamwork principles have relevance for all forms of neonatal health care delivery. Although the benefits are more challenging to quantify, system-wide generalized training may support teamwork within NICUs to a greater extent than task-specific training.[33]

To target system-wide benefit, The Agency for Healthcare Research and Quality has developed a teamwork tool kit in conjunction with the US Department of Defense. Named Team Strategies and Tools to Enhance Performance and Patient Safety (TeamSTEPPS), the intervention includes assessment, training, and sustainment phases focused on 4 core competencies: (1) team leadership, (2) situation monitoring, (3) mutual support, and (4) communication.[39] This approach has been used in multiple health care settings,[40,41] including one reported intervention that included NICU providers and showed an improvement in perceptions of teamwork.[42] Despite the heterogeneity of personal contributions, individual teamwork perception and teamwork climate are inextricably linked. The growing body of evidence regarding the ability to improve teamwork climate lends support for improved teamwork as a critical target of QI initiatives.

BURNOUT AND RESILIENCE IN THE NEONATAL INTENSIVE CARE UNIT

Another key contextual factor that may influence quality of care is provider burnout. Burnout describes a condition of fatigue, detachment, and cynicism resulting from prolonged high levels of stress.[43] In the critical care setting, burnout rates are likely driven predominantly by high workload, frequent changes in technology and guidelines, endeavors for high-quality care, and emotional challenges of dealing with critically ill patients and their families.[44–47] Burnout affects 27% to 86% of health care workers,[48–51] with more than half of physicians reporting moderate burnout[52] and around one-third of nurses and physicians meeting criteria for severe burnout.[48,53] The most commonly used instrument to measure burnout is the Maslach Burnout Inventory,[54] portions of which have been validated in multiple settings, including labor and delivery units and the NICU.[30,55] The emotional exhaustion subset has been used in isolation to provide a rapid assessment of an individual's burnout, consisting of 4 prompts: (1) I feel fatigued when I get up in the morning and have to face another day on the job, (2) I feel burned out from my work, (3) I feel frustrated by my job, and (4) I think I am working too hard on my job.[51] Responses to these questions, which cluster in the neutral or affirmative range, have been used as a marker for burnout.[43]

In contrast with burnout, resilience has been defined as a combination of characteristics that interact dynamically to allow an individual to bounce back, cope successfully, and function better than the norm in spite of significant stress or adversity.[43,56] Resilience has primarily been measured in the context of burnout avoidance. However, several key characteristics have been identified as directly contributing to resilience in qualitative research. These characteristics include optimism, adaptability, initiative, tolerance, organizational skills, being a team worker, keeping within professional boundaries, assertiveness, humor, and a sense of self-worth.[56]

Although often expressed as separate entities, the interpersonal aspects of resilience and teamwork are closely linked. Many of the characteristics identified as contributory to personal resilience are conceptually linked to those promoting a positive teamwork climate. Profit and colleagues[43] reported a negative association between burnout and teamwork climate among a large cohort of NICU providers, with the strongest association seen among providers reporting high levels of job frustration. In the same study, the proportion of NICU providers reporting low or very low burnout symptoms, calculated as the resilient proportion, was significantly associated with several domains relevant to quality. Strong correlation coefficients with teamwork climate (0.60), job satisfaction (0.65), safety climate (0.51), perceptions of management (0.61), and working conditions (0.53) were all highly significant.[43] A similar association has been observed in the pediatric ICU, with Lee and colleagues[57] describing a 7% increase in teamwork climate perception among providers with moderately high or high resilience scores.

The specific individual characteristics expected to drive these associations include adaptability, organizational skills, and a team-focused mindset, because these each carry profound implications for team functioning. Each individual's daily experience is an amalgamation of interactions that can each have positive or negative effects, creating a cumulative tide that may become substantial when taken in sum. Compared with smooth and coordinated interactions, effortful and inefficient interactions have been found to reduce self-regulation and performance on subsequent tasks.[58] As shown in **Fig. 3**, burned out individuals may be more prone to isolation, because they may have negative experiences with teamwork secondary to challenging interpersonal interactions. These negative interactions then drive further isolation and result in a positive feedback loop, resulting in escalating levels of burnout. Downward spirals in teamwork can have serious consequences; for example, nurses who

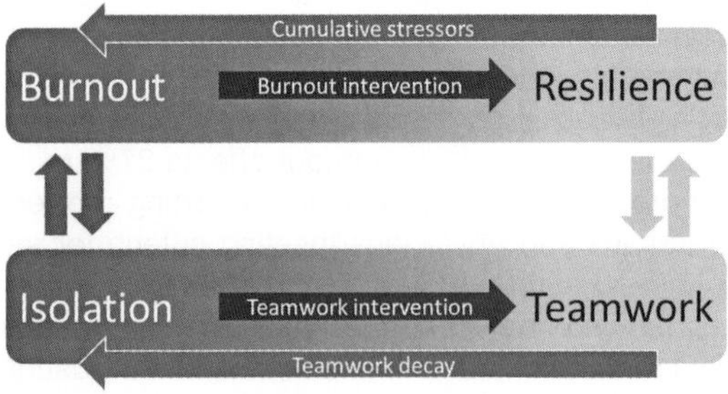

Fig. 3. Relationship of the burnout-resiliency continuum to the isolation-teamwork continuum. Burnout requires active intervention to achieve resilience, but can regress as the result of cumulative stressors. Similarly, isolation can be transformed to teamwork with interventions, but is prone to decay over time. Burned out individuals show reciprocity with isolated climates, but a positive teamwork climate can show positive feedback with resilience through affirmative interactions.

reported a serious lack of good teamwork had a 5-fold risk for intending to leave the profession.[59]

However, the converse also follows, with individuals showing higher resilience being more prone to positive teamwork interactions, which in turn feeds back to further improved resilience.[60] A qualitative study found that newly graduated nurses highlighted the importance of having nourishing interactions and good teamwork as integral to building workplace belongingness and staff empowerment.[61] The effects of better teamwork for resilience are just part of a large, overarching body of evidence that social connectedness significantly predicts better mental and physical well-being, and even lower rates of mortality.[62]

Burnout is a reversible condition, and resilience can be coached. Several strategies relevant to the health care setting have been developed to combat burnout and promote resilience. However, these strategies, such as mindfulness practice, are often time consuming and pragmatically challenging to administer.[63–66] Brief, widely distributable burnout interventions based on mindfulness strategies are currently being prospectively evaluated in multiple settings, including the NICU, with good benefit seen in pilot studies. The interventions focus on expressing thankfulness (gratitude), dwelling on positive events (3 good things), structured cultivation of awe and wonder (awe), random acts of kindness, identifying personal gifts (signature strengths), and relationship resilience. Profit and Sexton[67] have combined these interventions into a short resilience program called Web-based Implementation of the Science for Enhancing Resilience, which is funded by the National Institutes of Health for testing.

TEAMWORK-DRIVEN AND RESILIENCE-DRIVEN QUALITY IMPROVEMENT

Conceptually, improvements in teamwork climate and individual resilience can be expected to significantly contribute to improved quality of care. A single-center study by Rahn[68] reported a negative association between nursing teamwork and unassisted patient falls on a medical/surgical unit. Within the NICU setting, teamwork has been negatively associated with health care–associated infections among a diverse cohort of California NICUs, such that the odds of an infant contracting an infection decreased by 18% with each 10% increase in NICU survey respondents reporting good teamwork.[69]

In contrast, improvements in teamwork have been associated with reduced medication errors, decreased health care–associated infections,[70,71] and higher-quality newborn resuscitation.[35] Neily and colleagues[72] reported an 18% reduction in surgical mortality following implementation of team-based surgical checklists at Veterans' Affairs hospitals. In Michigan ICUs, Pronovost and colleagues[70,71] reported an 80% reduction in catheter-related bloodstream infections with the simultaneous introduction of a teamwork/unit safety intervention and an infection prevention intervention.

The association between provider resilience and quality of care has been largely unreported, but there is an increasing body of literature regarding burnout in relation to quality measures. A meta-analysis by Salyers and colleagues[73] evaluated 82 studies and reported a small to moderate negative association between provider burnout and quality of care measures, with 7% of quality measure variance and 5% of safety measure variance attributed to provider burnout. Notably, Aiken and colleagues[74] reported an observed 7% increase in patient mortality and 23% increase in the odds of nurse burnout for each additional patient added to a nurse's workload. Expounding on this work in multivariable analyses, Cimiotti and colleagues[75] reported that burnout carries a stronger association with health care–associated infections than does nurse staffing, with each 10% increase in burnout prevalence corresponding with 0.8 urinary tract infections and 1.6 surgical site infections per 1000 patients. Specific to neonatology, Tawfik and colleagues[51] reported a moderate correlation (r = 0.34) between health care worker burnout and increased rates of health care–associated infections among very-low-birthweight infants in high-volume NICUs in California, which was most pronounced among providers reporting feeling fatigued or overworked.

It remains to be proved that longitudinal increases in resilience can result in observable improvements in quality of care. However, the strength of associations repeatedly observed between high burnout and adverse events suggests that this domain of the quality microclimate is an appropriate target for QI endeavors.

SUMMARY

With the continued increasing recognition of the need for QI in health care, consideration of the context of the health care delivery system is of paramount importance. Aspects of context, including teamwork climate and personal resilience, are important factors in achieving optimal quality and safety outcomes and efforts to modify these aspects of context (eg, improve teamwork climate, build staff resilience) are a key QI strategy. Well-established tools, such as TeamSTEPPS, are available to improve teamwork for specific tasks or global applications. Similarly, burnout and, by extension, resilience, can be modified with specific interventions, such as cultivating gratitude, positivity, and awe. A growing body of literature has shown that teamwork and burnout relate to quality of care, with improved teamwork and decreased burnout expected to produce improved patient quality and safety metrics.

REFERENCES

1. Chassin MR, Loeb JM. High-reliability health care: getting there from here. Milbank Q 2013;91(3):459–90.
2. Kohn LT, Corrigan JM, Donaldson MS. To err is human: building a safer health system. Washington, DC: National Academy Press; 2000.
3. Makary MA, Daniel M. Medical error-the third leading cause of death in the US. BMJ 2016;353:i2139.
4. Shojania KG, Dixon-Woods M. Estimating deaths due to medical error: the ongoing controversy and why it matters. BMJ Qual Saf 2016;26(5):423–8.
5. Mangione-Smith R, DeCristofaro AH, Setodji CM, et al. The quality of care received by children and adolescents in the United States. Pediatric Academic Societies' Annual Meeting. San Francisco, 29 April-2 May, 2006.
6. McGlynn EA, Asch SM, Adams J, et al. The quality of health care delivered to adults in the United States. N Engl J Med 2003;348(26):2635–45.
7. Horbar JD, Badger GJ, Lewit EM, et al. Hospital and patient characteristics associated with variation in 28-day mortality rates for very low birth weight infants. Vermont Oxford Network. Pediatrics 1997;99(2):149–56.
8. Sankaran K, Chien L-Y, Walker R, et al. Variations in mortality rates among Canadian neonatal intensive care units. CMAJ 2002;166(2):173–8.
9. Rogowski JA, Staiger DO, Horbar JD. Variations in the quality of care for very-low-birthweight infants: implications for policy. Health Aff 2004;23(5):88–97.
10. Phibbs CS, Baker LC, Caughey AB, et al. Level and volume of neonatal intensive care and mortality in very-low-birth-weight infants. N Engl J Med 2007;356(21):2165–75.
11. Brodie SB, Sands KE, Gray JE, et al. Occurrence of nosocomial bloodstream infections in six neonatal intensive care units. Pediatr Infect Dis J 2000;19(1):56–65.

12. Stoll BJ, Hansen N, Fanaroff AA, et al. Late-onset sepsis in very low birth weight neonates: the experience of the NICHD Neonatal Research Network. Pediatrics 2002;110(2):285–91.
13. Olsen IE, Richardson DK, Schmid CH, et al. Intersite differences in weight growth velocity of extremely premature infants. Pediatrics 2002;110:1125–32.
14. Walsh-Sukys MC, Tyson JE, Wright LL, et al. Persistent pulmonary hypertension of the newborn in the era before nitric oxide: practice variation and outcomes. Pediatrics 2000;105(1):14–20.
15. Schulman J, Dimand RJ, Lee HC, et al. Neonatal intensive care unit antibiotic use. Pediatrics 2015;135(5):826–33.
16. Suresh G, Horbar JD, Plsek P, et al. Voluntary anonymous reporting of medical errors for neonatal intensive care. Pediatrics 2004;113(6):1609–18.
17. Van Spall H, Kassam A, Tollefson TT. Near-misses are an opportunity to improve patient safety: adapting strategies of high reliability organizations to healthcare. Curr Opin Otolaryngol Head Neck Surg 2015;23(4):292–6.
18. Sutcliffe KM, Paine L, Pronovost PJ. Re-examining high reliability: actively organising for safety. BMJ Qual Saf 2016;26(3):248–51.
19. Kaplan HC, Provost LP, Froehle CM, et al. The Model for Understanding Success in Quality (MUSIQ): building a theory of context in healthcare quality improvement. BMJ Qual Saf 2012;21(1):13–20.
20. Chassin MR, Loeb JM. The ongoing quality improvement journey: next stop, high reliability. Health Aff (Millwood) 2011;30(4):559–68.
21. Kaplan HC, Froehle CM, Cassedy A, et al. An exploratory analysis of the model for understanding success in quality. Health Care Manage Rev 2013;38(4): 325–38.
22. Vogus TJ. Safety climate strength: a promising construct for safety research and practice. BMJ Qual Saf 2016;25(9):649–52.
23. Schyve PM. Teamwork–the changing nature of professional competence. Jt Comm J Qual Patient Saf 2005;31(4):183–4.
24. Salas E, Rosen MA. Building high reliability teams: progress and some reflections on teamwork training. BMJ Qual Saf 2013;22(5):369–73.
25. Salas E, Almeida SA, Salisbury M, et al. What are the critical success factors for team training in health care? Jt Comm J Qual Patient Saf 2009;35(8):398–405.
26. Cooper S. Teamwork: what should we measure and how should we measure it? Int Emerg Nurs 2017;32:1–2.
27. Jones KJ, Skinner A, Xu L, et al. The AHRQ hospital survey on patient safety culture: a tool to plan and evaluate patient safety programs. In: Henriksen K, Battles JB, Keyes MA, et al, editors. Advances in patient safety: new directions and alternative approaches (Vol. 2: Culture and Redesign). Rockville (MD): Agency for Healthcare Research and Quality; 2008. p. 1–22.
28. Sexton JB, Helmreich RL, Neilands TB, et al. The safety attitudes questionnaire: psychometric properties, benchmarking data, and emerging research. BMC Health Serv Res 2006;6:44.
29. Profit J, Etchegaray J, Petersen LA, et al. The safety attitudes questionnaire as a tool for benchmarking safety culture in the NICU. Arch Dis Child Fetal Neonatal Ed 2012;97(2):F127–32.
30. Sexton JB, Sharek PJ, Thomas EJ, et al. Exposure to Leadership WalkRounds in neonatal intensive care units is associated with a better patient safety culture and less caregiver burnout. BMJ Qual Saf 2014;23(10):814–22.
31. Thomas EJ, Sexton JB, Helmreich RL. Discrepant attitudes about teamwork among critical care nurses and physicians. Crit Care Med 2003;31(3):956–9.

32. Profit J, Etchegaray J, Petersen LA, et al. Neonatal intensive care unit safety culture varies widely. Arch Dis Child Fetal Neonatal Ed 2012;97(2):F120–6.
33. Thomas EJ. Improving teamwork in healthcare: current approaches and the path forward. BMJ Qual Saf 2011;20(8):647–50.
34. Lerner S, Magrane D, Friedman E. Teaching teamwork in medical education. Mt Sinai J Med 2009;76(4):318–29.
35. Thomas EJ, Taggart B, Crandell S, et al. Teaching teamwork during the neonatal resuscitation program: a randomized trial. J Perinatol 2007;27(7):409–14.
36. Thomas EJ, Williams AL, Reichman EF, et al. Team training in the neonatal resuscitation program for interns: teamwork and quality of resuscitations. Pediatrics 2010;125(3):539–46.
37. Thomas EJ, Sexton JB, Helmreich RL. Translating teamwork behaviours from aviation to healthcare: development of behavioural markers for neonatal resuscitation. Qual Saf Health Care 2004;13(Suppl 1):i57–64.
38. Salas E, DiazGranados D, Klein C, et al. Does team training improve team performance? A meta-analysis. Hum Factors 2008;50(6):903–33.
39. Clancy CM, Tornberg DN. TeamSTEPPS: assuring optimal teamwork in clinical settings. Am J Med Qual 2007;22(3):214–7.
40. Mayer CM, Cluff L, Lin WT, et al. Evaluating efforts to optimize TeamSTEPPS implementation in surgical and pediatric intensive care units. Jt Comm J Qual Patient Saf 2011;37(8):365–74.
41. Sawyer T, Laubach VA, Hudak J, et al. Improvements in teamwork during neonatal resuscitation after interprofessional TeamSTEPPS training. Neonatal Netw 2013;32(1):26–33.
42. Beitlich P. TeamSTEPPS implementation in the LD/NICU settings. Nurs Manage 2015;46(6):15–8.
43. Profit J, Sharek PJ, Amspoker AB, et al. Burnout in the NICU setting and its relation to safety culture. BMJ Qual Saf 2014;23(10):806–13.
44. Braithwaite M. Nurse burnout and stress in the NICU. Adv Neonatal Care 2008; 8(6):343–7.
45. Rochefort CM, Clarke SP. Nurses' work environments, care rationing, job outcomes, and quality of care on neonatal units. J Adv Nurs 2010;66(10):2213–24.
46. van Mol MM, Kompanje EJ, Benoit DD, et al. The prevalence of compassion fatigue and burnout among healthcare professionals in intensive care units: a systematic review. PLoS One 2015;10(8):e0136955.
47. Portoghese I, Galletta M, Coppola RC, et al. Burnout and workload among health care workers: the moderating role of job control. Saf Health Work 2014;5(3): 152–7.
48. Shanafelt TD, West CP, Sloan JA, et al. Career fit and burnout among academic faculty. Arch Intern Med 2009;169(10):990–5.
49. Mealer M, Burnham EL, Goode CJ, et al. The prevalence and impact of post traumatic stress disorder and burnout syndrome in nurses. Depress Anxiety 2009; 26(12):1118–26.
50. Thomas EJ, Sherwood GD, Mulhollem JL, et al. Working together in the neonatal intensive care unit: provider perspectives. J Perinatol 2004;24(9):552–9.
51. Tawfik DS, Sexton JB, Kan P, et al. Burnout in the neonatal intensive care unit and its relation to healthcare-associated infections. J Perinatol 2016;37(3):315–20.
52. Shanafelt TD, Hasan O, Dyrbye LN, et al. Changes in burnout and satisfaction with work-life balance in physicians and the general us working population between 2011 and 2014. Mayo Clin Proc 2015;90(12):1600–13.

53. Bellieni CV, Righetti P, Ciampa R, et al. Assessing burnout among neonatologists. J Matern Fetal Neonatal Med 2012;25(10):2130–4.
54. Maslach C, Jackson SE. Maslach burnout inventory. Palo Alto (CA): Consulting Psychologists Press; 1981.
55. Block M, Ehrenworth JF, Cuce VM, et al. Measuring handoff quality in labor and delivery: development, validation, and application of the Coordination of Handoff Effectiveness Questionnaire (CHEQ). Jt Comm J Qual Patient Saf 2013;39(5): 213–20.
56. Matheson C, Robertson HD, Elliott AM, et al. Resilience of primary healthcare professionals working in challenging environments: a focus group study. Br J Gen Pract 2016;66(648):e507–515.
57. Lee KJ, Forbes ML, Lukasiewicz GJ, et al. Promoting staff resilience in the pediatric intensive care unit. Am J Crit Care 2015;24(5):422–30.
58. Finkel EJ, Campbell WK, Brunell AB, et al. High-maintenance interaction: inefficient social coordination impairs self-regulation. J Pers Soc Psychol 2006; 91(3):456–75.
59. Estryn-Behar M, Van der Heijden BI, Oginska H, et al. The impact of social work environment, teamwork characteristics, burnout, and personal factors upon intent to leave among European nurses. Med Care 2007;45(10):939–50.
60. Wahlin I, Ek AC, Idvall E. Staff empowerment in intensive care: nurses' and physicians' lived experiences. Intensive Crit Care Nurs 2010;26(5):262–9.
61. Cleary M, Horsfall J, Mannix J, et al. Valuing teamwork: insights from newly-registered nurses working in specialist mental health services. Int J Ment Health Nurs 2011;20(6):454–9.
62. Umberson D, Montez JK. Social relationships and health: a flashpoint for health policy. J Health Soc Behav 2010;51(Suppl):S54–66.
63. West CP, Dyrbye LN, Rabatin JT, et al. Intervention to promote physician well-being, job satisfaction, and professionalism: a randomized clinical trial. JAMA Intern Med 2014;174(4):527–33.
64. Rowe MM. Teaching health-care providers coping: results of a two-year study. J Behav Med 1999;22(5):511–27.
65. West CP, Dyrbye LN, Erwin PJ, et al. Interventions to prevent and reduce physician burnout: a systematic review and meta-analysis. Lancet 2016;388(10057): 2272–81.
66. Westermann C, Kozak A, Harling M, et al. Burnout intervention studies for inpatient elderly care nursing staff: systematic literature review. Int J Nurs Stud 2014;51(1):63–71.
67. Tawfik DS, Phibbs CS, Sexton JB, et al. Factors associated with provider burnout in the NICU. Pediatrics 2017;139(5):e20164134.
68. Rahn DJ. Transformational teamwork: exploring the impact of nursing teamwork on nurse-sensitive quality indicators. J Nurs Care Qual 2016;31(3):262–8.
69. Profit J, Sharek PJ, Kan P, et al. Teamwork in the NICU setting and its association with healthcare-associated infections in very low birth weight infants. Am J Perinatol 2017. [Epub ahead of print].
70. Pronovost P, Needham D, Berenholtz S, et al. An intervention to decrease catheter-related bloodstream infections in the ICU. N Engl J Med 2006;355(26): 2725–32.
71. Pronovost PJ, Berenholtz SM, Goeschel C, et al. Improving patient safety in intensive care units in Michigan. J Crit Care 2008;23(2):207–21.

72. Neily J, Mills PD, Young-Xu Y, et al. Association between implementation of a medical team training program and surgical mortality. JAMA 2010;304(15):1693–700.
73. Salyers MP, Bonfils KA, Luther L, et al. The relationship between professional burnout and quality and safety in healthcare: a meta-analysis. J Gen Intern Med 2016;32(4):475–82.
74. Aiken LH, Clarke SP, Sloane DM, et al. Hospital nurse staffing and patient mortality, nurse burnout, and job dissatisfaction. JAMA 2002;288(16):1987–93.
75. Cimiotti JP, Aiken LH, Sloane DM, et al. Nurse staffing, burnout, and health care-associated infection. Am J Infect Control 2012;40(6):486–90.

Family Involvement in Quality Improvement

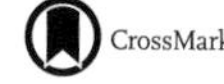

From Bedside Advocate to System Advisor

Joanna F. Celenza, MA, MBA[a], Denise Zayack, RN, MPH[b,*], Madge E. Buus-Frank, DNP, APRN-BC[c], Jeffrey D. Horbar, MD[d]

KEYWORDS

• Family advisors • Quality improvement (QI) • Family centered care (FCC)
• Quality improvement collaborative • Family integrated care
• Patient and family engagement (PFE) • Family engaged care (FEC) • Family leaders

KEY POINTS

- Involving families in neonatal intensive care unit (NICU) quality improvement is not a new concept, but recent developments in this partnership model have helped to shape the depth and breadth of family involvement in quality improvement.
- Families are more than stakeholders in NICU quality improvement and can serve as active partners in system design and improvement.
- Opportunities exist to enhance partnerships with families, and seeking to improve this key relationship is imperative to nurture a culture that ensures the best possible neonatal outcomes.

Video content accompanies this article at http://www.perinatology.theclinics.com.

INTRODUCTION

In 1992, Helen Harrison gathered a group of parents and physicians to initiate a dialogue addressing obstacles to meaningful participation for families of critically ill infants. This interaction resulted in the proclamation of 10 principles of family

---

Disclosure Statement: Consultant with Vermont Oxford Network (D. Zayack). Executive Vice President, Vermont Oxford Network (M.E. Buus-Frank). Chief Executive and Scientific Officer, Vermont Oxford Network (J.D. Horbar).

[a] Children's Hospital at Dartmouth-Hitchcock, One Medical Center Drive, Lebanon, NH 03756, USA; [b] Vermont Oxford Network, 33 Kilburn Street, Burlington, VT 05401, USA; [c] Vermont Oxford Network, Geisel School of Medicine and University of Vermont, 33 Kilburn Street, Burlington, VT 05401, USA; [d] Vermont Oxford Network, University of Vermont, 33 Kilburn Street, Burlington, VT 05401, USA

* Corresponding author.

E-mail address: dzayack@vtoxford.org

Clin Perinatol 44 (2017) 553–566

http://dx.doi.org/10.1016/j.clp.2017.05.008 **perinatology.theclinics.com** centered neonatal care, which, to this day, serve as the foundation for our understanding of patient and family centered care.

These guiding principles also serve as a context for delineating the potential impact family members who have the unique experience of care can have on the system of care. Family advisors can impact health care outcomes through meaningful and systematic engagement in quality improvement.[1]

Despite the dialogue that was initiated almost 25 years ago, potential remains for deeper and farther-reaching impact of family advisors as quality improvement agents in newborn intensive care. In this article, the authors review their experience as a field with family advisors in neonatal intensive care and particularly with regard to family involvement in quality improvement. After a brief historical context, the authors provide examples of opportunities for family engagement in neonatal care outside of quality improvement. The authors then outline different approaches and strategies for engaging families as partners in neonatal intensive care unit (NICU) quality improvement efforts. In much of this article, the authors use the experience of Vermont Oxford Network (VON) to illustrate principles of family engagement in quality improvement; although they recognize many other groups have made landmark contributions to this field, the authors are not reviewing those in detail.

Historical Perspective

Harrison's gathering of past NICU families with physicians in 1992 was instrumental in setting the stage for future quality improvement work. This gathering resulted in what has been called the Lake Champlain Manifesto because it was held in Burlington, Vermont. It was attended by several prominent neonatologists, including Dr Jerold F. Lucey, then Editor in Chief of *Pediatrics*, and Dr William Silverman who helped organize the meeting. The principles of family centered care were shared and are still relevant today. These principles and ideas include the following:

- There should be open and honest communication between families and health care professionals.
- Decision-making should be informed and balanced and decisions based on information that is unbiased and helpful to families.
- Parents and the health care team should work together to minimize pain in the neonate.
- The physical environment of the NICU should be as safe and developmentally appropriate as possible.
- Parents and professionals should ensure that medical interventions are effective and safe.
- Parents and professionals should collaborate on NICU policies and ensure parents' role is valued and supported.
- The follow-up of at-risk infants should be ensured.
- Shared decision-making, especially related to invasive and painful treatment options, should be carefully considered and health care outcomes shared with families.[1]

The group's broad-brush recommendations for a developmentally supportive environment for the infant and psychologically supportive environment for families were reinforced by suggestions that families and health care professionals work together to operationalize these principles and systematically apply them.

In 2001, the Institute of Medicine released its report on requirements to achieve quality in health care. It identified 6 aims for improvement, including patient-centered care.[2] The Institute for Patient- and Family-Centered Care (IPFCC) developed core concepts of patient and family centered care.[3] These core concepts are described in **Box 1** and mirror many of the concepts suggested earlier by Harrison.

Family Involvement in Neonatal Intensive Care Unit Improvement (via Methods Other than Quality Improvement)

Although the focus of this article is family engagement in quality improvement, there are numerous other ways in which families have played and can play essential roles in helping to define and shape clinical care of their infant.

First, family involvement may help ensure the clinical environment of the neonate provides the optimal setting and best possible long-term outcome for the infant and family. NICUs were historically designed in open bays, reminiscent of traditional multi-bed wards. Inadequate space at the bedside and lack of privacy are 2 of the barriers cited by staff to achieving family centered care. Recent designs have embraced single rooms and small pods that encourage family presence, which, given a supportive culture, may facilitate their participation in all aspects of care. The perspective and participation of graduate families is recommended in the design of NICUs.[4]

In 2004, Dr Robert White of Memorial Hospital in South Bend, Indiana, a champion of family centered NICU design, challenged the neonatal care community to move the locus of care from the isolette to the mother's arms.[5] In a NICU in Sweden, at Akademiska Barnsjukhuset University Children's Hospital, Uppsala, each care space includes an adult bed, located immediately adjacent to the intensive care equipment ensuring infants can be cared for in their parents' arms or while kangarooing (Video 1). In 2014, Dr Uwe Ewald partnered with VON, Burlington, Vermont, to create a virtual video visit to their Care by Parent NICU. In step-down care, parents provide most care to their infants (Video 2).

Box 1
Core concepts of patient- and family-centered care

Respect and dignity

Health care practitioners listen to and honor patient and family perspectives and choices. Patient and family knowledge, values, beliefs, and cultural backgrounds are incorporated into the planning and delivery of care.

Information sharing

Health care practitioners communicate and share complete and unbiased information with patients and families in ways that are affirming and useful. Patients and families receive timely, complete, and accurate information in order to effectively participate in care and decision-making.

Participation

Patients and families are encouraged and supported in participating in care and decision-making at the level they choose.

Collaboration

Patients and families are also included on an institution-wide basis. Health care leaders collaborate with patients and families in policy and program development, implementation, and evaluation; in health care facility design; and in professional education as well as in the delivery of care.

From Johnson BH, Abraham MR. Partnering with patients, resident and families: a resource for leaders of hospitals, ambulatory care settings, and long-term care communities. Institute for Patient- and Family-Centered Care; 2012. Available at: http://www.ihi.org/education/conferences/APACForum2012/Documents/I1_Presentation_Johnson.pdf. Accessed July 10, 2017.

Skin to skin or kangaroo care is a family centered practice that has been the focus of recent quality improvement projects and is a core care concept in the Uppsala NICU (Video 3). The role of NICU fathers is less often reported on and supported. In the Uppsala unit, fathers are active in the care of their infants and report feeling more like parents (Video 4).

Participation in the design of research presents a second example of the impact of families' roles in achieving improvement. The Family Integrated Care (FICare) research project in Canada included graduate families as partners in its design. Families enrolled in the study were encouraged to provide their infants' care and were fully engaged as decision-makers. Ongoing educational opportunities reinforced their role as caregivers. Graduate parents were key participants in the design of the FICare program and also provided peer support.[6]

THE CURRENT PRACTICE

What Has Been Achieved for Family Involvement in Quality Improvement

Numerous groups have developed resources to help define and guide potentially better practices for family involvement in quality improvement. Here, the authors focus on the work done by VON and then share resources developed by other national organizations.

In 2004, the IPFCC partnered with VON to develop a self-assessment resource for teams to help determine their status related to family advisor engagement in quality improvement. Teams, including family advisors, were encouraged to assess their culture and jointly develop strategies to improve. The goal was to deepen and enhance the involvement of families in quality improvement.[7]

VON modeled this collaboration by not only encouraging quality improvement teams to identify family advisors but also appointing family faculty to partner with faculty from other disciplines to lead quality improvement collaborative groups. Each family leader coleads the improvement activities with the other faculty from unique disciplines to ensure comprehensive representation. A family advisor has also served on the overarching advisory board to shape future collaboratives.

The 2007 VON e-book *NICQ 2007 Improvement in Action*[8] highlights some key findings from the quality improvement work not only within VON but also from publicly available examples of innovative projects and methods of partnering with families.

In the most recent VON intensive quality improvement initiative, NICQ Next^2, it has been a goal to ensure every test of change includes a measurement of its impact on families because every change impacts the family, either directly or indirectly. The family faculty (family leaders) within each group of hospitals work closely with the participating teams to identify measures to assess the impact of tests of change on families and to explore opportunities to codesign quality improvement projects. Family advisors may be able to identify opportunities that the clinical team members might not consider, thus, allowing for more robust improvements.

Each comprehensive toolkit created to support the improvement projects included family leaders as coauthors. Many participating teams developed at least one aim focused explicitly on family centered care or enhancing the culture to support a family centered approach to care. Some of the potentially better practices authored include

- Ensure family integration in care to improve outcome, build confidence, and promote attachment.
- Develop, test, implement, and continually refine standardized processes designed to integrate family centered care into all documented protocols for surgical care.

In September 2016, VON NICQ Next[2] teams gathered in Chicago to advance their collaborative improvement work. Of 61 teams attending, 59 acknowledged in their quality improvement abstract the inclusion of at least one family advisor as a member of their VON team and 36 teams sponsored the attendance of a family advisor at the meeting. More than 250 quality improvement posters were presented, and attendees assessed the 26 family advisor stories as exceptionally impactful. Families identified opportunities for future improvement by including the section *what I wish I had known* when their infants were in the NICU. See **Box 2** for a summary of themes that emerged.

Box 2
Reflection on neonatal intensive care unit experience by quality improvement family advisors: a few excerpts

What I Wish I Had Known While in the NICU
—Vermont Oxford Network Annual Quality Congress Poster Fair, Chicago 2016.

That my presence makes a difference to my baby (Family presence, participation, and caregiving are valuable variables to the outcome of infant and parents desire knowledge about their value to the team.)

- "{I wish I had known} what I could do to help my babies and why my presence mattered."
- "{I wish I had known} that my presence in the NICU was important."
- "{I wish I had known} that my loving touch was actually therapeutic and meaningful. For both of us!"

How it could feel to be a parent in the NICU (Parental roles can feel tenuous and need to be supported/encouraged.)

- "I wish I would've felt like a mom sooner than I did."
- "I wish I would've felt confident enough to ask for help—help in understanding what was happening to my babies, help in navigating the NICU, and help with how to feel like a parent."
- "{I wish I had known} that it was my right and responsibility to advocate for my children."
- "I wish I would have known that it was okay to request to touch, kiss, hold or assist in providing daily care, without fearing that I was interfering or that I would do something wrong."
- "I wish I would've known that I wasn't as powerless as I felt."

That I would experience so much guilt (Parental guilt can be an overriding emotion, and psychosocial support is crucial throughout the journey, including after discharge from the NICU.)

- "{I wish I had known} years later I would still feel at fault for his early delivery."
- "{I wish I had} felt less guilty and believed this wasn't my fault."
- "I wish my daughter would have felt comfort during painful care procedures."
- "I wanted to cry, yet I didn't know if my tears were supposed to be tears of joy or tears of sorrow. Or did I have no right to cry at all; was this somehow all my fault?"
- "I experienced PTSD from everything I had gone through, and have had dreams and flashbacks of my hours spent by his bedside. I wish I had known that his first birthday, and even his second, would be an extremely difficult and emotional day and not one I would want to celebrate like most other moms."

That I too would be the subject of assessment (Parents have a keen awareness of environment.)

- "They Talk About Parents, Too –change of shift is used for more than just reporting on the medical status of the patient."

That the journey can be full circle and serve as a way to improve others' experience

- "{I wish I had known}...that someday we would embrace our journey and use it to help others."

Abbreviation: PTSD, posttraumatic stress disorder.

In 2013, the Agency for Healthcare Research and Quality (AHRQ) developed a guide to achieve patient engagement as a means to advance hospital quality and safety. This guide provides specific recommendations, including evidence on how families can enhance quality and safety efforts. Best practices are identified, including tips for leadership on ensuring a collaborative environment to enhance patient partnerships, including transitions of care.[9]

In 2015, the National Perinatal Association partnered with parents and interdisciplinary representatives to establish recommendations for the psychosocial support of NICU families. The recommendations are supported by a series of principles, including interdisciplinary collaboration, continuity of care, varied family responses to traumatic events, and an imperative for a universal level of support for all families with additional supports where accessible.[10]

Examples of Family Involvement in Quality Improvement Achieved

The authors provide examples based on the *Framework for Family Involvement in Quality Improvement*, developed by the IPFCC and a VON family advisor and detailed in **Boxes 3** and **4**.[7]

Box 3
Framework for family involvement in quality improvement

Level I

Families complete surveys or engage in other evaluative activities as respondents (for example, focus groups). The level of participation is time limited and may be cursory but can be helpful to guide practices and identify needs and themes that improvement teams can then address. This level of involvement may be appealing for those families interested in sharing their insight, yet may not wish to commit to long-term projects.

Level II

Family advisory councils serve as a resource to the quality improvement team (for example, review projects, documents). Having an established advisory council as well as sustaining the council is a prerequisite to this type of collaboration. This level can provide a more cohesive and consistent approach to gathering feedback from family advisors.

Level III

Families participate as occasional reviewers and consultants during an improvement project. Identifying family advisors to serve as consultants and engaging them throughout the project can be a way to enhance patient- and family centered care practices. Families can be called on to help identify opportunities as well as inform practice changes and enhancements.

Level IV

Families participate as active members of improvement teams and/or may serve on unit-based task forces and committees and faculty for staff and clinician education. Identifying family advisors to serve as ongoing full members of the team is a requirement. Sustaining this involvement by providing diverse and flexible opportunities to participate can be a way to ensure consistent and ongoing involvement.

Level V

Families are coleaders of improvement initiatives. At this level, family advisors are on equal footing with other leaders of quality improvement initiatives. Families have equal responsibilities related to leadership of quality improvement projects. Compensation would be comparable with other leaders at this same level.

From Abraham M, Nickerson J. Framework for involving patients and families in research. Institute for Patient and Family-Centered Care. October 20, 2009; with permission. Available at: http://www.ipfcc.org.

Box 4
Requirements to establish level V family advisor involvement

Recognize the family as an essential partner in CARE and support quality improvement efforts:

- Support families at the bedside (at the clinical level of care).
- Ensure the parental role is honored and supported through education and peer support.
- Ensure family presence is supported with open and unrestricted NICU access and clarify that families have the opportunity to designate who they consider to be family.
- Consider the importance of the physical space that provides the best developmental environment for the baby and also allows for privacy and family bonding time (ie, kangaroo care and so forth).
- Provide educational information that is helpful, timely, and affirming.
- Ensure a feedback loop is provided to assess the care experience of families.

Recognize the family as an essential partner on the QUALITY IMPROVEMENT team:

- Support families in a family advisor role in quality improvement.
- Establish visual identification of family advisors (ie, name tags that are different color, recognition at plenary sessions) at meetings and conferences.
- Ensure introductions of family advisors to the team and vice versa.
- Consider providing stipends for volunteer family advisors on the team.
- Consider identifying more than one family advisor for each project/committee.
- Develop systems, such as advisory councils, that ensure continuity and sustainability of family advisors.
- Provide similar quality improvement training for family advisors as for other disciplines.
- Provide opportunities for family advisors to engage in peer networking and support.

Recognize the family as LEADERS OF QUALITY IMPROVEMENT INITIATIVES:

- Support families as leaders in quality improvement.
- Establish paid faculty roles for family leaders to coordinate family related activities.
- Provide a feedback loop (ie, advisory board) to gather ideas and inform future direction of quality improvement work.
- Provide opportunities for presenting the family perspective at any and all presentations.
- Provide authorship opportunities for materials and articles.
- Engage family advisors in research opportunities.

Recognize the role and responsibility of the quality improvement LEADERSHIP TEAM: establish principles and consistent processes to guide teams

- Set the expectation that every team will include at least one family advisor as a fully supported and realized quality improvement team member.
- Provide resources to teams and family advisors to achieve role clarity and understanding.
- Follow through on expectations and provide consultative support to teams that are challenged in achieving family inclusion goals.
- Embed family centeredness in clinical quality improvement projects by measuring the impact of tests of change on families, partnering with families to codesign tests of change and collaborating with families who will lead tests of change.

Data from Pragmatic tips to structure and systematically integrate family involvement in quality improvement – lessons from Vermont Oxford Network collaboratives, 1999–2016.

Examples of Level I Family Involvement in Quality Improvement

Families complete surveys or engage in other evaluative activities as respondents (for example, focus groups)

There are numerous examples of level I participation, including focus groups and surveys.[11,12] Providing an opportunity for families to share their experiences can lead to a better understanding of the health care system and identify opportunities for improvement. A recent qualitative research project to explore the hospital experience of families with infants being treated for neonatal abstinence syndrome (NAS) led to key insight in the treatment of this group of infants and their families. Through interviews with the research team, families articulated their clear desire to be part of the care team; desired clear communication with the health care team, especially during care transitions; and valued education that reinforced their role as parents and decision-makers during the course of their stay.[13]

Examples of Level II Family Involvement in Quality Improvement

Family advisory councils serve as a resource to the quality improvement team (for example, review projects, documents)

Family advisory councils composed of family members whose children had been cared for in the NICU are in place in many hospitals.[14] The councils typically provide feedback on proposals and projects that are initiated by members of the NICU staff. Quality improvement projects may be presented for review and the irreplaceable perspective of NICU families sought.

During the most recent VON quality improvement collaborative, NICQ Next[2], a team from the UMass Memorial Medical Center, was seeking to improve the rates of human milk provision for oral care to infants in their NICU. The team developed a multifaceted approach to improving this, including the development of colostrum collection kits to be distributed to mothers. When the NICU Parent and Family Advisory Council was presented with the proposed project, the group of graduate parents rejected the wording on the kits, offering valuable feedback and suggestions. The value of engaging a family advisory council is directly aligned with the humility of those seeking its feedback.

Examples of Level III Family Involvement in Quality Improvement

Families participate as occasional reviewers and consultants during an improvement project

VON's quality improvement collaboratives have provided many examples of family advisor participation as reviewers and consultants. Some improvement collaborative teams included families who provided feedback on multiple projects. One that focused specifically on family centered care was the creation and pilot implementation of a family centered care map (FCC map) providing potentially better practices with examples aligned with phases of care in the NICU (http://www.fccmap.org/).[15,16]

In a different setting, family advisors participated in the refinement of a survey to be administered to graduate NICU families to better understand and design services based on family perceptions of barriers to fully assuming their roles in the NICU.[17]

Examples of Level IV Family Involvement in Quality Improvement

Families participate as active members of improvement teams and/or may serve on unit-based task forces and committees and faculty for staff and clinician education

Families as full participants in quality improvement are evidenced in unit-based projects and as regular committee members at all levels within organizations. One example of level IV work is family advisor participation on patient safety committees.[18]

Family advisors bring fresh eyes to patient safety rounds and powerful advocacy for future infants and families.

From 1998 to 2000, a VON quality improvement collaborative, with faculty from The IPFCC developed potentially better practices for NICU family centered care.[19] Family advisors were full members of the team that evaluated practices and made site visits to centers with strong self-reported family centered care. Among the important assessments made was that collaboration with NICU families depends less on the physical facilities and depends more on the attitudes of the staff. Readiness to advance family centered care often hinged on cultural prerequisites, such as cohesive multidisciplinary teamwork.

A team at The Children's Hospital at Dartmouth-Hitchcock Medical Center, Lebanon, New Hampshire conducted a quality improvement project from 2013 to 2015 focused on NAS. This project included a family advisor on the team and sought feedback repeatedly from families to improve iterative tests of change. By supporting families rooming-in with their NAS newborns, the use of pharmacologic agents and length of stay were decreased while optimizing family centered care.[20]

A systematic review of family involvement in health care systems revealed that collaboration at this level led to changes in the health care delivery systems in several different ways. Results varied, but some reported outcome improvements and improvement related to access to services.[21]

Examples of Level V Family Involvement in Quality Improvement

Families are coleaders of improvement initiatives

At level V, families are fully integrated as critical members of the quality improvement team at all levels. One example at the NICU level was achieved by the family advisor at Helen DeVos Children's Hospital in Grand Rapids, Michigan. As a member of VON's NICQ Next[2] quality improvement collaborative, the family advisor codesigned and led tests of change for staff education. The family advisor and nurse educator designed a very impactful educational module in support of their team's Small Baby Unit, addressing the needs of micropremature infants. Graduate families contributed to informed conversations, included in a staff education video providing parental insight into the NICU experience and life after the NICU.

All staff who viewed the educational video assessed it as extremely impactful. Some reported intentions to change their practice of interaction and use of language with families. An excerpt of the video is provided (Video 5).

MAJOR RECOMMENDATIONS

Socioeconomic determinants of health impact infants as the trajectory of their lives is directly impacted by the degree to which they establish and maintain physical, psychological, and emotional well-being.[22] It is critical to facilitate, support, and deepen involvement of families in quality improvement. Family members who have the unique experience of newborn intensive care see the health care system through a different lens. By collaborating with families serving as equal partners in quality improvement, opportunities for improvement can more readily be identified and acted on.

The Model for Improvement[23] prompts the following question: What are we trying to improve? Clinicians have valuable insight into the physiologic requirements of the infant's care. Families have exclusive insight into the needs of their family unit. Everything that happens to an infant in the NICU impacts the family. That impact should be acknowledged, respected, and measured. Some organizations have done this on a system level, such as the Institute for Healthcare Improvement, VON, AHRQ,

Patient-Centered Outcomes Research Institute, and others. The IPFCC published a resource highlighting tangible examples of partnerships at all levels of involvement.[24]

The authors suggest a model whereby engaged family advisors are active at every level and in every aspect of the hospital system. The levels of engagement enable teams to build on their achievements, thus, ensuring different opportunities and mechanisms for partnership. At level V, for example, families are codesigning and coleading quality improvement projects and have representation on committees and may leverage advisory councils for feedback and assistance. They are members of organization-wide planning and review teams, and the quality of care and interactions are being continuously improved through repeated feedback and individualization of care planning and assessment with every family entering the nursery.

The Controversies

Barriers

As a sociologic imperative, infants will thrive as members of strong, loving, supportive, and supported families. Failure to establish this as the goal of neonatal intensive care limits the contributions the dedicated professional team is able to make. Effective neonatal care requires clinical excellence, psychosocial support and services, family education, staff support and education, and a culture that includes a shared vision and a commitment to respect and empathize with every interaction.

Researchers have observed that conditions in the NICU fail to invite and support families in full participation and care of their infant. Barriers include lack of privacy, inadequate space for families to remain with their infant, priority given to technical activities, inadequate educational support provided to families, staffing constraints, and unit culture.[25]

Competing interests

Demands on the clinical health care team impact family centered care. Staffing may be determined based solely on technical requirements for care and fails to provide time and educational resources to mentor families in the care of their infant. Budgetary constraints impact on funded family advisor roles and provision of psychosocial support. The participation of senior leaders is critical to aligning organizational goals with leveraging of resources. Length of stay and family satisfaction are key organizational indicators, both of which can be positively impacted with family centered resources and staffing ratios.

In an evaluation of NICU family presence on rounds, medical trainees were least supportive, as it was interpreted as interfering with the pattern of education on rounds.[26] Family presence and participation on rounds presents unique educational and learning opportunities. Physician mentors have the opportunity to model family centered rounds by demonstrating effective communication and resultant shared decision-making, which contributes to empowered, functional families.

Changes in Practices That Are Likely to Improve Outcomes

What is required to establish level V

All neonatal care providers should seek to establish level V family advisor involvement. In **Box 4**, the authors offer detailed steps that will help an institution achieve level V using the framework described earlier. Here, the authors offer an additional framework for achieving full family centered care as a health care system.

Microsystem (the neonatal intensive care unit)

In 1992, Helen Harrison provided us with the building blocks to support family involvement in quality improvement by noting that family-staff partnership was necessary to establish and develop programs, which include quality improvement. The features of interdisciplinary collaboration, effective communication, shared goals, and conflict resolution processes all contribute to patient outcomes in the NICU.[27,28] All of these features coalesce in unit culture. When the culture includes accountability for the patient and family experience, the health care team is free to partner effectively with those it serves to improve the quality of care and experience.

Fully implementing family centered care will enable family integrated care wherein parents provide both the locus for care and most of the care itself. Newborn intensive parenting units will become the new norm. Fully supported and integrated families will both inform bedside quality improvement and demonstrate it.

Mesosystem (the program level = perinatal/neonatal-obstetrics/mother-baby, as examples)

Opportunities for families to participate in neonatal quality improvement begin with their first interaction with the perinatal team. Some pregnancies are identified as high risk; expectant mothers are referred to obstetric specialists, genetic counselors, or diagnostic services. In cases whereby the mother is hospitalized antenatally, regular communication between the obstetric and neonatal team should occur with the family and families should be educated and oriented to the NICU. Understanding and respecting the unique needs of families before admission to the NICU facilitates an optimal transition of care.

Macrosystem (the organization)

The Institute of Medicine identified in *Crossing the Quality Chasm* that although organizations make the commitment to embrace rules and principles to achieve quality, there must remain a commitment to individualize care based on patient preference and informed choice.[2]

Although much of the work to design NICU environments occurs within the microsystem (NICU), the expectations and guiding principles are determined at the level of the organization and its charter sponsored by senior leaders. Ensuring those principles are respectful of family centered care will invite family partnership and tests of concept.[29]

Metasystem (networks, health systems, and collaboratives)

In addition to ensuring family involvement throughout the organization, family centered care is fostered by considering metasystems beyond the hospital. These metasystems include metasystems around the individual patient, focused on care after neonatal hospitalization, and metasystems around the individual hospital, such as state and national collaboratives.

At the individual patient level, metasystems must recognize the family's needs beyond the hospital setting to achieve the highest quality care, particularly for NICU graduates. Neonatal follow-up programs provide standardized developmental assessments and service referral, but this commitment is not sufficient. In 2002, the American Academy of Pediatrics redefined its policy statement on the medical home.[30] In addition to other aspects of family centered care, key recommendations are for provision of care coordination and the maintenance of a central record. Families face recurring challenges in effectively navigating the health service environment, advocating for their NICU graduate children. For those children with complex needs, quality care may be supported by pediatric mental health models, such as high-fidelity wraparound care, which operationalizes care coordination and individualization to meet underlying needs.[31] Given that the relationship between the professional team and the family is unquestionably focused on the best possible outcome for the infant, fulfilling that commitment requires a reset from the provision of traditional follow-up to follow through.

Perinatal/neonatal quality improvement collaboratives are metasystems that involve families in the design, testing, and evaluation of care improvements at health system, state, and multi-state levels. The Ohio Perinatal Quality Collaborative (https://www.opqc.net/) provides relevant patient resources as well as an open invitation for patients and families to become engaged in the quality improvement work. The Perinatal Quality Collaborative of North Carolina is an example of a statewide quality improvement collaborative that has engaged family advisors. Videos with family stories are included as part of the resources shared publicly for many of the initiatives (PQCNC initiatives).

SUMMARY STATEMENT

A culture of accountability to those served is required at the highest levels, manifested by partnership with families in the design, assessment, and prioritization of quality improvement. Intending to serve is not sufficient. Without the fully empowered voice of the family recognized from the bedside to the boardroom at the organization and health system level, all efforts in the programmatic and NICU milieu are diminished in legitimacy.

As caregivers, providers, administrators, and supporters, we are challenged to demonstrate a noble commitment the interests of those we serve, over our own desire for control. Advances continue to be made in family centered, family integrated, and family engaged care. If quality improvement is a method we embrace, learning what is important to those served is vital to achieving quality. Partnering with families to improve quality will optimize our success at every level of the health care system.

ACKNOWLEDGMENTS

The authors wish to acknowledge the inspiring contributions of the families of NICU infants everywhere. The authors also thank the following individuals for their leadership in neonatal family centered care and quality improvement:

Ewe Ewald, MD, PhD former Head and Adjunct Professor, Department of Neonatology, University Children's Hospital, Uppsala, Sweden: Dr Ewald's unit is featured in video clips demonstrating family integrated care and parents' arms as the locus of care.

Amy Nyberg, BS, March of Dimes NICU Family Support Coordinator, Helen DeVos Children's Hospital, Grand Rapids, Michigan: Amy, along with her hospital team, produced impactful family videos for staff education for their Small Baby Unit and generously shared those videos.

Marybeth Fry, MEd, NICU Family Care Coordinator, Akron Children's Hospital, Akron, Ohio for her leadership within Vermont Oxford Network's NICQ Next^2 quality improvement collaborative, which invited posters from improvement team family advisors for presentation at Vermont Oxford Network's Annual Quality Congress in 2016.

Kate Robson, MEd, Family Support Specialist, Sunnybrook Health Sciences Centre, Toronto, Ontario, Canada and Executive Director, Canadian Premature Babies Foundation: Kate's leadership in the improvement community in both the United States and Canada inspires us to continue this important work.

Julia Sullivan Burns, BA, Program Assistant, Vermont Oxford Network, Burlington, Vermont. Julia provided skilled assistance in the collection of resources and the formatting of this article.

Andy Warner, Webinar Producer and Multimedia Producer, Vermont Oxford Network, Burlington, Vermont: Andy made it possible for the authors to share video clips with the readers.

The authors' editors, Drs Munish Gupta and Heather Kaplan, for their guidance, support, and thoughtful feedback.

SUPPLEMENTARY DATA

Supplementary data related to this article can be found at http://dx.doi.org/10.1016/j.clp.2017.05.008.

REFERENCES

1. Harrison H. The principles for family-centered neonatal care. Pediatrics 1993;92:643–50.
2. Institute of Medicine. Crossing the quality chasm: a new health system for the 21st century; 2001. Available at: http://www.ihi.org/education/conferences/APACForum2012/Documents/I1_Presentation_Johnson.pdf. Accessed July 10, 2017.
3. Johnson BH, Abraham MR. Partnering with patients, resident and families: a resource for leaders of hospitals, ambulatory care settings, and long-term care communities. Institute for Patient- and Family-Centered Care; 2012. Available at: http://www.ihi.org/education/conferences/APACForum2012/Documents/I1_Presentation_Johnson.pdf. Accessed July 10, 2017.
4. White RD, Smith JA, Shepley MM. Recommended standards for newborn ICU design, eighth edition. J Perinatol 2013;33:S2–16.
5. White RD. Mothers' arms - the past and future locus of neonatal care? Clin Perinatol 2004;31:383–7.
6. Macdonell K, Christie K, Robson K, et al. Implementing family-integrated care in the NICU: engaging veteran parents in program design and delivery. Adv Neonatal Care 2013;13(4):262–9.
7. Abraham M, Nickerson J. Framework for family involvement in quality improvement. Bethesda (MD): Institute for Family-Centered Care; 2009 (revised).
8. Conway JB, Celenza J, Abraham MR. Advancing patient- and family-centered newborn intensive care in: NICQ 2007: improvement in action. In: Horbar JD, Leahy K, Handyside J, editors. Burlington (VT): Vermont Oxford Network; 2010. p. 1-1-1-9.
9. Agency for Healthcare Research and Quality. Internet citation: guide to patient and family engagement in hospital quality and safety. Rockville (MD): Agency for Healthcare Research and Quality; 2013. Available at: http://www.ahrq.gov/professionals/systems/hospital/engagingfamilies/index.html.
10. Hynan MT, Hall SL. Psychosocial program standards for NICU parents. J Perinatol 2015;35:S1–4.
11. Steflox HT, Boyd JM, Straus SE, et al. Developing a patient and family-centered approach for measuring the quality of injury care: a study protocol. BMC Health Serv Res 2013;13:31.
12. Sydnor-Greenberg N, Dokken D. Coping and caring in different ways: understanding and meaningful involvement. Pediatr Nurs 2000;26(2):185–90.
13. Atwood EC, Sollender G, Hsu E, et al. A qualitative study of family experience with hospitalization for neonatal abstinence syndrome. Hosp Pediatr 2016;6(10):626–32.

14. McMullan C, Parker M, Sigward J. Developing a unit-based family advocacy board on a pediatric intensive care unit. Perm J 2009;13(4):28–32.
15. Dunn MS, Reilly MC, Johnston AM, et al. Development and dissemination of potentially better practices for the provision of family-centered care in neonatology: the family-centered care map. Pediatrics 2006;188:S95.
16. Johnston AM, Bullock CE, Graham JE, et al. Implementation and case-study results of potentially better practices for family-centered care: the family-centered care map. Pediatrics 2006;118:S108.
17. Dobbins N, Bohlig C, Sutphen J. Partners in growth: implementing family-centered changes in the neonatal intensive care unit. Child Health Care 1994; 3(2):115–26.
18. Institute for Family-Centered Care. Partnering with patients and families to enhance safety and quality: a mini toolkit. Bethesda (MD): Institute for Family-Centered Care; 2008.
19. Saunders RP, Abraham MR, Crosby MJ, et al. Evaluation and development of potentially better practices for improving family-centered care in neonatal intensive care units. Pediatrics 2003;4:S111.
20. Holmes AV, Atwood EC, Whalen B, et al. Rooming-in to treat neonatal abstinence syndrome: improved family-centered care at lower cost. Pediatrics 2016;137(6) [pii:e20152929].
21. Crawford MJ. Systematic review of involving patients in the planning and development of health care. BMJ 2002;325(7375):1263.
22. Braveman PA, Egerter SA, Mockenhaupt RE. Broadening the focus: the need to address the social determinants of health. Am J Prev Med 2011;40(1S1):S4–18.
23. Langley GL, Moen R, Nolan KM, et al. The improvement guide: a practical approach to enhancing organizational performance. 2nd edition. San Francisco (CA): Jossey-Bass Publishers; 2009.
24. Johnson B, Abraham M, Conway J, et al. Partnering with patients and families to design a patient- and family-centered health care system: recommendations and promising practices. Bethesda (MD): Institute for Patient- and Family-Centered Care; 2008.
25. Wigert H, Berg M, Hellstrom A-L. Health care professionals' experiences of parental presence and participation in neonatal intensive care unit. Int J Qual Stud Health Well Being 2007;2:45–54.
26. Grzyb MJ, Coo H, Ruhland L, et al. Views of parents and health-care providers regarding parental presence at bedside rounds in a neonatal intensive care unit. J Perinatol 2014;34:143–8.
27. Mitchell P, Shortell SM. Adverse outcomes and variations in organization of care delivery. Med Care 1977;35:NS19–32.
28. Pollack MM, Koch MA, The NIH-District of Columbia Neonatal Network. Association of outcomes with organizational characteristics of neonatal intensive care units. Crit Care Med 2003;31(6):1620–9.
29. Robson K, MacMillan-York E, Dunn MS. Celebration in the face of trauma: supporting NICU families through compassionate facility design. Newborn Infant Nurse Rev 2016;16:226–9.
30. American Academy of Pediatrics. The medical home. Pediatrics 2002;110:184–6.
31. Rosenblatt A. Bows and ribbons, tape and twine: wrapping the wraparound process for children with multi-system needs. J Child Fam Stud 2012;(5):101.

Improving Neonatal Care

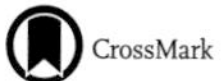

A Global Perspective

Danielle Yerdon Ehret, MD, MPH[a,b,*], Jacquelyn Knupp Patterson, MD[c], Carl Lewis Bose, MD[c]

KEYWORDS

• Quality improvement • Low-resource setting • Neonatal mortality • Coverage gap • Quality gap • Quality of care • Indicators • Education

KEY POINTS

- Each year, approximately 2.7 million babies die during the neonatal period; more than 90% of these deaths occur in developing countries.
- Prevention of mortality from the 3 major causes of death (complications of preterm birth, intrapartum-related causes, and sepsis) is possible with the implementation of simple, low-cost interventions, even in countries with limited resources.
- Mortality may result from a gap in coverage or a gap in quality of essential interventions and services. Both coverage and quality gaps may be amenable to improvement strategies.
- A variety of international organizations, including the World Health Organization and United Nations Children's Fund, have recommended key indicators of quality and established roadmaps for improving neonatal outcomes.
- The use of quality improvement methods is not yet part of standard educational training or routine health care delivery in developing countries.

INTRODUCTION

Poor perinatal outcomes are a significant global health burden. Each year, approximately 300,000 women die during or after childbirth, 2.6 million babies are stillborn, and 2.7 million babies die within the first month of life. More than 90% of these deaths occur in developing countries.[1,2] Until the late twentieth century, maternal and neonatal mortality were considered an expected and unavoidable outcome of many pregnancies in developing countries. It is now recognized that most of these deaths are preventable, and reducing perinatal mortality is now a priority in the world

---

Disclosure: The authors have nothing to disclose.

[a] Department of Pediatrics, Robert Larner M.D. College of Medicine at the University of Vermont, 89 Beaumont Avenue, Burlington, VT 05405, USA; [b] Vermont Oxford Network, 33 Kilburn Street, Burlington, VT 05401, USA; [c] Department of Pediatrics, University of North Carolina School of Medicine, 321 S. Columbia Street, Chapel Hill, NC 27516, USA

* Corresponding author. Department of Pediatrics, Robert Larner M.D. College of Medicine at the University of Vermont, 89 Beaumont Avenue, Burlington, VT 05405.

E-mail address: Danielle.Ehret@uvmhealth.org

Clin Perinatol 44 (2017) 567–582
http://dx.doi.org/10.1016/j.clp.2017.05.002

community. Strategies to improve perinatal health in developing countries have ranged from educating health care workers, to providing commodities essential for quality health care, to improving monitoring and evaluation. Continuous quality improvement (QI) methods have been used to a lesser degree.

This article discusses applications of QI science in developing countries. It reviews:

- The current state of global neonatal health
- Metrics to identify and monitor quality of care
- The role and limitations of education in reducing mortality
- The use of QI methods: international to facility-level initiatives
- Future needs

The focus in this article is on strategies to improve neonatal care and reduce neonatal mortality. In many cases, similar and concurrent strategies are being used to improve maternal care and reduce fetal and maternal mortality.

THE CURRENT STATE OF GLOBAL NEONATAL HEALTH

A new and intense focus on reducing neonatal mortality in developing countries began in 2000 when world leaders adopted a United Nations declaration that established goals to reduce extreme poverty and improve health: the Millennium Development Goals (MDGs). The MDGs covered a broad array of health goals; within perinatal care and pediatrics, MDG number 4 was reduction of mortality of children less than 5 years of age by two-thirds from 1990 to 2015, with a target under–5 years old mortality (U5M) of 30 per 1000 live births by 2015. Although this target was not reached, substantial progress was made, with the U5M decreasing by 53% from 91 to 43 per 1000 live births over this period (**Fig. 1**). This improvement was primarily caused by

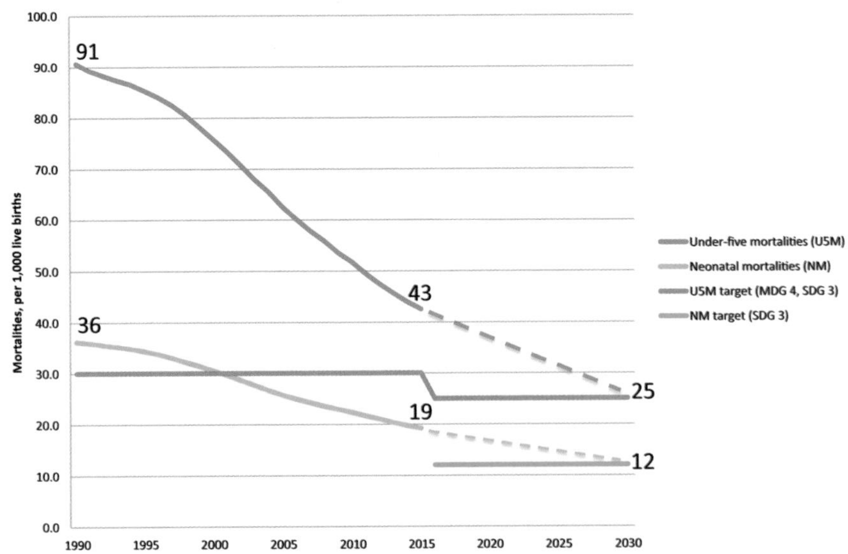

Fig. 1. Global U5M and neonatal mortality (NM) per 1000 live births from 1990 to 2015, and projected decline (*dashed line*) in mortality required to reach 2030 Sustainable Development Goal 3 (SDG 3). SDG 3 targets include U5M of 25 per 1000 live births and NM of 12 per 1000 live births. (*Data from* http://data.unicef.org.)

a decline in postneonatal mortality; less improvement in neonatal survival occurred over the same period, with the global neonatal mortality (NM) declining 47%, from 36 to 19 per 1000 live births. Because of this disproportionate decline in U5M and NM, deaths during the neonatal period now account for an increasing proportion of U5M.[2,3] Therefore, further reductions in the U5M will increasingly depend on reductions in NM. Recently, a new set of goals was adopted: the Sustainable Development Goals (SDGs). These goals document the world community's continued commitment to ending preventable deaths of newborns and children less than 5 years old by 2030. The new SDGs include goals to reduce the global U5M to 25 per 1000 live births and the global NM to 12 per 1000 live births by 2030. As a reference, the NM goal of 12 deaths per 1000 live births is the highest rate among nearly all developed countries.[4]

The 3 most common causes of neonatal deaths worldwide are complications of preterm birth (35%), intrapartum-related causes (24%), and sepsis (15%)[2] (**Fig. 2**A). However, the proportion of deaths attributed to these causes is highly dependent on the baseline NM. The worldwide proportions reflect the proportions in developing countries where most neonatal deaths occur. In developing countries with an NM greater than 30 per 1000 live births, approximately 40% of neonatal deaths are caused by complications of preterm birth, 22% have intrapartum-related causes, 15% are caused by sepsis, and 5% by congenital anomalies. By contrast, in high-resource, developed countries with a baseline NM less than 5 per 1000 live births, deaths caused by complications of preterm birth and congenital anomalies account for more than 75% of deaths; deaths with intrapartum-related causes are uncommon.[5] Likewise, the relative risk of death from these causes is also highly dependent on the baseline NM. The relative risks of death caused by preterm birth, intrapartum-related causes, and sepsis are 10, 36, and 34 times greater, respectively, in settings with NM greater than 30 compared with settings with NM less than 5.[6]

Many neonatal deaths in developing countries could be avoided with simple, low-cost interventions that address the needs of women and newborns across the continuum of care, with an emphasis on care around the time of birth. Prevention of most deaths does not require intensive care. It is estimated that 71% of newborn deaths are preventable with evidence-based care practices.[7] Many of these practices are in the category of essential care recommended for all newborns, often called essential newborn care (ENC), and include immediate drying and stimulation, delayed cord clamping, thermal care, support for immediate breastfeeding, infection prevention, the early assessment of newborns, and identification of problems presenting at birth.[8–18] The births of all newborns should be attended by a birth attendant proficient in the knowledge base and skills of neonatal resuscitation to reduce intrapartum-related deaths.[19] Complications of preterm birth may be amenable to preventive therapy with administration of antibiotics and/or antenatal corticosteroids to the mother with preterm labor in some settings,[20–23] and support of small and preterm infants with kangaroo mother care (KMC).[24] For neonates presenting with signs or symptoms of infection, prompt recognition and administration of antibiotics is important to prevent sepsis-related mortality[25,26] (see **Fig. 2**B).

In areas with high NMs, there remains a substantial gap in the availability of these basic and potentially lifesaving treatments, often termed a coverage gap.[7] Coverage is defined as the percentage of the intended population that receives an intervention or service. A coverage gap therefore represents the percentage of newborns that do not receive an essential intervention. **Fig. 3** shows the availability of a variety of basic interventions to reduce NM, showing a significant coverage gap for all of these interventions.[7] Since 2005, a group of international investigators has periodically reported the progress in closing coverage gaps in 75 developing countries with the highest burden of preventable neonatal deaths (the Countdown project).[3,27]

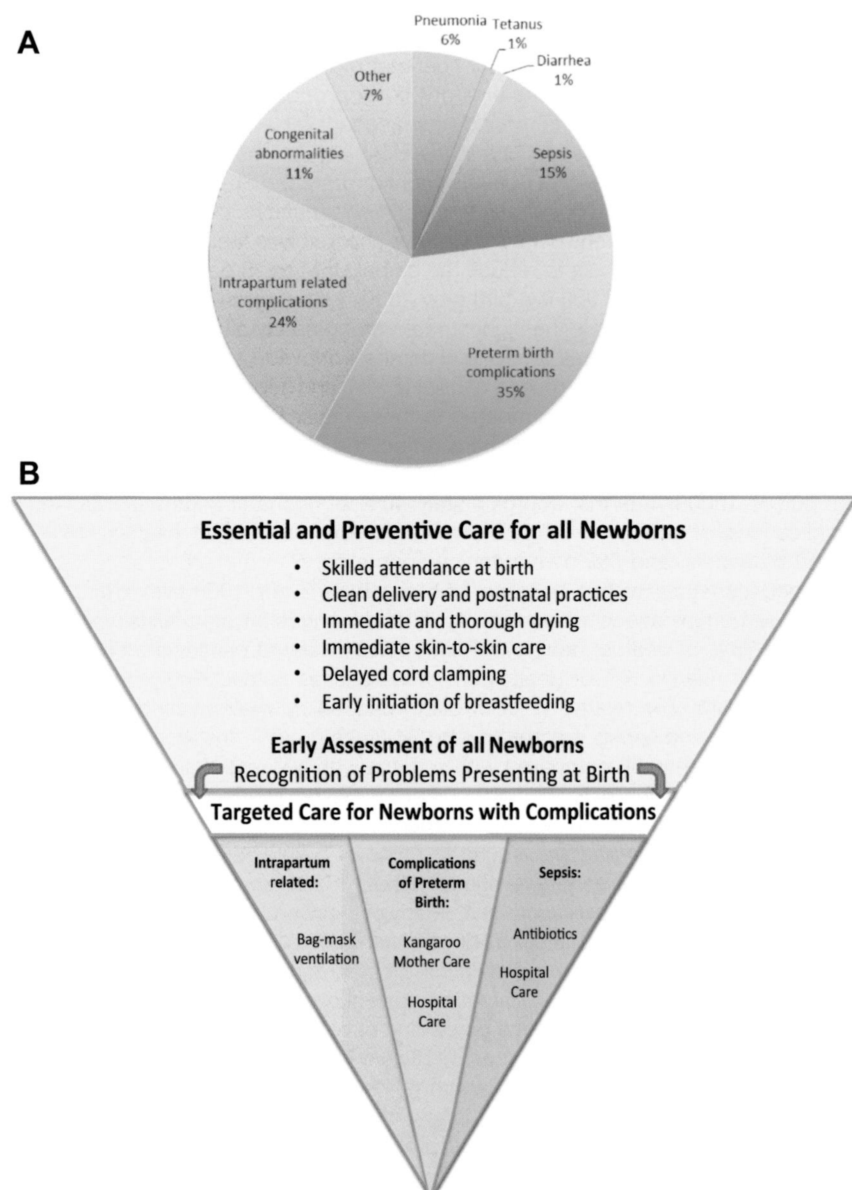

Fig. 2. (*A*) Causes of global neonatal mortality in 2015, as a percentage of deaths in live-born infants within first 28 days of life. (*B*) Prevention and treatment of the main causes of newborn mortality. Essential and preventive care for all newborns (*top section in yellow*) is the first step in prevention of neonatal mortality. The hierarchy of this graphic denotes the importance of prevention, followed by specific evidence-based treatments available for the 3 main causes of neonatal mortality: intrapartum-relation complications (*orange*), complications of preterm birth (*blue*), and sepsis (*purple*). An estimated 71% of newborn deaths are preventable with an approach that includes high-quality essential preventive care for all newborns, followed by targeted care for newborns with complications. ([*A*] *Data from* WHO and Maternal Child Epidemiology Estimation Group. 2015. Available at: http://data.unicef.org.)

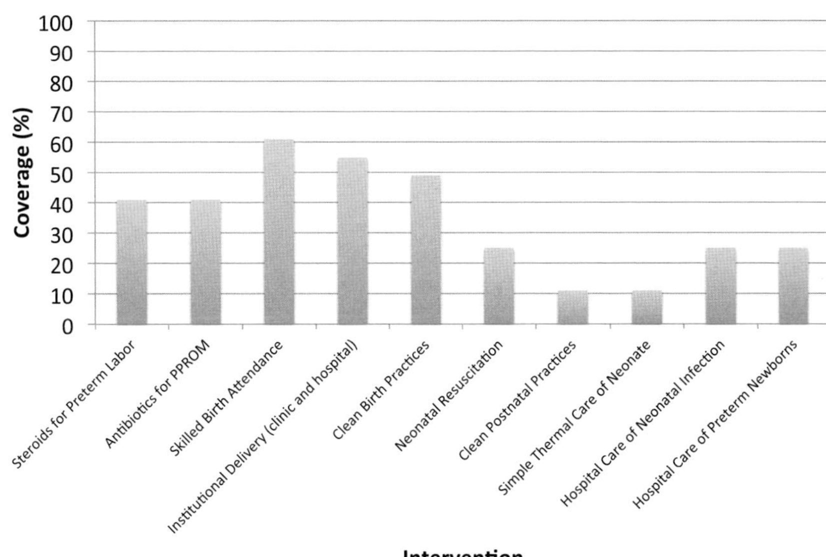

Fig. 3. Coverage of selected interventions to improve neonatal survival in the 75 Countdown countries. PPROM, preterm premature rupture of fetal membranes. (*Data from* Bhutta ZA, Das JK, Bahl R, et al. Can available interventions end preventable deaths in mothers, newborn babies, and stillbirths, and at what cost? Lancet 2014;384(9940):347–70.)

Historically, a major focus in global health has been to increase access to care in an effort to close these coverage gaps. However, access to a service or intervention does not necessarily ensure that care is received, nor does it ensure that an intervention is of adequate quality. A quality gap exists when services are available but care is of inadequate quality or is ineffective.[26,28] For example, in the 75 countries in the Countdown project, 55% of infants are born in facilities. However, clean postnatal practices are available in only about 10% of these facilities. Therefore, in these countries, in addition to the coverage gap in facility births of 45%, there is an additional quality gap of 45% caused by the lack of clean postnatal practices in facility births[26,29] (**Fig. 4**). Quality gaps represent missed opportunities to provide evidence-based high-quality care to patients already using the health care system. The cause of a quality gap may be multifactorial. A quality gap may be caused by a lack of essential commodities, such as clean water, soap, gloves and alcohol-based hand gel for proper hand hygiene, sterile razors and clean cord ties for clean cord care, clean towels and blankets for drying infants and temperature maintenance, self-inflating bags with neonatal and preterm-sized masks for ventilation, and antibiotics for treatment of infections. A quality gap may also be caused by limitations of the environment, such as inadequate staffing or insufficient physical space to serve the needs of all patients, and inadequate knowledge and skills of providers. Both coverage and quality gaps may be amenable to improvement strategies. However, structural changes in the health system may be required to close coverage gaps in contrast with quality gaps, which may be modifiable using facility-based continuous QI methods.

Often in developing countries, data describing the availability of services and quality of care provided are lacking. These data gaps make it impossible to quantify coverage

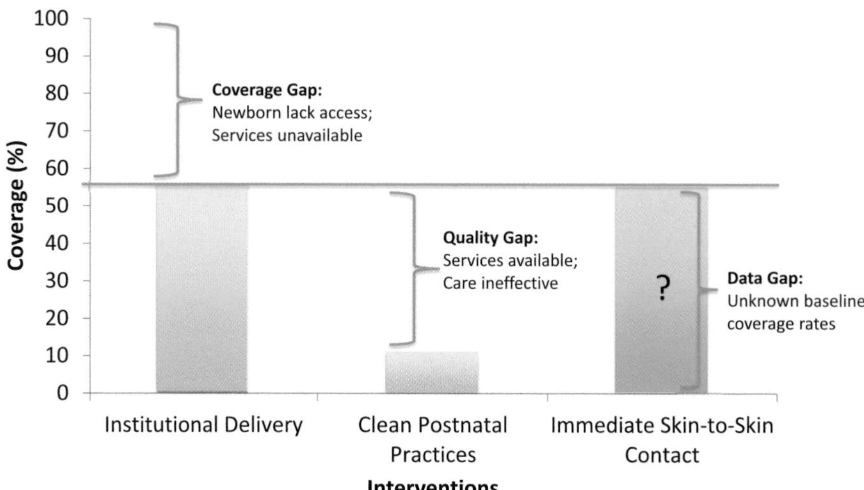

Fig. 4. Coverage of selected interventions to improve neonatal survival in the 75 Countdown countries. A coverage gap represents the percentage of newborns that do not receive an essential intervention. A quality gap represents availability of services, but care is of inadequate quality or ineffective. Data gaps (*light blue*) represent interventions with unknown baseline coverage rates. (*Data from* Bhutta ZA, Das JK, Bahl R, et al. Can available interventions end preventable deaths in mothers, newborn babies, and stillbirths, and at what cost? Lancet 2014;384(9940):347–70; and *Adapted from* Dickson KE, Kinney MV, Moxon SG, et al. Scaling up quality care for mothers and newborns around the time of birth: an overview of methods and analyses of intervention-specific bottlenecks and solutions. BMC Pregnancy Childbirth 2015;15(Suppl 2):S1; and Lawn JE, Davidge R, Paul VK, et al. Born too soon: care for the preterm baby. Reprod Health 2013;10 Suppl 1:S5.)

and quality gaps[26,28] (see **Fig. 4**). Closing data gaps has been a major focus of many international improvement efforts, often using new and creative data collection schemes.

METRICS TO IDENTIFY AND MONITOR QUALITY OF CARE

The international community has long understood the value of data. The lack of registration of births has been and remains a major data gap. At present, half of the world's babies do not receive a birth certificate, and almost all stillbirths and most neonatal deaths lack a death certificate.[5] In recognition of the importance of vital registration, as well as documenting contextual factors contributing to these deaths, many developing countries have devised strategies to register all pregnancies and determine all birth outcomes.[30] These efforts, along with other strategies for tracking pregnancies (eg, periodic national surveys), have provided fairly accurate data about mortality, and have highlighted the serious problem of high maternal and perinatal mortality. To date, data for the morbidities among preterm infants commonly reported in developed countries, such as chronic lung disease, intracranial hemorrhage, necrotizing enterocolitis, and neurodevelopmental impairment, have not been collected in developing countries. This omission is understandable and appropriate given the more urgent need to reduce mortality. In addition to pregnancy outcomes, data collection now often includes other indicators of the quality of care, such as essential commodities and processes of care.

Current Metrics

In addition to the mortality targets established by the SDGs, the international community has recommended input, process, and coverage indicators to provide important information about quality of care and system performance.[31] For example, the Every Newborn Action Plan (ENAP), led jointly by the United Nations Children's Fund (UNICEF) and the World Health Organization (WHO), was launched in 2014 with the aim of supporting countries in ending preventable newborn death. The ENAP recommends maternal and newborn care based on the best available evidence-based practices and is described in a sentinel publication, the *Lancet* Every Newborn series. The ENAP aims to "improve the quality of maternal and newborn care, to reach every woman and newborn with universal coverage, and to strengthen measurement capacity and count every death to drive improvement and accountability."[32] A key feature of the ENAP is the development of objective indicators of quality so that gaps in quality can be identified. The ENAP includes 10 core impact and coverage indicators and 10 additional indicators[33,34] (**Table 1**). Among the impact indicators are 3 outcomes (maternal mortality ratio, stillbirth rate, and NM) that track progress toward the health-related SDGs. Some of the indicators are not currently routinely tracked globally, whereas others lack consistent definitions and require additional testing. The core coverage metrics that are available for immediate use include skilled attendant at birth, postnatal care for newborns within 48 hours of birth, and early initiation of breastfeeding. Early initiation of breastfeeding serves as a tracer indicator or proxy for all of the elements of essential newborn care under the assumption that the presence or absence of early initiation of breastfeeding accurately reflects the receipt of all of the elements of ENC. Some indicators describe rates of specific high-risk groups

Table 1
Every Newborn Action Plan (ENAP) core and additional indicators

	Core ENAP Indicators	Additional Indicators
Impact	1. Maternal mortality ratio	
	2. Stillbirth rate[a]	Intrapartum stillbirth rate[a]
	3. Neonatal mortality rate	Low birth weight rate
		Preterm birth rate[a]
		Small for gestational age[a]
		Neonatal morbidity rates[a,b]
		Disability after neonatal conditions[a,b]
Coverage: Care for all Mothers and Newborns	4. Skilled attendant at birth	Antenatal care
	5. Early postnatal care for mothers and babies	
	6. Early initiation of breastfeeding	Exclusive breastfeeding up to 6 mo
Coverage: Care for Newborns at Risk or with Complications	7. Antenatal corticosteroid use[a,b]	Cesarean section rate
	8. Neonatal resuscitation[a,b]	
	9. Kangaroo mother care[a,b]	
	10. Treatment of severe neonatal infections[a,b]	Chlorhexidine cord cleansing[a,b]

Indicators to be disaggregated to assess equity such as urban/rural, regional, wealth quintile, and education.

[a] Not currently routinely tracked at global level.

[b] Indicator requiring additional testing to inform consistent measurement.

Adapted from Refs.[33,34,70]

(eg, low-birth-weight infants) or the care of neonates with complications (eg, infected infants), whereas others provide information that informs issues such as equity of care and morbidity. Several indicators still require validation and testing for feasibility.[34]

Facility-Level Quality-of-Care Indicators

The metrics described earlier are intended to portray the quality of care of populations. These metrics may be challenging to track consistently at the country level and do not provide specific information about the features of the site of care that might inform improvement efforts. An alternative or additional approach is to collect indicators that describe the quality of care provided by individual facilities. Indicators describing contact with the health system, such as facility delivery, are imperfect proxy measures of the care provided. There is an increased emphasis on collecting more granular and informative data, specifically examining the care provided. By using the denominator of all births in a facility over a specific time period, these metrics can be reported and used to guide improvement efforts at each facility.

The WHO issued quality-of-care indicators for maternal, newborn, and child health care in facilities. These indicators were intended to be action focused, important, operational, feasible, simple, and valued. Five core newborn health indicators were included, of which 3 describe care capabilities at the facility level, and 2 are population metrics reported at the facility-level[35]:

- Proportion of health facilities with maternity services that have functional bag and masks (2 neonatal mask sizes) in the delivery area
- Proportion of health facilities where KMC is operational, by level of facility
- Proportion of health facilities offering maternity services that have Baby Friendly Hospital Initiative certification, not more than 2 years old
- Proportion of newborns who received all 4 elements of ENC
    - Immediate and thorough drying
    - Immediate skin-to-skin contact
    - Delayed cord clamping
    - Initiation of breastfeeding in the first hour
- Facility NM, disaggregated by birth weight category

Of note, for the 4 elements of ENC, as mentioned earlier, breastfeeding in the first hour may be considered a tracer indicator or proxy measure for all 4 components. If this proxy measure is used, receipt of all 4 elements of ENC is reported at the patient level in a binary fashion, based on initiation of breastfeeding in the first hour.

Challenges of Data Describing Public Health

Because of limited resources and lack of informatics infrastructure in most developing countries, continuous collection of quality indicators is either challenging or impossible. An alternative is to measure health services at the country level using periodic household surveys.[34] The 2 largest and best-known household surveys are the Multiple Indicator Cluster Survey (MICS) funded by UNICEF[35,36] and the Demographic and Health Surveys (DHS) program funded by the United States Agency for International Development (USAID).[37] Both data sets are free and publicly available. These surveys use trained field workers who conduct interviews with household members. The frequency of survey administration varies by country. The current versions of both surveys include important neonatal coverage indicators, such as skilled attendant at birth, early initiation of breastfeeding, early postnatal care, and exclusive breastfeeding.

Although the MICS and DHS may accurately describe the general availability of services, they are not well designed to measure treatments for newborns at risk for specific problems or with complications. The sample size of surveys may be inadequate to measure infrequent outcomes in small populations. Reliance on parental recall may require less rigorous definitions of outcomes and reporting may be inaccurate. For the core indicators under development regarding coverage of care intended solely for newborns at risk or with complications, facility-based data are necessary to accurately describe the percentage of the intended population that receive interventions or services with high-quality, or effective, coverage.

Innovative Methods of Facilitating Data Collection

Several innovative tools have been developed to assist an improvement team in establishing local baseline data and identifying opportunities for improvement. To supplement the DHS survey, the program has developed the Service Performance Assessment (SPA), which provides important information on input and process indicators at the facility level. SPA surveys measure service readiness indicators and several other key maternal and child health indicators, including the availability of functional neonatal bag and masks in labor and delivery service areas, as well as availability of gentamicin for treatment of severe neonatal infection. The SPA modules include observation protocols, patient exit interviews, and health worker interviews. Before use in-country, the core questionnaires are adapted to the information and health needs of each country by local experts. The inventory questionnaire includes all questions in the WHO Service Availability and Readiness Assessments (SARA) tool.[34]

In addition to the SPA and SARA tools, the Newborn Services Rapid Health Facility Assessment is a newborn-specific health facility audit and health worker interview developed by the interagency Newborn Indicators Technical Working Group to identify potential gaps in policy or implementation.[38] An audit may be used simply to identify an opportunity for improvement, or followed serially over time to assess changes and their effect on improvement.

Developed specifically with the aim of improving quality of care in the perinatal period for mothers and newborns delivering in facilities, the WHO Safe Childbirth Checklist can be used to track processes of care, and effective coverage of interventions in facilities, over time.[39–41] The checklist is divided into 4 sections, representing natural pause points in care: on admission, just before delivery, soon after birth, and before discharge. To date, use of this checklist in India has shown improvement in the quality of care delivered at birth, with an ongoing cluster-randomized controlled trial assessing the effectiveness of the checklist program in reducing severe maternal, fetal, and newborn harm. The checklist and its corresponding implementation guide are publicly available.[42]

THE ROLE AND LIMITATIONS OF EDUCATION IN REDUCING MORTALITY

In developing countries, quality gaps are often identified, either by use of one of the tools described earlier or from locally derived data collection strategies. A common cause of a quality gap is a lack of knowledge and skills among providers. Under these circumstances, it is often assumed that education of health care workers will close this gap and improve health outcomes. Toward these ends, many programs have been developed to teach evidence-based care to providers in developing countries.[43–47] Designed for low-resource settings, these programs use inexpensive materials and do not rely on extensive technology. Many of the programs reinforce learning through simulation using low-fidelity models. Helping Babies Breathe (HBB), an educational program designed to teach newborn resuscitation in low-resource settings, is a prime example.[48]

Although these programs have shown that education can improve knowledge and skills, they have also highlighted the limitations of one-time training as a strategy for reducing mortality. For example, formative field testing of HBB showed high efficacy with good learner satisfaction and gains in knowledge and skills of providers.[45] Subsequent effectiveness testing of HBB in a variety of low-resource settings further supported these gains.[49,50] However, despite improved resuscitation skills as shown in simulation exercises after HBB training, translation into clinical management did not consistently ensue.[51]

One reason that a single educational experience does not translate into a change in practice is that knowledge and skills may decline over time. This decline was reported with Neonatal Resuscitation Program (NRP) training of nurse-midwives in Zambia.[52] More recently, implementation of HBB in Tanzania showed significant declines in knowledge and skills at 4 to 6 weeks after training, with ongoing declines out to 4 to 6 months.[53] One strategy to prevent this decline is to conduct refresher training.[54,55] However, the optimal frequency and duration of this training is unknown.

Another reason that one-time training may not translate into care at the bedside is that complex skills may require repeated practice before they can be used effectively. For example, effectiveness testing of HBB showed that perfect performance of bag-mask ventilation following a one-time training is unattainable for most participants.[49,50] One strategy to enhance learning of complex skills is to conduct periodic on-the-job simulation practice (referred to as low-dose, high-frequency practice). This strategy supported improved bag-mask ventilation skills in Sudanese village midwives at 1 year following HBB training.[56]

More recent implementation of HBB has included both refresher training and low-dose, high-frequency simulation practice with improved results. This implementation package in Tanzania resulted in good retention of knowledge and skills at 2 years following training, and ultimately decreased fresh stillbirths and early newborn mortality.[57,58] A similar implementation strategy in Nepal also significantly reduced intrapartum stillbirths and first-day NM.[54]

In addition, changes in practice and subsequent changes in outcome may not occur immediately after a training course. A period of use and reinforcement of training may be necessary before a decline in mortality occurs. Among deliveries attended by both skilled and traditional birth attendants in a rural region of the Democratic Republic of Congo, there was no decline in perinatal mortality immediately following ENC training of birth attendants.[59] However, there was a gradual but significant decline in perinatal mortality during the year following training, which was independently associated with time following training.

Although education of providers has contributed to improvements in neonatal care and reductions in mortality, it has become increasingly clear that education alone does not permit developing countries to reach their desired reductions in mortality. Education must be supplemented with strategies that facilitate the translation of education into evidence-based clinical practice.

THE USE OF QUALITY IMPROVEMENT METHODS: INTERNATIONAL TO FACILITY-LEVEL INITIATIVES

The value of QI science in reducing mortality in the developing world is increasingly being recognized at the international, national, and facility levels as a critical strategy for reducing NM. In 2016, the WHO published a quality-of-care framework for pregnant women and newborns, emphasizing both provision and experience of care.[60] In addition, the WHO developed a guide for auditing stillbirths and neonatal deaths in order to learn from and respond to preventable deaths.[30]

At the national level, the ENAP has spurred many ministries of health to action with 15 of the 18 countries that were categorized with the highest newborn mortalities or highest number of neonatal deaths taking specific steps to improve newborn care. Progress has included developing national newborn plans or a newborn component in the reproductive maternal newborn child health plan, developing a budget for the plan, and defining target NM and stillbirth rates.[61] Additional improvement efforts by ministries of health have included sponsoring national hospital collaboratives and facility audits.[62,63]

Although there is increasing emphasis on improving quality at the international and national levels, local activities to improve quality in health care facilities have been adopted more slowly.[64] This slow adoption may be caused by the unique challenges of implementing QI activities in these settings compared with in the highly resourced, developed world where facility-level infrastructure, electronic health records, and QI expertise support improvement activities. In contrast, in low-resource settings, health care workers are frequently too busy to devote time to improvement activities. Support from health facility and national leadership is also lacking.[65] In the absence of electronic record keeping, QI in low-resource settings relies on data extraction from paper charts, often with adaptation of local records to capture needed metrics.[31] In addition, QI expertise within institutions in these settings is rare, thus successful QI often requires coaching from an external QI expert.

Despite these limitations, there is an increasing body of literature describing the use of QI methodology to address local barriers in low-resource settings (as well as much work that goes unreported). Common features to successful initiatives include:

1. The use of an outside QI expert or coach to facilitate QI activities
2. Involvement of front-line health care workers in developing and testing solutions to quality gaps
3. Selection of low-cost solutions such as restructuring staff roles or reorganizing processes of care

For example, the Institute for Healthcare Improvement's Project Fives Alive! in Ghana identified barriers to facility provision of care, and then tested and implemented local solutions using improvement collaboratives and coaching from a quality expert. The intervention showed impact at scale for early antenatal care, skilled delivery, and facility level U5M.[66] United States Agency for International Development through Applying Science to Strengthen and Improve Systems has also supported implementation of QI in low-resource settings such as Niger and Mali with the formation of local QI teams, periodic supportive supervision, and collaborative learning sessions.[67] Changes implemented by QI teams included restructuring work hours and staff roles, placing essential commodities at the point of care delivery, and reorganizing processes of care with resulting improvements in early newborn care provision and postpartum monitoring.

FUTURE NEEDS

The international community has confirmed its continued commitment to improving the quality of neonatal care and reducing newborn mortality. This commitment has prompted many countries with high NMs to make this same commitment by allocating both resources and political will to improve the health of newborns. Despite this will to improve outcomes, change will not occur at the pace desired unless critical unmet needs are addressed, including the need for more data describing details of care and outcomes and the development of local expertise in QI methodology.

Accurate data describing neonatal outcomes are largely available through DHS and other sources. Health authorities are increasingly prioritizing documentation and review of maternal deaths, with 51 of the priority countries having a formal policy on maternal death notification. This prioritization must expand to include newborns because only 17 of the priority countries have a formal policy on reporting stillbirths and neonatal deaths.[30] However, beyond tracking outcomes, there is an ongoing need to collect accurate data on processes of care at the facility level in order to improve care delivery. The WHO has proposed a minimum perinatal data set, and several international and national organizations have identified additional key indicators, but many of these indicators still require validation and testing. Furthermore, data collection remains a burdensome task in low-resource settings, and one that is less frequently supported by health authorities. Also, data are often used to identify errors and are used in a punitive manner. Improving data collection and the utility of data at the local level will require a paradigm shift from data collection as a burden to data collection as empowerment. Data will be most empowering when effectively placed in the hands of providers at the bedside as a tool to inform and improve the quality of care. A new Web-based QI database, designed specifically for neonatal units in resource-limited settings with quality of care indicators and real-time reporting, is under development by the Vermont Oxford Network.[68] Future work to assess the feasibility and value for improvement teams, as well as scalability, will be important.

As data become more readily available, efforts at educating providers in evidence-based practices must be paired with QI methods at the local facility level. QI expertise at the facility level must be built with practical education in QI methodology. To be most effective, this education will incorporate a multidisciplinary team approach, recognizing the value that families add as improvement team members. QI education must be incorporated into preservice training and recertification. Ministries of health must build national-level QI expertise and provide targeted coaching to facilities to do quality work.

Ideally, efforts to increase expertise at the facility level should be supported by training programs designed for providers in resource-limited areas. There are several existing QI training programs, such as the Institute for Healthcare Improvement's Certificate in Quality and Safety, and Lean Six-Sigma. Although these programs have been effective in the developed world, there is less literature supporting their successful use in low-resource, QI-naive environments. The newly released American Academy of Pediatrics QI guide, *Improving Care of Mothers and Babies*,[69,70] represents an alternative QI education program designed specifically for resource-limited settings. Although this program may be a useful alternative, its effectiveness has not been tested, and it is not known whether it can be used without considerable support from a mentor or coach with QI expertise.

SUMMARY

Each year, approximately 2.7 million babies die during the neonatal period; more than 90% of these deaths occur in developing countries. Reducing NM is a priority of international health organizations. Prevention of mortality from the 3 major causes of death (complications of preterm birth, intrapartum-related causes, and sepsis) is possible with the implementation of simple, low-cost interventions, even in countries with limited resources.

Mortality may result from a coverage gap or the lack of availability of a critical intervention. It may also result from a quality gap when a critical intervention is not delivered consistently or effectively. Both coverage and quality gaps may be amenable to improvement strategies. However, often these gaps are not easily identified because of data gaps (the lack of data describing processes of care and outcomes).

A variety of international organizations, including the WHO and UNICEF, have established roadmaps for improving neonatal outcomes. The ENAP outlines strategies to close data gaps and improve the quality of maternal and newborn care. A component of the ENAP is the establishment of recommended key indicators of quality. Many developing countries have used the ENAP as a guide to establish country plans for reducing NM.

The use of QI methods, in which quality gaps are identified and strategies to overcome barriers to quality are tested, has become a routine part of health care in developed countries, but not in developing countries. Although QI methods have been endorsed at the national level in many of these countries, the use of QI methods at the facility level is rare, and local improvement projects are often supported by external experts. New databases and teaching programs designed specifically for providers in resource-limited facilities may increase the use of QI methods and improve outcomes.

REFERENCES

1. Levels and trends in child mortality, report 2015, United Nations Children's Fund. Available at: https://www.unicef.org/publications/files/Child_Mortality_Report_2015_Web_9_Sept_15.pdf. Accessed December 1, 2016.
2. The millennium development goals report 2015. Available at: http://www.un.org/millenniumgoals/2015_MDG_Report/pdf/MDG%202015%20rev%20(July%201).pdf. Accessed February 1, 2017.
3. Countdown to 2015 for maternal newborn and child survival. A decade tracking progress maternal, newborn, child survival: the 2015 Report. Available at: http://countdown2030.org/reports-and-articles/2015-final-report. Accessed February 1, 2017.
4. The sustainable development goals. Available at: https://sustainabledevelopment.un.org/sdg3. Accessed June 6, 2017.
5. Lawn JE, Blencowe H, Oza S, et al. Every newborn: progress, priorities, and potential beyond survival. Lancet 2014;384(9938):189–205.
6. Oza S, Lawn JE, Hogan DR, et al. Neonatal cause-of-death estimates for the early and late neonatal periods for 194 countries: 2000-2013. Bull World Health Organ 2015;93(1):19–28.
7. Bhutta ZA, Das JK, Bahl R, et al. Can available interventions end preventable deaths in mothers, newborn babies, and stillbirths, and at what cost? Lancet 2014;384(9940):347–70.
8. McDonald SJ, Middleton P, Dowswell T, et al. Effect of timing of umbilical cord clamping of term infants on maternal and neonatal outcomes. Cochrane Database Syst Rev 2013;(7):CD004074.
9. Garofalo M, Abenhaim HA. Early versus delayed cord clamping in term and preterm births: a review. J Obstet Gynaecol Can 2012;34(6):525–31.
10. Barros FC, Bhutta ZA, Batra M, et al. Global report on preterm birth and stillbirth (3 of 7): evidence for effectiveness of interventions. BMC Pregnancy Childbirth 2010;10(Suppl 1):S3.
11. Blencowe H, Cousens S, Mullany LC, et al. Clean birth and postnatal care practices to reduce neonatal deaths from sepsis and tetanus: a systematic review and Delphi estimation of mortality effect. BMC Public Health 2011;11(Suppl 3):S11.
12. Bhutta ZA, Ahmed T, Black RE, et al. What works? Interventions for maternal and child undernutrition and survival. Lancet 2008;371(9610):417–40.
13. Lamberti LM, Fischer Walker CL, Noiman A, et al. Breastfeeding and the risk for diarrhea morbidity and mortality. BMC Public Health 2011;11(Suppl 3):S15.
14. Garcia CR, Mullany LC, Rahmathullah L, et al. Breast-feeding initiation time and neonatal mortality risk among newborns in South India. J Perinatol 2011;31(6):397–403.
15. Mullany LC, Katz J, Li YM, et al. Breast-feeding patterns, time to initiation, and mortality risk among newborns in southern Nepal. J Nutr 2008;138(3):599–603.

16. WHO. Essential newborn care course, 2010. Available at: http://www.who.int/maternal_child_adolescent/documents/newborncare_course/en/. Accessed February 1, 2017.
17. WHO, U.N.P.F, UNICEF. Pregnancy, childbirth, postpartum and newborn care: a guide for essential practice. 3rd edition. 2015. Available at: http://apps.who.int/medicinedocs/documents/s23076en/s23076en.pdf. Accessed February 1, 2017.
18. WHO. Towards a grand convergence for child survival and health: a strategic review of options for the future building on lessons learnt from IMNCI, 2016. Available at: http://apps.who.int/iris/bitstream/10665/251855/1/WHO-MCA-16.04-eng.pdf. Accessed February 1, 2017.
19. Lee AC, Cousens S, Wall SN, et al. Neonatal resuscitation and immediate newborn assessment and stimulation for the prevention of neonatal deaths: a systematic review, meta-analysis and Delphi estimation of mortality effect. BMC Public Health 2011;11(Suppl 3):S12.
20. Mwansa-Kambafwile J, Cousens S, Hansen T, et al. Antenatal steroids in preterm labour for the prevention of neonatal deaths due to complications of preterm birth. Int J Epidemiol 2010;39(Suppl 1):i122–33.
21. Kenyon S, Boulvain M, Neilson JP. Antibiotics for preterm rupture of membranes. Cochrane Database Syst Rev 2013;(12):CD001058.
22. Flenady V, Hawley G, Stock OM, et al. Prophylactic antibiotics for inhibiting preterm labour with intact membranes. Cochrane Database Syst Rev 2013;(12):CD000246.
23. Roberts D, Dalziel S. Antenatal corticosteroids for accelerating fetal lung maturation for women at risk of preterm birth. Cochrane Database Syst Rev 2006;(3):CD004454.
24. Lawn JE, Mwansa-Kambafwile J, Horta BL, et al. 'Kangaroo mother care' to prevent neonatal deaths due to preterm birth complications. Int J Epidemiol 2010;39(Suppl 1):i144–54.
25. Zaidi AK, Ganatra HA, Syed S, et al. Effect of case management on neonatal mortality due to sepsis and pneumonia. BMC Public Health 2011;11(Suppl 3):S13.
26. Dickson KE, Kinney MV, Moxon SG, et al. Scaling up quality care for mothers and newborns around the time of birth: an overview of methods and analyses of intervention-specific bottlenecks and solutions. BMC Pregnancy Childbirth 2015;15(Suppl 2):S1.
27. Victora CG, Requejo JH, Barros AJ, et al. Countdown to 2015: a decade of tracking progress for maternal, newborn, and child survival. Lancet 2016;387(10032):2049–59.
28. Marchant T, Bryce J, Victora C, et al. Improved measurement for mothers, newborns and children in the era of the sustainable development goals. J Glob Health 2016;6(1):010506.
29. Lawn JE, Davidge R, Paul VK, et al. Born too soon: care for the preterm baby. Reprod Health 2013;10(Suppl 1):S5.
30. WHO. Making every baby count: audit and review of stillbirths and neonatal deaths, 2016. Available at: http://www.who.int/maternal_child_adolescent/documents/stillbirth-neonatal-death-review/en/. Accessed February 1, 2017.
31. Hill K, Clark PA, Narayanan I, et al. Improving quality of basic newborn resuscitation in low-resource settings: a framework for managers and skilled birth attendants. Bethesda (MD): 2014. Available at: http://www.healthynewbornnetwork.org/hnn-content/uploads/newbornresuscitationqualityframework_aug2014.pdf. Accessed February 1, 2017.
32. WHO. Every newborn: an action plan to end preventable deaths, 2014. Available at: http://www.who.int/maternal_child_adolescent/topics/newborn/enap_consultation/en/. Accessed December 1, 2016 – February 1, 2017.

33. Mason E, McDougall L, Lawn JE, et al. From evidence to action to deliver a healthy start for the next generation. Lancet 2014;384(9941):455–67.
34. Moxon SG, Ruysen H, Kerber KJ, et al. Count every newborn; a measurement improvement roadmap for coverage data. BMC Pregnancy Childbirth 2015; 15(Suppl 2):S8.
35. WHO. Consultation on improving measurement of the quality of maternal, newborn and child care in health facilities 2014. Available at: http://www.who.int/maternal_child_adolescent/documents/measuring-care-quality/en/. Accessed February 1, 2017.
36. UNICEF. The multiple indicators cluster survey program. Available at: http://mics.unicef.org.
37. USAID. The demographic and health surveys. Available at: http://dhsprogram.com/data. Accessed December 12, 2016.
38. Newborn services rapid health facility assessment. Available at: http://www.healthynewbornnetwork.org/resource/newborn-services-rapid-health-facility-assessment/. Accessed December 12, 2016.
39. Spector JM, Agrawal P, Kodkany B, et al. Improving quality of care for maternal and newborn health: prospective pilot study of the WHO Safe Childbirth Checklist program. PLoS One 2012;7(5):e35151.
40. Hirschhorn LR, Semrau K, Kodkany B, et al. Learning before leaping: integration of an adaptive study design process prior to initiation of BetterBirth, a large-scale randomized controlled trial in Uttar Pradesh, India. Implement Sci 2015;10:117.
41. Kumar S, Yadav V, Balasubramaniam S, et al. Effectiveness of the WHO SCC on improving adherence to essential practices during childbirth, in resource constrained settings. BMC Pregnancy Childbirth 2016;16(1):345.
42. WHO. Safe childbirth checklist. Available at: http://www.who.int/patientsafety/implementation/checklists/childbirth-checklist/en/. Accessed December 12, 2016.
43. Chomba E, McClure EM, Wright LL, et al. Effect of WHO newborn care training on neonatal mortality by education. Ambul Pediatr 2008;8(5):300–4.
44. Thukral A, Lockyer J, Bucher SL, et al. Evaluation of an educational program for essential newborn care in resource-limited settings: essential care for every baby. BMC Pediatr 2015;15:71.
45. Singhal N, Lockyer J, Fidler H, et al. Helping babies breathe: global neonatal resuscitation program development and formative educational evaluation. Resuscitation 2012;83(1):90–6.
46. Walker D, Cohen S, Fritz J, et al. Team training in obstetric and neonatal emergencies using highly realistic simulation in Mexico: impact on process indicators. BMC Pregnancy Childbirth 2014;14:367.
47. Nelissen E, Ersdal H, Mduma E, et al. Helping mothers survive bleeding after birth: retention of knowledge, skills, and confidence nine months after obstetric simulation-based training. BMC Pregnancy Childbirth 2015;15:190.
48. Helping Babies Breathe. Available at: http://www.helpingbabiesbreathe.org. Accessed December 12, 2016.
49. Musafili A, Essén B, Baribwira C, et al. Evaluating Helping Babies Breathe: training for healthcare workers at hospitals in Rwanda. Acta Paediatr 2013;102(1):e34–8.
50. Seto TL, Tabangin ME, Josyula S, et al. Educational outcomes of Helping Babies Breathe training at a community hospital in Honduras. Perspect Med Educ 2015; 4(5):225–32.
51. Ersdal HL, Vossius C, Bayo E, et al. A one-day "Helping Babies Breathe" course improves simulated performance but not clinical management of neonates. Resuscitation 2013;84(10):1422–7.

52. Carlo WA, Wright LL, Chomba E, et al. Educational impact of the neonatal resuscitation program in low-risk delivery centers in a developing country. J Pediatr 2009;154(4):504–8.e5.
53. Arlington L, Kairuki AK, Isangula KG, et al. Implementation of "Helping Babies Breathe": a three-year experience in Tanzania. Pediatrics 2017;139(5) [pii: e20162132].
54. Kc A, Wrammert J, Clark RB, et al. Reducing perinatal mortality in Nepal using Helping Babies Breathe. Pediatrics 2016;137(6) [pii:e20150117].
55. Reisman J, Arlington L, Jensen L, et al. Newborn resuscitation training in resource-limited settings: a systematic literature review. Pediatrics 2016;138(2) [pii:e20154490].
56. Arabi AM, Ibrahim SA, Ahmed SE, et al. Skills retention in Sudanese village midwives 1 year following Helping Babies Breathe training. Arch Dis Child 2016; 101(5):439–42.
57. Mduma E, Ersdal H, Svensen E, et al. Frequent brief on-site simulation training and reduction in 24-h neonatal mortality–an educational intervention study. Resuscitation 2015;93:1–7.
58. Msemo G, Massawe A, Mmbando D, et al. Newborn mortality and fresh stillbirth rates in Tanzania after Helping Babies Breathe training. Pediatrics 2013;131(2):e353–60.
59. Matendo R, Engmann C, Ditekemena J, et al. Reduced perinatal mortality following enhanced training of birth attendants in the Democratic Republic of Congo: a time-dependent effect. BMC Med 2011;9:93.
60. WHO. Standards for improving quality of maternal and newborn care in health facilities, 2016. Available at: http://www.who.int/maternal_child_adolescent/documents/improving-maternal-newborn-care-quality/en/. Accessed February 1, 2017.
61. WHO. Every Newborn action plan progress report, 2015. Available at: http://www.who.int/pmnch/ewec_progressreport.pdf. Accessed February 1, 2017.
62. Linnander E, McNatt Z, Sipsma H, et al. Use of a national collaborative to improve hospital quality in a low-income setting. Int Health 2016;8(2):148–53.
63. Sahel A, DeBrouwere V, Dujardin B, et al. Implementing a nationwide quality improvement approach in health services. Leadersh Health Serv (Bradf Engl) 2015;28(1):24–34.
64. National Academies of Science, Engineering, and Medicine. Improving quality of care in low- and middle-income countries: workshop summary. Washington, DC: The National Academies Press; 2015.
65. Bouchet B, Francisco M, Ovretveit J. The Zambia quality assurance program: successes and challenges. Int J Qual Health Care 2002;14(Suppl 1):89–95.
66. Singh K, Brodish P, Speizer I, et al. Can a quality improvement project impact maternal and child health outcomes at scale in northern Ghana? Health Res Policy Syst 2016;14(1):45.
67. Boucar M, Hill K, Coly A, et al. Improving postpartum care for mothers and newborns in Niger and Mali: a case study of an integrated maternal and newborn improvement programme. BJOG 2014;121(Suppl 4):127–33.
68. Vermont Oxford Network global health initiatives. Available at: https://public.vtoxford.org/about-us/global-health-initiatives/. Accessed February 1, 2017.
69. Helping Babies Survive; quality improvement. Available at: http://www.aap.org/en-us/advocacy-and-policy/aap-health-initiatives/helping-babies-survive/Pages/Quality-Improvement.aspx. Accessed December 12, 2016.
70. WHO, UNICEF. Every Newborn action plan. Geneva (Switzerland): World Health Organization; 2014. Available at: http://www.everynewborn.org/.

Using Health Information Technology to Improve Safety in Neonatal Care

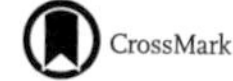

A Systematic Review of the Literature

Kristin R. Melton, MD[a,*], Yizhao Ni, PhD[b],
Heather L. Tubbs-Cooley, PhD, RN[c], Kathleen E. Walsh, MD, MSc[d]

KEYWORDS

• Health information technology • Patient safety • Neonatology • NICU
• Quality improvement • Medical errors

KEY POINTS

- Health information technology (HIT) interventions have been increasingly used in the provision of neonatal care. They are often moved into neonatal settings with little evaluation, however, and should be adequately tested before full adoption.
- We identified 4 qualities characterizing HIT interventions that achieved patient safety improvements: addresses a critical clinical need and leverages unique IT capabilities, and can be rigorously evaluated and generalized beyond the initial site.
- Quality improvement methodology can facilitate meaningful testing and implementation of HIT interventions.

INTRODUCTION

Issues in patient safety were brought to the forefront by the Institute of Medicine reports "To Err is Human"[1] and "Crossing the Quality Chasm."[2] Compared with adults, children experience higher rates of patient safety events, such as central line–associated blood stream infections and medication errors with potential for harm.[3,4] Within

Disclosure Statement: The authors have nothing to disclose.
[a] Division of Neonatology, Department of Pediatrics, Cincinnati Children's Hospital Medical Center, 3333 Burnet Avenue, MLC 7009, Cincinnati, OH 45229, USA; [b] Division of Biomedical Informatics, Department of Pediatrics, Cincinnati Children's Hospital Medical Center, 3333 Burnet Avenue, MLC 7024, Cincinnati, OH 45229, USA; [c] Research in Patient Services, Division of Nursing, Cincinnati Children's Hospital Medical Center, 3333 Burnet Avenue, MLC 11016, Cincinnati, OH 45229, USA; [d] Department of Pediatrics, James M. Anderson Center for Health Systems Excellence, Cincinnati Children's Hospital Medical Center, 3333 Burnet Avenue, MLC 7014, Cincinnati, OH 45229, USA
* Corresponding author.
E-mail address: Kristin.Melton@cchmc.org

Clin Perinatol 44 (2017) 583–616
http://dx.doi.org/10.1016/j.clp.2017.04.003
perinatology.theclinics.com

the pediatric population, neonates are uniquely vulnerable to errors primarily because of their physiologic immaturity, medication dosing that is influenced by weight and age, and the need for intensive care.[3,5] Some errors occur more commonly in the neonatal population, including identification errors due to multiple births and breast milk errors.[6–8]

Health information technology (HIT) has been used to streamline clinical workflow and improve patient safety in inpatient settings. In some studies, technology has been used to identify errors, prevent medication errors, assist with medical decision-making, improve communication, and detect early clinical deterioration.[9–13] For example, early studies of Computerized Physician Order Entry (CPOE) showed that it reduced errors by several methods, including forcing inclusion of key pieces of information in orders (eg, route) while allowing ready access to dosing recommendations.[14,15] Links to clinical guidelines and individual laboratory results may facilitate decision-making and streamline care.[16,17] Conversely, the introduction of new technology has also been shown to introduce new errors into the environment by changing clinician work flow and task performance, introducing unfamiliar systems, and by adding to workload.[18–20] As such, HIT interventions need to be carefully tested in different populations and environments, because the interaction of the technology with the health care environment will produce different clinical impact in different populations.[21] Several HIT-based interventions have demonstrated improvements in patient safety among adults and have subsequently been adopted in the neonatal intensive care environment. In this systematic review, we sought to evaluate the specific evidence for use of HIT interventions to improve patient safety in neonatal care.

METHODS

Search Strategy

A search strategy was designed to identify all potential publications related to the intersection of "health IT," "patient safety," and "neonatology" (see Appendix 1 for complete search queries). A search of MEDLINE, Cumulative Index of Nursing and Allied Health Literature, Scopus, and Embase was conducted for all articles published from 2000 to 2016, with key words and topic categories (eg, MeSH terms) related to the listed topics. A second key word search was then applied on the titles and abstracts of the returned articles to exclude articles that did not contain the key words of all 3 topics. The identified articles were manually reviewed by title and abstract to exclude studies that did not meet inclusion criteria. Finally, the remaining articles and a set of studies identified by reference searches were reviewed for findings and themes.

Inclusion and Exclusion Criteria

We included articles with a focus on neonatology, safety, and HIT conducted in settings caring for newborns and infants 30 days old or younger. For patient safety articles, we included studies that sought to optimize safe patient care and prevent medical errors and adverse events. We included studies that examined the impact of HIT on safety outcomes such as medical errors and adverse events and those that reported the usability, feasibility, and acceptability of HIT interventions. We did not consider studies that used HIT to identify disease in asymptomatic patients (newborn screening or retinopathy of prematurity screening) to be related to patient safety, but we did include studies that used HIT for early detection of disease or critical events based on a patient's current signs and symptoms. We also included studies that improved care through reduced variation or enhanced communication and situational awareness. HIT was defined as interventions that use information technology (IT) to promote health care, including but not limited to CPOE systems, Clinical Decision Support (CDS) algorithms, Electronic Health Record (EHR) systems, electronic prescribing, Bar-Coded Medication Administration (BCMA) systems, smart infusion pumps, health information exchange, personal health records, and telemedicine. If an electronic system was used only for data documentation or extraction, it was not considered HIT. We included original research articles encompassing multiple study designs including retrospective and prospective studies of HIT in clinical care, surveys, reports of quality improvement (QI) interventions, and studies of HIT in simulated environments. We excluded publications that were abstracts or case reports. We also excluded non-English language articles and articles focused solely on adult or pediatric populations without neonates.

Abstract and Article Review Process

Two authors reviewed each abstract to determine if the full article should be reviewed. The 2 authors then reviewed the selected article to determine inclusion or exclusion. Disagreements were discussed by all 4 authors and consensus reached regarding inclusion. We abstracted information from each article, including the study author, title, dates, design, setting, patient population/age, number of included patients, HIT topic, description of the HIT intervention, categorization of HIT development or application, and results/conclusions. Authors searched reference lists for additional relevant articles.

RESULTS

Our database search identified 2659 potentially relevant citations. Following key word filtering, we identified and manually reviewed 939 abstracts. We found 97 relevant articles for review and identified an additional 16 articles by searching references in reviews, commentaries, and original research articles. **Table 1** summarizes these articles.

Computerized Provider Order Entry

CPOE is a HIT application that allows providers to directly enter medical orders into a computer system. CPOE is defined primarily by the electronic order system itself, but may include components such as order sets that group associated orders. CPOE has the potential to decrease prescribing errors by requiring information entry, constraining choices regarding medication dose or route, providing dosing decision support, and by performing calculations. This is particularly important for weight-based dosing in neonates. CPOE also has the potential to decrease errors of omission by grouping orders and setting order defaults.

In our review, CPOE was the most investigated HIT intervention for neonates. Several studies have shown that CPOE systems reduced errors in prescription of total parenteral nutrition (TPN), which is prescribed frequently for neonates.[10,22–26] The developed systems all sought to avoid common prescribing errors, such as ordering calcium-phosphorous ratios that result in precipitation. All were pre-post studies that found a reduction in errors, and the 4 articles that performed statistical tests found these reductions to be statistically significant. Lehmann and colleagues[10] demonstrated that use of an online TPN order system and TPN calculator reduced errors by 61%, from 10.8 errors per 100 TPN orders to 4.2 errors in the first year of use, with a further 89% reduction of errors following 2 years of use.

Table 1
Summary of included articles

HIT Intervention	Reference	Type(s) of Safety Risk	Aim	Design	Sample	Results
CPOE	Bissinger et al,[31] 2013	Medication errors (delayed dispensing and administration)	Evaluate effect of CPOE and CDS implementation on antibiotic timing	Quality improvement (pre/post)	551 antibiotic orders for VLBW infants in 1 NICU	Delays reduced by process standardization, implementation of CPOE, and use of CDS
	Brown et al,[23] 2007	Medication errors (prescribing)	To describe epidemiology of TPN error rates; to assess the impact of electronic TPN worksheet to reduce TPN error rate; to assess TPN ordering and processing time when using the TPN worksheet	Quality improvement (pre/post)	480 TPN orders written by medical residents and NNPs	Implementation of a TPN CPOE system reduced TPN errors
	Chapman et al,[30] 2012	Delayed medication administration	To evaluate length of time between admission and administration of antibiotics before and after CPOE implementation	Pre-post	376 NICU infants preimplementation; 341 NICU infants postimplementation	No significant difference in time between admission and antibiotic administration between the groups; mean time to pharmacy order verification for a subset of patients was significantly shorter

Chuo and Hicks,[35] 2008	Medication errors (prescribing, dispensing)	To analyze computer-related NICU medication errors and CPOE errors reported to the MEDMARX database	Descriptive quantitative; retrospective analysis	343 medication errors in 48 institutions	One-third of CE errors reached patients vs fewer than one-fourth of CPOE errors; most CE errors occurred during transcription, whereas most CPOE errors occurred during prescribing; most common error type in CE is improper dose/ quantity, most common error in CPOE is prescribing error; major factors contributing to CPOE errors include distractions and inexperience; most errors resulted in no action to patient
Cordero et al,[33] 2004	Medication errors (prescribing, medication delay)	To study the impact of CPOE on medication error rates and order to completion time intervals for pharmacy orders and radiology procedures	Pre-post	111 VLBW infants born 6 mo before CPOE implementation; 100 VLBW infants born within 6 mo after CPOE implementation	CPOE resulted in reduced turnaround time for administration of caffeine loading dose and increased accuracy of gentamicin dosing; radiology response time decreased significantly after CPOE implementation

(*continued on next page*)

Table 1
(continued)

HIT Intervention	Reference	Type(s) of Safety Risk	Aim	Design	Sample	Results
	Giannone,[28] 2005	Medication errors (prescribing)	To describe the development of a computer application enabling weight-based medication infusion calculation for neonates within the CPOE information system	Case report	N/A	A health system was able to work with vendor before implementation to produce an add-on to the technology that met the information needs of the NICU clinicians
	Huston et al,[24] 2013	Medication errors (prescribing)	To evaluate the effectiveness of a computerized neonatal TPN calculator order program in reducing errors and optimizing nutrient intake	Retrospective analysis; pre/post	All infants with BW $\leq$1500 g, as well as larger infants with GI abnormalities requiring surgical intervention who received TPN for at least 5 d and also survived until at least DOL 8 were included	Ordering errors were reduced from 4.6 per 100 in 2007 to 0.1 per 100 in 2009
	Kazemi et al,[27] 2011	Medication errors (prescribing)	To compare the effect of CPOE without and with CDS in reducing nonintercepted medication dosing errors in antibiotics and anticonvulsants	Retrospective cohort design	Medication orders for 288 neonates during study period	No reduction in medication dosing errors after CPOE implemented but significant decline after decision support added to CPOE

Kazemi et al,[34] 2010	Medication errors (prescribing)	To evaluate whether a collaborative order entry method with nurse order entry and physician verification is as effective as physician order entry	Prospective observational	Medication orders for 158 neonates	The rate of nonintercepted medication errors was 40% lower during the nurse order period than the physician order period; prescription orders decreased from 10.3% during physician order period to 4.6% during nurse order period
Lehman et al,[10] 2004	Medication errors (prescribing)	To describe the development of a pragmatic low-cost online TPN calculator designed to reduce TPN ordering errors in the NICU at the Johns Hopkins Hospital	Quality improvement (pre/post)	1684 TPN orders (557 pre, 471 intervention period 1, 656 intervention period 2)	Significant reduction in TPN ordering errors after implementation of the online calculator; errors reduced 89% to 1.2 errors/100 orders
Lehman et al,[22] 2002	Medication errors (prescribing)	To describe the development of a pragmatic low-cost online TPN calculator designed to reduce TPN ordering errors in the NICU at the Johns Hopkins Hospital and evaluate impact on errors and user satisfaction	Quality improvement (pre/post)	1028 TPN orders (557 before and 471 after implementation)	Ordering errors were significantly reduced 61% from 10.8 errors/100 orders to 4.2 errors/100 orders; users were supportive of the program

(*continued on next page*)

Table 1
(continued)

HIT Intervention	Reference	Type(s) of Safety Risk	Aim	Design	Sample	Results
	Luton et al,[8] 2015	Breast milk and formula errors (prescribing, administration)	To describe the development of a program to improve processes surrounding infant feeding	Quality improvement (pre/post)	All infant feeding orders over a 2-year period	Errors were reduced by 83% after a multistep improvement program was implemented
	Peverini et al,[25] 2000	Medication errors (prescribing)	To describe the design, development, and implementation of a neonatal TPN decision support system	Pre-post	556 TPN orders (266 before implementation, 290 after)	By incorporating a display of the relationship between solution volume, protein, calcium and phosphorus, calcium-phosphorus precipitation TPN errors were eliminated
	Skouroliakou et al,[26] 2005	Medication errors (prescribing)	To compare extent of error occurrence between manual TPN calculation and use of computer-based method of TPN calculation; to examine difference in personnel time required for manual vs computer-based TPN prescribing	Pre-post	96 preterm and term neonates requiring 941 TPN prescriptions	Computer prescribing of TPN reduced clinician time and eliminated TPN calculation errors

	Taylor et al,[29] 2008	Medication errors (prescribing, medication delay)	To study the impact of CPOE on medication administration errors, especially wrong-time and wrong-route errors	Pre-post	526 NICU medication administrations (254 before CPOE, 272 after)	Medication administration errors were reduced from 19.8% pre to 11.6% post; wrong-time errors decreased from 9.9% to 6.7% and wrong-route errors were eliminated
	Walsh et al,[18] 2008	Medication errors (all types)	To evaluate the effect of CPOE on the rate of inpatient pediatric medication errors	Pre-post, interrupted time series	627 pediatric admissions and 12,672 medication orders in NICU, PICU, and inpatient pediatric units at 1 general hospital	156 medication errors were detected overall; there was a 7% decrease in the rate of nonintercepted serious medication errors after CPOE implementation; no change in rate of injuries secondary to medication error after CPOE implementation
CDS	Heermann and Thompson,[36] 1997	Neonatal transport	Report on the development of a CDS to assist with stabilization of neonates before transport; logic-rules (if-then rules) were developed based on the guidelines and standards presented in The STABLE Assistant	Structural testing on the correctness of the rules based on user survey	Patient data from 19 charts were used to evaluate the rules	Prototype CDS was successfully developed

(*continued on next page*)

Table 1
(continued)

HIT Intervention	Reference	Type(s) of Safety Risk	Aim	Design	Sample	Results
	Hum et al,[17] 2014	Antibiotic prescription	To develop and implement a CDS tool to improve antibiotic prescribing in the NICU and evaluate use and acceptance of the tool	Prospective observational	1303 CDS activations for 452 patients	Prescribing recommendations viewed during 15% of activations; respondents considered most useful features to be summarized culture results (43%) and antibiotic recommendations (48%)
	Longhurst et al,[11] 2009	Jaundice treatment decisions	To describe the development of a Web-based decision support tool to increase use of neonatal hyperbilirubinemia guidelines	Prospective observational	469 clinician survey responders' 25,000 hits to BiliTool daily	63% of clinicians surveyed are BiliTool users; 25,000 Web site hits daily
	Mani et al,[13] 2014	Early detection of neonatal late-onset sepsis	To develop noninvasive, predictive models for late-onset neonatal sepsis from existing data using machine learning algorithms	Observational design; retrospective analysis of existing data	Records from 299 infants evaluated for late-onset sepsis in 1 NICU	Predictive models developed from existing data using machine learning exceeded the treatment sensitivity and specificity of clinicians

Maat et al,[32] 2013	Medication (glucose) prescribing	To evaluate the effect of a computerized prescribing and calculating system on hypoglycemia and hyperglycemia and on prescribing time efficiency in neonatal intensive care patients	Interrupted time series, crossover design for time	2040 patients with assessment of hypoglycemia and hyperglycemia per 100 hospital days	Faster prescribing calculations with no loss of accuracy
Pallás et al,[37] 2008	Medication errors (prescribing)	To estimate the prevalence of violations of GPP before and after GPP education and implementation of pocket PC-based automatic calculation system	Pre-post quasiexperimental	6320 handwritten prescriptions in the first period and 1435 in the second period	Incorrect prescriptions decreased from 39.5% before intervention to 11.9% after; the number of wrongly specified items on a single prescription decreased from 11.1% to 1.3%
Vergano et al,[38] 2013	Early detection of hyperammonemia	To design and implement an EMR-based tool to assist detection of hyperammonemia	Retrospective review; prospective evaluation of intervention	27 hospitalized infants in discovery cohort; all infants in institution after tool implementation from January–December 2012	Implementation of an EMR-based warning system can improve surveillance for hyperammonemia in a susceptible population
Zabidi et al,[39] 2012	Early detection of asphyxia	To design a tool that automatically detects asphyxia in infants based on analysis of their cry	Technical report	Infants birth to 6 mo of age	Classification accuracy of 96.03% reported

(*continued on next page*)

Table 1
(continued)

HIT Intervention	Reference	Type(s) of Safety Risk	Aim	Design	Sample	Results
BCMA	Dougherty and Nash,[7] 2009	Breast milk administration errors	To evaluate reductions in breast milk administration errors after introduction of a bar-coding system for breast milk	Quality improvement (pre-post)	All breast milk administrations over a 3-year period	NICU breast milk errors decreased from 3% to 0.4% of administrations; number of errors decreased from 11 per year to 1.3 per year
	Morriss et al,[42] 2009	Medication administration errors	To understand nurses' opinions about patient safety, use, acceptance, and occupational effects after implementation of BCMA	Prospective; survey study	46 NICU nurses	Almost all respondents stated that the system helped them avoid making a medication error, and most reported that the system helped them avoid an ADE; most nurses believed that the system improved their professionalism, and approximately one-half said that it contributed to their job satisfaction
	Morriss et al,[41] 2009	Preventable ADEs	To evaluate reductions in ADEs after implementation of BCMA	Prospective, observational cohort study	475 infants before BCMA and 483 infants after BCMA	BCMA reduced risk of targeted preventable ADEs by 47%, controlling for number of medication doses/ subject/day

	Morriss et al,[40] 2011	Preventable ADEs	To examine the effect of BCMA on risk of ADE in neonates treated with opioids	Prospective, observational cohort study	618 infants in 1 NICU	32 preventable ADEs occurred; infants treated with an opioid were 4.74 times more likely to have preventable ADE compared with infants not receiving opioids; patients treated with opioid in absence of BMCA system had 10% probability of ADE after hospitalization for 6 d
	Steele and Bixby,[43] 2014	Breast milk administration errors	To describe changes in breast milk misadministration after implementation of breast milk bar code scanning	Quality improvement (pre-post)	7000 breast milk feedings per month evaluated over 16 mo	Breast milk administration errors decreased to zero; during first 6 mo after bar coding, 55 attempts to feed the wrong milk to the wrong infant occurred and 127 attempts to feed expired breast milk were prevented

(*continued on next page*)

Table 1
(*continued*)

HIT Intervention	Reference	Type(s) of Safety Risk	Aim	Design	Sample	Results
Smart pumps	Bergon-Sendin et al,[44] 2015	Medication errors	To use random safety audits to assess and compare the frequency of appropriate use of infusion pump safety systems before and after QI interventions	Prospective, observational	Information from 44,924 infusions during 2 time periods	Frequency of appropriate pump programming/pump use was 0% in the first time period and 73% in second time period; 46% of infusions had drug names recorded into the pump; 2.5% of applicable cases there was an attempt to exceed the absolute limit
Error/event detection	Dickerman et al,[54] 2011	Medication-related adverse events	To describe the use of an automated adverse-event detection system to detect and categorize hypoglycemia-related adverse events in pediatric inpatients	Retrospective cohort	1254 hypoglycemia triggers over 1 y for inpatient pediatric population (including neonates)	Most hypoglycemia-related adverse events (68%) occurred in the NICU; 83% of total adverse events in the NICU occurred in infants receiving insulin therapy

Li et al,[53] 2015	Medication/infusion-related adverse events	To report on the development of novel algorithms to detect adverse events and compare to current error detection systems, including trigger tool and voluntary incident-reporting systems	Retrospective cohort	753 NICU patient EHRs from 2011	12 severe IV infiltrates detected, 1 narcotic over-sedation, 17 narcotic errors; computerized algorithms demonstrated significantly better sensitivity and specificity than current detection systems
Li et al,[9] 2015	Medication/infusion-related adverse events	To evaluate rates of medication administration errors in neonatal care and to compare the performance of computerized algorithms with traditional incident reporting for error detection	Retrospective cohort	Data from all infants in a Level IV NICU in 2011 (16,388 patient days) and 2012 (16,685 patient days)	Error rates varied from 0.3% to 12.8% for continuous medications; MAE rates were higher for medications that were adjusted frequently and fluids administered concurrently; the algorithms performed better than currently used incident-reporting systems

(*continued on next page*)

Table 1
(*continued*)

HIT Intervention	Reference	Type(s) of Safety Risk	Aim	Design	Sample	Results
Telemedicine	Garingo et al,[46] 2012	Telemedicine	To describe the use of a wireless mobile robotic telecommunications system in the NICU and assess agreement between patient assessments of an on-site and off-site neonatologist	Case report	304 NICU patient encounters	Excellent or intermediate agreement noted for most examination assessments except for breath, heart, and bowel sound assessment and capillary refill time; duration of encounters was similar
	Garingo et al,[45] 2016	Telemedicine	To investigate the feasibility of telerounding in the NICU and compare patient outcomes for patients cared for by on-site and off-site neonatologists	Case report	20 NICU patient pairs matched by gestation, diagnosis, and disease severity; with 373 patient encounters	No differences in length of stay, age at discharge, hospital charges, nutrition, respiratory support, days of antibiotics, days of phototherapy, or number of radiologic studies; median time of visit was 5 min for control and 8 min for telemedicine

McGregor et al,[47] 2007	Telemedicine	To describe the architecture developed to deliver On-Demand Virtual NICU support for rural, remote and urban Australia; to describe the application of the architecture to a pilot collaboration between 2 hospitals	Case report	N/A	Physiologic data and images can be delivered real-time to off-site neonatologists for assessment
Minton et al,[48] 2014	Telemedicine	To describe a telecommunications system used for family engagement and physician-family communication and the use of teleresuscitation beds	Case report	N/A	Physiologic data and images can be delivered real-time to off-site neonatologists and similar systems can be used to promote family communication and engagement

(*continued on next page*)

Table 1
(continued)

HIT Intervention	Reference	Type(s) of Safety Risk	Aim	Design	Sample	Results
Communication	Gray et al,[12] 2000	Parent-provider communication	To evaluate an Internet-based telemedicine program to reduce cost and provide better medical, informational, and emotional support to NICU families	Randomized observational	Parents of 56 VLBW infants in the one NICU, 30 control and 26 study patients	Parents with CareLink reported higher overall quality of care, fewer problems with care quality (3% vs 13%) and greater satisfaction; no difference in frequency of visits, telephone calls, or length of stay
	Phillips,[51] 1999	Parent-provider communication	To describe the development of an Internet-based telemedicine program to provide better medical, informational, and emotional support to NICU families	Technical report	Parents of VLBW infants in 1 NICU	Brief report about development, components and goals of Baby Care Link
	Safran,[52] 2003	Parent-provider communication	To describe a computerized tool, Baby CareLink, to support communications between parents, patients and clinicians and to assess generalizability to different populations	Case report	370 parents in 2 different institutions and regions of the country with 11,600 activations of Baby CareLink	The use of Baby CareLink successfully provides communication and customized education for parents, even though remote from the NICU

	Taylor and El-Kafrawy,[49] 2012	Parent and visitor communication	To describe a novel audiovisual computerized system to improve adherence to hand hygiene and infection-control practices	Quality improvement (pre-post)	24 NICU visitors before intervention and 58 visitors after intervention	Hand-washing compliance and appropriate technique improved in visitors from 79% to 100%
	Weyand et al,[50] 2011	Parent-provider communication and parent decision tool	To describe the development of the Physician and Parent Decision Support (PPADS), a tool to help parents make more informed decisions and improve physician-parent communication	Usability testing	8 parents of NICU patients	Surveyed parents found the tool very easy to use and learn, and indicated that they would use the tool
Monitoring and Care processes	Burke and Downes,[53] 2006	Monitoring and detection of apnea events	To describe the development of an apnea monitor that integrates physiologic measures and processes them with a fuzzy logic algorithm to reliably detect life-threatening events	Simulation (bench testing using signal generator, oscilloscope, patient simulator and a data recording system)	Signals generated from signal generators	After some fine-tuning during development, the monitor was successful in detecting all apnea scenarios generated by the simulator

(*continued on next page*)

Table 1
(continued)

HIT Intervention	Reference	Type(s) of Safety Risk	Aim	Design	Sample	Results
	Gray,[61] 2011	Provider-provider communication (handoff)	To describe the development and application of the Digital Crumb Investigator; the tool was used to analyze and visualize the handoffs between clinicians for a patient and patient-provider care interactions	Observational design; retrospective analysis of existing data	4498 mothers and 4678 infants (4130 well newborns and 548 infants receiving intermediate or intensive care)	Network analysis using digital crumbs can provide understanding of clinical team structure and dynamics (number of providers involved, providers most closely associated with a patient's care, provider handoffs)
	Griffin,[57] 2003	Sepsis prediction	To develop and validate a predictive statistical model using clinical data to yield a heart rate characteristic index used to predict sepsis and sepsis-like illness	Prospective, observational	316 neonates in the derivation cohort with 155 episodes of sepsis and 317 neonates in the validation cohort with 118 episodes of sepsis	The heart rate characteristic index showed significant association with sepsis and added significantly to demographic information like birth weight and gestational age in predicting sepsis

	Liu,[59] 2009	Noise reduction	To describe the development of 2 multichannel active noise control algorithms; the algorithms were used to reduce the noise inside an infant incubator	Simulation	Evaluation of noise level on 520 points inside the incubator	Noise reduction of 5–40 dB at all measuring points in the incubator
	Moorman,[58] 2011	Sepsis prediction	To test the ability of heart rate characteristic monitoring to improve neonatal outcomes and reduce mortality	Randomized controlled clinical trial	3003 VLBW neonates in 9 NICU centers	Mortality was reduced in infants with displayed heart rate characteristic monitoring from 10.2% to 8.1% (hazard ratio 0.78 [CI: 0.61–0.99])
	Palma,[62] 2011	Provider-provider communication (handoff)	To evaluate the impact of integrating a handoff tool into the EHR on sign-out accuracy, satisfaction and workflow	Pre/post quasiexperimental	52 clinicians (attendings, NNPs, fellows, residents, charge nurses, and managers) responded to pre survey; 46 responded to post survey	The integration of a handoff tool specific to neonatal care within an EHR resulted in improvements in perceived sign-out accuracy, satisfaction, and at least 1 aspect of workflow; customization of commercially available EHRs to meet NICU demands is possible

(*continued on next page*)

Table 1
(continued)

HIT Intervention	Reference	Type(s) of Safety Risk	Aim	Design	Sample	Results
	Saria,[56] 2010	Risk prediction of mortality	To describe the development of a risk stratification method that predicts morbidity for preterm infants by integrating multiple continuous physiologic signals from the first 3 h of life	Retrospective cohort	138 preterm neonates that were 34 wk gestational age or less and <2000 g without major congenital malformations	The ability to interpret patterns in patient data and automate morbidity prediction was demonstrated; the algorithm provided better accuracy in prediction of overall morbidity than other neonatal scoring systems, including the standard Apgar score

Abbreviations: ADE, adverse drug event; BCMA, bar-coded medication administration; BW, birth weight; CDS, clinical decision support; CE, computer entry; CI, confidence interval; CPOE, Computerized Physician Order Entry; DOL, day of life; EHR, electronic health record; EMR, electronic medical record; GI, gastrointestinal; GPP, good prescribing practices; IV, intravenous; MAE, medication administration error; N/A, not applicable; NICU, neonatal intensive care unit; NNP, neonatal nurse practitioner; PICU, pediatric intensive care unit; TPN, total parenteral nutrition; VLBW, very low birth weight.

Some studies have shown decreased ordering errors using CPOE for weight-based dosing in neonates.[27,28] Taylor and colleagues[29] found that the use of CPOE led to significantly fewer medications being given at the wrong time, and also eliminated wrong-route administrations.

Others have shown beneficial effects of CPOE on the timing of drug delivery for important medications like antibiotics, caffeine, and glucose infusions.[30–33] Bissinger and colleagues[31] demonstrated that use of CPOE for antibiotic ordering in neonates with suspected infection decreased the time for antibiotic delivery and reduced variation. By developing electronic order sets that automatically entered STAT antibiotic orders transmitted directly to pharmacy to avoid administration delay, they showed that the percentage of antibiotics delivered within 2 hours of evaluation was improved from 66% to 85%.

Although most reports have focused on physicians as ordering providers, Kazemi and colleagues[34] specifically compared nurse order entry with physician order entry in the neonatal ward. In this system, nurses electronically entered orders that were given by physicians, and physicians verified and countersigned the orders. Prescriber warnings were still presented to physicians at the time of signature. A lower rate of nonintercepted medication errors was seen during the nurse order entry period, which the authors felt was secondary to a higher rate of prescriber compliance with electronic warnings during this period.

Few available studies have evaluated the effect of CPOE on patient harm, in part because errors resulting in harm are rare.[18] Walsh and colleagues[18] demonstrated that implementation of CPOE alone, without an electronic medication administration record or bar coding, reduced the rate of nonintercepted serious errors by just 7% in a pediatric population. There were 6 children injured by ordering errors before CPOE and 7 after. In the neonatal intensive care unit (NICU), there was no significant change in error rates, with 12.8 nonintercepted serious medication errors per 1000 patient days before CPOE and 14.7 after. Similarly, Chuo and Hicks[35] evaluated CPOE errors for NICU medications reported voluntarily to a national error-reporting program and warned that although CPOE decreased the errors that reached patients, proper implementation of CPOE systems required significant support and flawed implementation could fail quickly.

Overall, there is a sizable body of evidence that evaluates the effect of CPOE on patient outcomes and demonstrates that CPOE is effective for reducing prescription errors and wrong-time/wrong-route administration errors in neonates. There is no evidence, however, demonstrating a meaningful reduction in harm.

Clinical Decision Support

Electronic clinical decision support is a key functionality of HIT in which knowledge and patient information is presented at appropriate times to support health care decisions. CDS includes a variety of tools that assist in clinical decision-making and may reduce errors by providing access to pertinent information at the time of ordering and during pharmacist review. The literature on CDS for neonates demonstrates its use for a wide spectrum of clinical decision-making in prescribing and treatment, in transport of neonates, and in prediction of critical events. Our search identified 8 articles that used HIT for decision support.[11,13,17,32,36–39] For treatment decisions, the development of the BiliTool, an extremely popular Web-based CDS tool to support decisions regarding neonatal jaundice treatment, was described by Longhurst and colleagues.[11] In the tool, patient age and the time of bilirubin collection are manually entered, and the tool returns phototherapy recommendations based on risk. In a survey of 469 respondents regarding BiliTool, Longhurst and colleagues[11] showed high marks for usability and frequency of use, with 71% of those surveyed frequently or always consulting the hour-specific nomogram when seeing a jaundiced infant. Hum and colleagues[17] demonstrated the use of a CDS tool to improve antibiotic prescribing in a NICU. The tool aggregated select laboratory results and provided recommendations for antimicrobial selection based on algorithms that took culture results, clinical situation, and antimicrobial susceptibility patterns into account. When prescribers were surveyed, they considered the most useful features to be the summarized culture results (43%) and antibiotic recommendations (48%).

Regarding use of CDS in transport of neonates, Heermann and Thompson[36] described the STABLE Assistant (S-blood glucose, T-body temperature, A-artificial breathing, B-blood pressure, L-lab work, E-emotional support of infant and family), which is a prototype rule-based system assessing stability for transport. The user enters clinical information and receives recommendations based on STABLE guidelines for safely transporting neonates. In a simulated review of 19 clinical cases, a group of neonatologists and neonatal transport experts answered a 7-point Likert scale regarding the degree of safety and judged the STABLE Assistant to be safe.

Finally, several CDS tools used machine learning algorithms to identify critical clinical events, including sepsis, hyperammonemia, asphyxia, and glucose abnormalities.[13,32,38,39] Mani and colleagues[13] described the use of machine learning–based algorithms to predict neonatal sepsis. Nine computerized algorithms that took into account culture results, laboratory results, and specific clinical conditions were tested for sepsis prediction. The sensitivity of all algorithms and the specificity of 8 algorithms exceeded that of the physician for predicting sepsis. To expedite the treatment of hypoglycemia and hyperglycemia, Maat and colleagues[32] created CDS for calculation of glucose doses in CPOE. In an interrupted time series study, they found that there was no change in rates of hypoglycemia or hyperglycemia, but the amount of time needed to calculate doses was significantly reduced.

In summary, although there are many articles that address CDS use in neonates, many evaluate the usability, feasibility, or acceptability of the HIT interventions rather than effect on patient outcomes. The few that do evaluate patient outcomes support the use of CDS tools to identify disease, reduce variation, and optimize safe neonatal care.

Bar-Coded Medication Administration Technology

BCMA is a nurse-driven point-of-care process that uses bar-coding technology to accurately match in-hand medications with medication orders and patient identity immediately before administration. Our search yielded 5 articles on the use of BCMA technology in neonatal settings.[7,40–43] Morriss and colleagues[40–42] authored 3 articles, each focused on the effect of BCMA on different staff and medication safety outcomes. In their first article, Morriss and colleagues[41] found the risk of preventable adverse drug events was reduced by 47% after BCMA implementation. In a second article on adverse drug events, they found that infants treated with opioids in the absence of BCMA had a 10% probability of an adverse event after hospitalization for 6 days but that use of a BCMA system significantly decreased the risk of harm associated with opioid administration.[40] Last, the study team examined NICU nurses' opinions about safety, use, acceptance, and workflow effects of BCMA.[42] Most nurses reported comfort with the technology within 2 weeks and believed that the system had prevented errors, although they did believe that workarounds had occurred.

Some neonatal units have also adopted the use of a bar-coding system for breast milk administration.[7,43] Steele and Bixby[43] studied the effects of bar coding on breast milk administration errors. Within the first 6 months, total breast milk errors dropped from a baseline of 45 to 4. Bar coding assisted with identification and prevention of near-miss attempts to feed the wrong milk to the wrong infant (n = 55) and to administer expired breast milk (n = 127). In total, the literature suggests a beneficial role for BCMA in reducing errors associated with the administration of neonatal medications and fluids, but there is only a small number of existing studies evaluating patient outcomes.

Smart Pumps

Smart pumps are infusion pumps that contain a population-specific drug library with defined limits for medication and fluid administration. We identified only 1 article describing the use of smart pumps for intravenous drug and fluid infusion in neonatal settings. Bergon-Sendin and colleagues[44] reported on the use of random safety audits to evaluate appropriate use of infusion pump systems before and after QI interventions. Over a 2-year period, appropriate smart pump programming increased from 0% to 73%. Despite this progress, multiple safety risks persisted during and after the intervention phase: only 46% of infusions had the drug names recorded in the pump and in 2.5% of cases, there was an attempt to exceed the absolute dosing limit, particularly for administration of fentanyl and midazolam. Although the investigators did not measure direct harm to patients as a result of these risks, the results suggest that smart pumps, which prevent attempts to exceed maximum dosing limits, may be able to prevent dosing and administration errors if used appropriately every time. Although the evidence from this single study is promising, the use of smart pumps has increased dramatically without evidence that this HIT intervention prevents harm.

Telemedicine

Telemedicine is defined as the use of IT to provide remote evaluation, diagnosis, and treatment of patients. Transmission of audio, visual, and electronic data can be used to facilitate assessment of neonates at a distance, improving patient safety by enhancing accurate diagnosis, standardizing care, and increasing early recognition of clinical deterioration or critical events. Telemedicine may help to mitigate such events while also preventing unnecessary transport of neonates. Telemedicine has previously been used to support physician-to-physician consultation, but its application has grown as telecommunication systems have improved. Using telemedicine technology, Garingo and colleagues[45] demonstrated no significant differences in care or outcomes between patients cared for by on-site or off-site neonatologists, including no differences in length of stay, age at discharge, hospital charges, number of tests or consults, or days of TPN, respiratory support, antibiotics, or phototherapy. There was a small but statistically significant difference in the amount of time spent on encounters (5 minutes for controls vs 8 minutes for telemedicine). Several other reports described the architecture needed to provide telemedicine support that allows a neonate to receive specialty evaluation yet remain at their birth facility.[45–48] Minton and colleagues[48] described the development of remotely monitored neonatal resuscitation beds to provide feedback during active neonatal resuscitations as a way to provide expertise in resource-limited or rural areas. Overall, there are few studies on neonatal telemedicine, and much of the literature focuses on feasibility of use and architecture needs rather than patient outcomes (eg, the number of patients remaining safely at their birth hospital). Although the use of telemedicine appears promising for the provision of remote care in a number of different clinical scenarios, the effect of its use on neonatal outcomes has not been well studied.

Family Communication

There were multiple articles that described and evaluated patient-facing and family-facing HIT. The types of interventions included here are technologies to inform parents about neonatal care, to support decisions, and to allow parents to video monitor their child remotely. Taylor and El-Kafrawy[49] developed a novel audiovisual computerized intervention to improve NICU visitors' adherence to hand hygiene and infection-control procedures. The intervention was a continuously running instructional video about hand washing supplemented by an audio announcement that ran whenever the NICU doorbell rang. Visitor compliance with correct hand-washing technique improved from 19 (79%) of 24 visitors before intervention to 58 (100%) of 58 visitors after the HIT implementation ($P<.0016$). In another example of family-facing HIT, Weyand and colleagues[50] described usability testing of a decision support tool for parents of patients in the NICU. The computerized tool was designed to augment discussions with clinical staff and inform parents regarding ethically challenging situations in the NICU. In a study by Gray and colleagues,[12] an Internet-based videoconferencing system called Baby CareLink, designed for parents at home to have virtual house calls, distance monitoring, and virtual learning, was associated with significant improvements in parent satisfaction with care.[51] Another study of Baby CareLink found that both rural and inner-city Medicaid families used the system, demonstrating that families were interested in technology solutions and able to access them in multiple environments.[52] In summary, the few studies on family communication assess heterogenous HIT interventions, and most studies assess HIT usability and acceptability rather than effects on patient outcomes.

Error Detection and Adverse Event Detection

Several studies used HIT to detect and analyze adverse events in neonates, using electronic algorithms to identify medication errors as well as trigger tools to detect adverse events.[9,53,54] Li and colleagues[53] developed computerized algorithms to detect intravenous infiltrates and narcotic overdoses and found that the algorithm identified more of these events than both trigger tools and incident reporting. In a second study, Li and colleagues[9] developed novel computerized algorithms to detect medication administration errors in the NICU. Compared with incident reporting, the algorithms had improved sensitivity (5% vs 82%) and precision (50% vs 70%). Dickerman and colleagues[54] used EHR-based algorithms to detect hypoglycemia in children. Of 198 adverse events detected, 62% occurred in the NICU. Few in number, these studies all assess the ability to detect, but not prevent, errors and adverse events. This small body of literature demonstrates the ability of computerized algorithms to identify adverse patient events but does not assess the effect of identification on patient harm.

Improved Monitoring and Care Processes in the Neonatal Intensive Care Unit

New IT development was most apparent in publications that sought ways to improve monitoring of neonatal patients or means to improve processes of care in the NICU, such as the use of early warning systems or tools to improve handoff. Burke and Downes[55] used fuzzy logic to improve the reliability of monitoring in patients undergoing physiologic monitoring for apnea and found that their system that assessed respiration, electrocardiogram, and oxygen saturation in combination was able to successfully detect all apnea scenarios in a test environment. Although the article describes the development of a novel system, the clinical impact has not been evaluated. Saria and colleagues[56] demonstrated that routinely captured physiologic data could be used to predict clinical morbidity in premature infants. They created a probability score for illness severity based on physiologic signals, including heart rate, respiratory rate, and oxygen saturation in the first 3 hours of life, in combination with gestational age and weight. Physiologic parameters that were electronically captured, such as short-term variability in respiratory and heart rates, contributed more significantly to morbidity predictions than invasive laboratory tests. Their probability score demonstrated 86% sensitivity and 96% specificity for predicting overall morbidity in preterm infants. Similarly, Griffin and colleagues[57] mathematically characterized abnormal heart rate characteristics, including reduced variability and transient decelerations in heart rate that precede late-onset sepsis, and developed a heart rate characteristic index that represents the fold-increase in risk of sepsis during the next 24 hours. A monitoring system, called the HeRO monitoring system, which obtains heart rate characteristics from the cardiac monitor and displays the heart rate characteristic index, was used in a large clinical trial in neonates which demonstrated that the mortality rate was reduced by 22% in very low birth weight infants whose heart rate characteristics were monitored.[58]

Processes for better care delivery and better communication were also enhanced by IT developments. In a test environment, Liu and colleagues[59] demonstrated the ability to reduce noise exposure by 5 to 40 dB in a neonatal isolette using an active noise control system. Given that NICU noise levels often exceed the American Academy of Pediatrics recommended noise levels of less than 45 dB, small noise reductions may be significant.[60] Others have shown the ability of HIT to improve neonatal care through improvements in communication, including the use of digital crumbs, the detailed audit trail left by care providers in the EHR, to identify the care team and understand how team structure influences patient/family satisfaction[61] and the use of an EHR-integrated handoff tool to improve handoff accuracy and provider workflow and efficiency.[62] Integration of the handoff tool into the EHR decreased the percentage of total handoff preparation time dedicated to transcribing data from the EHR from 25% to 49% to less than 25% after implementation (P = .0006).

Overall, there are only a few studies assessing the effect of HIT on care processes, and the studies assess different HIT interventions and outcomes. Because most of these HIT interventions are newly developed, the studies primarily assess their feasibility and acceptability, and with the exception of the heart rate characteristic index, have not been studied in terms of their effects on patient outcomes.

QUALITY IMPROVEMENT AND HEALTH INFORMATION TECHNOLOGY IMPLEMENTATION

QI projects designed to improve outcomes and processes of care for neonates frequently include HIT interventions as one of the many interventions that are tested and implemented. For example, in a QI effort to decrease breast milk administration errors, Dougherty and Nash[7] implemented an HIT solution to improve their feeding-management processes. Following use of a Failure Modes and Effects Analysis tool to examine their system, the decision was made to implement a bar-coding system to identify patients for appropriate breast milk administration as a final step in their improvement program. Use of the system ultimately decreased the number of errors from 3% to 0.4% of breast milk administrations.

In a similar effort to improve the safety of breast milk administration, Luton and colleagues[8] used a QI approach incorporating elements from the Model for Improvement, Lean, and Six Sigma methodologies, along with principles of high reliability organizations, to drive their improvement strategies. Among many interventions that were tested and adopted, they identified variation in their electronic ordering as a significant contributor to errors and waste, especially when free text was used in CPOE orders. As part of their interventions, orders were simplified and clarified through the use of discrete data fields and defined prepopulated selections. Over a 12-month period, the NICU achieved an 83% reduction in breast milk administration errors.

In another example using CPOE as part of a QI intervention, Bissinger and colleagues[31] used QI techniques to reduce the time from decision to evaluate for sepsis to administration of antibiotics to less than 2 hours. Several CPOE interventions were implemented, including automated weight-based calculations for antibiotics, automatic STAT orders for antibiotics, and the use of standardized sepsis order sets. The number of patients receiving antibiotics in less than 2 hours increased from 45% to 85% (P<.001).

In addition to using HIT interventions as change strategies to improve processes and outcomes, QI approaches also may be useful to facilitate the appropriate implementation of HIT interventions. For example, Bergon-Sendin and colleagues[44] used random safety audits as part of a QI effort to improve the appropriate use of smart pumps in the NICU. Interventions directed at increasing the appropriate use of smart pumps included adoption of a new drug library, utilization of relative and absolute drug infusion rate limits, and development of a detailed protocol for pump programming. Following testing of interventions, the frequency of appropriate NICU smart pump use significantly increased from 0% (0/52) to 73% (117/160) of infusions (P<.0001).

DISCUSSION

HIT interventions are increasingly used in the provision of neonatal care (**Fig. 1**). Technology development for neonatology started with tools that implemented practical rule-based algorithms. Due to the rudimentary infrastructure of EHRs, the early algorithms used limited resources and patient information to support simple clinical tasks, such as oxygen saturation monitoring,[63] transport safety monitoring,[36] and dosage calculation.[10,22,28] More recently, the adoption of EHRs across the nation has grown as a result of the enactment of the American Recovery and Reinvestment Act of 2009. The rapid adoption has resulted in advances in EHR infrastructure and access to more granular information, such as physiologic signals,[39,56] laboratory and microbiology results,[13] and physician assessments.[9] As the EHR has advanced, so have HIT applications (see **Fig. 1**). In the past 10 years, advanced technologies, including signal processing,[39,59] machine learning,[13,56] and natural language processing,[53] have been leveraged to analyze the data and facilitate application development. Recent applications have gone beyond traditional logic-rules and started exploiting bigger data to generate new clinical knowledge. Nevertheless, at the time of our literature search, many of these technologies are still in their development stage and are being tested on retrospective data or through simulation.[9,13,53,59] However, compared with the estimated 17-year delay for research evidence to be implemented into clinical practice,[64] the rapid evolution of IT technologies results in a much shorter time lag between research and production.[65] As such, we anticipate that a large volume of HIT applications will emerge and be integrated into clinical practice in the next few years.

With the potential explosion of HIT applications in clinical practice over the next few years, we must keep in mind that the introduction of new technologies can introduce new safety challenges. In fact, studies in the adult and pediatric populations, including those reviewed here, have demonstrated some of these safety concerns.[18–20] Those looking to implement HIT interventions in neonatal populations should keep in mind that safety risks may be different in the NICU compared with other environments, and new interventions must be thoughtfully implemented and tested before integrating

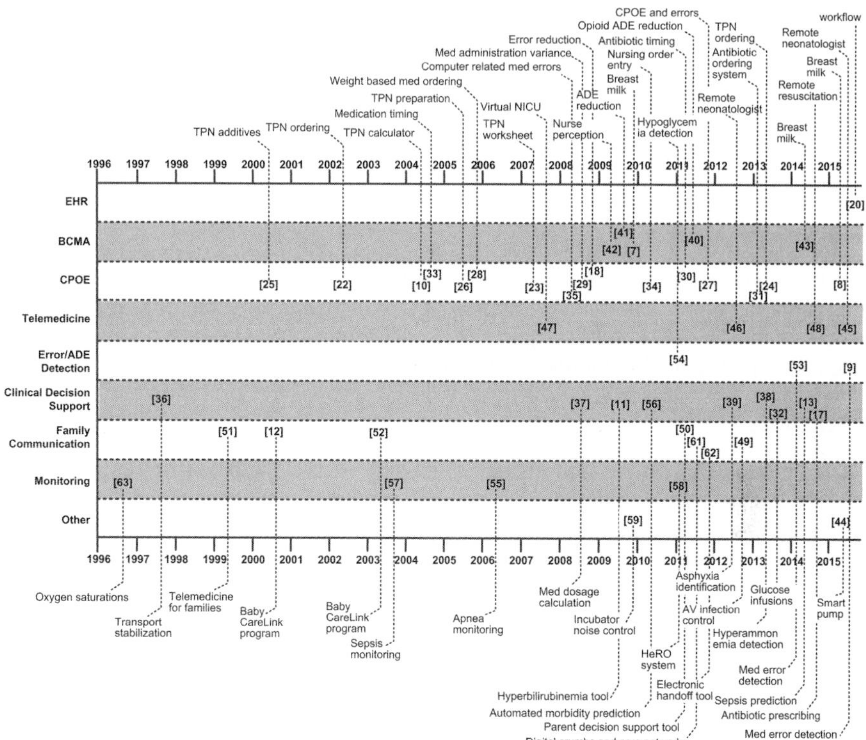

Fig. 1. Major publications reviewed in the study. Study publications are listed by publication year, research category, and reference number, with the main contribution of the publication described. ADE, adverse drug event.

into clinical workflow.[35] Only a few HIT interventions, like CPOE, have been well tested for the neonatal population. QI methodology appears to be one way to facilitate meaningful testing and implementation of HIT interventions.

The current literature on HIT interventions in neonatal care suffers from several weaknesses. Current studies focus on single-center interventions, with limited applicability beyond the initial site. Most published studies focus on the application of the HIT intervention rather than the effect on patient outcomes. Many studies evaluate error reduction based on an HIT intervention, but fail to assess the effect on patient harm. We found that there was a paucity of outcomes data about the impact of some interventions, such as electronic medication administration records and smart pumps in the neonatal population, although these interventions are used widely in practice. Finally, current evidence focuses on the phase of medication prescription/ordering, and no studies evaluate the full medication cycle from prescription to administration in neonates.

Through literature review, we identified 4 qualities that we believe characterize a successful technology-based intervention. First, the HIT intervention solves a critical clinical need. Two examples are clinical decision supports for parenteral nutrition calculations and jaundice treatment decisions.[10,11] Without CDS technologies, these decisions are complex and error-prone. Second, the HIT intervention leverages unique IT capabilities, for example by performing complex calculations or by connecting people who are at a distance. In the example of Baby CareLink, technology links distant parents to their infants. Third, the impact of the technology can be rigorously evaluated, including both its benefits and risks. Finally, the HIT intervention can be easily generalized and spread. The final characteristic is true of the BiliTool intervention, but not of the several different parenteral nutrition calculators. We found 6 different TPN calculators in the reviewed articles, indicating a need for this intervention but a failure of these interventions to spread outside of local application. On the other hand, the BiliTool intervention has been widely used because of its clinical utility and ease of access and use.[11]

Ultimately, technology, when adequately tested and appropriately implemented, has the potential to help us optimize care to this vulnerable pediatric population. Although new interventions are emerging, gaps in evaluation of impact remain. This review identifies some of these gaps and can inform future studies and strategies to safely implement HIT interventions in neonatal care.

REFERENCES

1. Institute of Medicine, Committee on Quality Health Care in America. Kohn LT, Corrigan JM, Donaldson MS, editors. To err is human: building a safer health system. Washington, DC: National Academy Press; 2000.
2. Institute of Medicine, Committee on Quality Health Care in America. Crossing the quality chasm—a new health system for the 21st century. Washington, DC: National Academy Press; 2001.
3. Kaushal R, Bates D, Landrigan C, et al. Medication errors and adverse drug events in pediatric inpatients. JAMA 2001;285(16):2114–20.
4. Miller MR, Griswold M, Harris JM 2nd, et al. Decreasing PICU catheter-associated bloodstream infections: NACHRI's quality transformation efforts. Pediatrics 2010;125(2):206–13.
5. Gray JE, Goldmann DA. Medication errors in the neonatal intensive care unit: special patients, unique issues. Arch Dis Child Fetal Neonatal Ed 2004;89(6):F472–3.
6. Gray JE, Suresh G, Ursprung R, et al. Patient misidentification in the neonatal intensive care unit: quantification of risk. Pediatrics 2006;117(1):e43–7.
7. Dougherty D, Nash A. Bar coding from breast to baby: a comprehensive breast milk management system for the NICU. Neonatal Netw 2009;28(5):321–8.
8. Luton A, Bondurant PG, Campbell A, et al. Got (the right) milk? How a blended quality improvement approach catalyzed change. Adv Neonatal Care 2015;15(5):345–53.
9. Li Q, Kirkendall ES, Hall ES, et al. Automated detection of medication administration errors in neonatal intensive care. J Biomed Inform 2015;57:124–33.
10. Lehmann CU, Conner KG, Cox JM. Preventing provider errors: online total parenteral nutrition calculator. Pediatrics 2004;113(4 I):748–53.
11. Longhurst C, Turner S, Burgos AE. Development of a Web-based decision support tool to increase use of neonatal hyperbilirubinemia guidelines. Jt Comm J Qual Patient Saf 2009;35(5):256–62.
12. Gray JE, Safran C, Davis RB, et al. Baby CareLink: using the Internet and telemedicine to improve care for high-risk infants. Pediatrics 2000;106(6):1318–24.
13. Mani S, Ozdas A, Aliferis C, et al. Medical decision support using machine learning for early detection of late-onset neonatal sepsis. J Am Med Inform Assoc 2014;21(2):326–36.
14. Bates DW, Teich JM, Lee J, et al. The impact of computerized physician order entry on medication error prevention. J Am Med Inform Assoc 1999;6(4):313–21.

15. Potts AL, Frederick EB, Gregory DF, et al. Computerized physician order entry and medication errors in a pediatric critical care unit. Pediatrics 2004;113(1):59–63.
16. Stockwell MS, Fiks AG. Utilizing health information technology to improve vaccine communication and coverage. Hum Vaccin Immunother 2013;9(8):1802–11.
17. Hum RS, Cato K, Sheehan B, et al. Developing clinical decision support within a commercial electronic health record system to improve antimicrobial prescribing in the neonatal ICU. Appl Clin Inform 2014;5(2):368–87.
18. Walsh KE, Landrigan CP, Adams WG, et al. Effect of computer order entry on prevention of serious medication errors in hospitalized children. Pediatrics 2008;121(3):e421–7.
19. Koppel R, Metlay JP, Cohen A, et al. Role of computerized physician order entry systems in facilitating medication errors. JAMA 2005;293(10):1197–203.
20. Carayon P, Wetterneck TB, Alyousef B, et al. Impact of electronic health record technology on the work and workflow of physicians in the intensive care unit. Int J Med Inform 2015;84(8):578–94.
21. Harvey G, Kitson A. PARIHS revisited: from heuristic to integrated framework for the successful implementation of knowledge into practice. Implement Sci 2016;11:33.
22. Lehmann CU, Conner KG, Cox JM. Provider error prevention: online total parenteral nutrition calculator. Proc AMIA Symp 2002;435–9.
23. Brown CL, Garrison NA, Hutchison AA. Error reduction when prescribing neonatal parenteral nutrition. Am J Perinatol 2007;24(7):417–27.
24. Huston RK, Markell AM, McCulley EA, et al. Computer programming: quality and safety for neonatal parenteral nutrition orders. Nutr Clin Pract 2013;28(4):515–21.
25. Peverini RL, Beach DS, Wan KW, et al. Graphical user interface for a neonatal parenteral nutrition decision support system. Proc AMIA Symp 2000;650–4.
26. Skouroliakou M, Konstantinou D, Papasarantopoulos P, et al. Computer assisted total parenteral nutrition for pre-term and sick term neonates. Pharm World Sci 2005;27(4):305–10.
27. Kazemi A, Ellenius J, Pourasghar F, et al. The effect of computerized physician order entry and decision support system on medication errors in the neonatal ward: experiences from an Iranian teaching hospital. J Med Syst 2011;35(1):25–37.
28. Giannone G. Computer-supported weight-based drug infusion concentrations in the neonatal intensive care unit. Comput Inform Nurs 2005;23(2):100–5.
29. Taylor JA, Loan LA, Kamara J, et al. Medication administration variances before and after implementation of computerized physician order entry in a neonatal intensive care unit. Pediatrics 2008;121(1):123–8.
30. Chapman AK, Lehmann CU, Donohue PK, et al. Implementation of computerized provider order entry in a neonatal intensive care unit: impact on admission workflow. Int J Med Inform 2012;81(5):291–5.
31. Bissinger RL, Mueller M, Cox TH, et al. Antibiotic timing in neonates with suspected hospital-acquired infections. Adv Neonatal Care 2013;13(1):22–8.
32. Maat B, Rademaker CM, Oostveen MI, et al. The effect of a computerized prescribing and calculating system on hypo- and hyperglycemias and on prescribing time efficiency in neonatal intensive care patients. JPEN J Parenter Enteral Nutr 2013;37(1):85–91.
33. Cordero L, Kuehn L, Kumar RR, et al. Impact of computerized physician order entry on clinical practice in a newborn intensive care unit. J Perinatol 2004;24(2):88–93.

34. Kazemi A, Fors UG, Tofighi S, et al. Physician order entry or nurse order entry? Comparison of two implementation strategies for a computerized order entry system aimed at reducing dosing medication errors. J Med Internet Res 2010; 12(1):e5.
35. Chuo J, Hicks RW. Computer-related medication errors in neonatal intensive care units. Clin Perinatol 2008;35(1):119–39.
36. Heermann LK, Thompson CB. Prototype expert system to assist with the stabilization of neonates prior to transport. Proc AMIA Annu Fall Symp 1997;213–7.
37. Pallás CR, De-La-Cruz J, Del-Moral MT, et al. Improving the quality of medical prescriptions in neonatal units. Neonatology 2008;93(4):251–6.
38. Vergano SA, Crossette JM, Cusick FC, et al. Improving surveillance for hyperammonemia in the newborn. Mol Genet Metab 2013;110(1–2):102–5.
39. Zabidi A, Khuan LY, Mansor W. Asphyxia screening kit. Conf Proc IEEE Eng Med Biol Soc 2012;2012:1298–301.
40. Morriss FH Jr, Abramowitz PW, Nelson SP, et al. Risk of adverse drug events in neonates treated with opioids and the effect of a bar-code-assisted medication administration system. Am J Health Syst Pharm 2011;68(1):57–62.
41. Morriss FH Jr, Abramowitz PW, Nelson SP, et al. Effectiveness of a barcode medication administration system in reducing preventable adverse drug events in a neonatal intensive care unit: a prospective cohort study. J Pediatr 2009;154(3): 363–8, 368.e1.
42. Morriss FH Jr, Abramowitz PW, Carmen L, et al. "Nurses Don't Hate Change"–survey of nurses in a neonatal intensive care unit regarding the implementation, use and effectiveness of a bar code medication administration system. Healthc Q 2009;12 Spec No Patient:135–40.
43. Steele C, Bixby C. Centralized breastmilk handling and bar code scanning improve safety and reduce breastmilk administration errors. Breastfeed Med 2014;9(9):426–9.
44. Bergon-Sendin E, Perez-Grande C, Lora-Pablos D, et al. Smart pumps and random safety audits in a neonatal intensive care unit: a new challenge for patient safety. BMC Pediatr 2015;15:206.
45. Garingo A, Friedlich P, Chavez T, et al. "Tele-rounding" with a remotely controlled mobile robot in the neonatal intensive care unit. J Telemed Telecare 2016;22(2): 132–8.
46. Garingo A, Friedlich P, Tesoriero L, et al. The use of mobile robotic telemedicine technology in the neonatal intensive care unit. J Perinatol 2012;32(1):55–63.
47. McGregor C, Kneale B, Tracy M. On-demand virtual neonatal intensive care units supporting rural, remote and urban healthcare with bush babies broadband. J Netw Comput Appl 2007;30(4):1309–23.
48. Minton S, Allan M, Valdes W. Teleneonatology: a major tool for the future. Pediatr Ann 2014;43(2):e50–5.
49. Taylor RJ, El-Kafrawy U. A simple inexpensive audio-visual reminder of infection control procedures on entry to a neonatal intensive care unit. J Hosp Infect 2012; 82(3):203–6.
50. Weyand SA, Frize M, Bariciak E, et al. Development and usability testing of a parent decision support tool for the neonatal intensive care unit. Conf Proc IEEE Eng Med Biol Soc 2011;2011:6430–3.
51. Phillips M. Telemedicine in the neonatal intensive care unit. Pediatr Nurs 1999; 25(2):185–6, 189.
52. Safran C. The collaborative edge: patient empowerment for vulnerable populations. Int J Med Inform 2003;69(2–3):185–90.

53. Li Q, Melton K, Lingren T, et al. Phenotyping for patient safety: algorithm development for electronic health record based automated adverse event and medical error detection in neonatal intensive care. J Am Med Inform Assoc 2014;21(5):776–84.
54. Dickerman MJ, Jacobs BR, Vinodrao H, et al. Recognizing hypoglycemia in children through automated adverse-event detection. Pediatrics 2011;127(4):e1035–41.
55. Burke MJ, Downes R. A fuzzy logic based apnoea monitor for SIDS risk infants. J Med Eng Technol 2006;30(6):397–411.
56. Saria S, Rajani AK, Gould J, et al. Integration of early physiological responses predicts later illness severity in preterm infants. Sci Transl Med 2010;2(48):48ra65.
57. Griffin MP, O'Shea TM, Bissonette EA, et al. Abnormal heart rate characteristics preceding neonatal sepsis and sepsis-like illness. Pediatr Res 2003;53(6):920–6.
58. Moorman JR, Carlo WA, Kattwinkel J, et al. Mortality reduction by heart rate characteristic monitoring in very low birth weight neonates: a randomized trial. J Pediatr 2011;159(6):900–6.e1.
59. Liu L, Gujjula S, Kuo SM. Multi-channel real time active noise control system for infant incubators. Conf Proc IEEE Eng Med Biol Soc 2009;2009:935–8.
60. Lasky RE, Williams AL. Noise and light exposures for extremely low birth weight newborns during their stay in the neonatal intensive care unit. Pediatrics 2009;123(2):540–6.
61. Gray JE, Feldman H, Reti S, et al. Using Digital Crumbs from an Electronic Health Record to identify, study and improve health care teams. AMIA Annu Symp Proc 2011;2011:491–500.
62. Palma JP, Sharek PJ, Longhurst CA. Impact of electronic medical record integration of a handoff tool on sign-out in a newborn intensive care unit. J Perinatol 2011;31(5):311–7.
63. Wolf M, Keel M, von Siebenthal K, et al. Improved monitoring of preterm infants by fuzzy logic. Technol Health Care 1996;4(2):193–201.
64. Morris ZS, Wooding S, Grant J. The answer is 17 years, what is the question: understanding time lags in translational research. J R Soc Med 2011;104(12):510–20.
65. Office of Technology Assessment, Congressional Board of the 99th U.S. Congress. Information Technology R&D: critical trends and issues. February 1985; Available at: http://files.eric.ed.gov/fulltext/ED261643.pdf. Accessed March 9, 2016.

APPENDIX 1: SEARCH STRATEGY

An article should contain at least 1 of the key words for each category.

- *Health IT*: "EHR", "electronic medical record", "information system", "medical order entry systems", "medical records system", "computerized", "medical record system", "decision support system", "biomedical", "clinical informatics", "user-computer", "user computer", "pharmacy information system", "computer-assisted", "computer assisted", "algorithm".
- *Patient safety*: "medical error", "quality of health care", "health care quality", "safety management", "quality improve", "quality assurance", "health care", "patient safety", "error prevention", "error control".
- *Neonatology*: "neonatal", "intensive care", "infant", "newborn", "neonatal nursing", "neonatology", "neonate", "neonatology", "NICU".

Improving Value in Neonatal Intensive Care

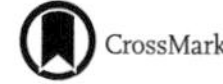

Timmy Ho, MD, MPH[a,*], John A.F. Zupancic, MD, ScD[a], DeWayne M. Pursley, MD, MPH[a], Dmitry Dukhovny, MD, MPH[b]

KEYWORDS

• Quality improvement • Value • Value equation • Costs • Outcomes • Neonatology

KEY POINTS

- Increasing value using quality improvement methods is fundamental to improving the US health care system.
- Quality improvement teams can improve value by either improving outcomes or reducing costs, but measuring both is essential.
- Value-based improvement is challenging for multiple reasons, including the investment of time and effort in producing sustainable change and the lack of training of health care providers.

Health care costs in the United States continue to rise.[1] Press coverage of rising health care premiums[2] and monopoly-driven precipitous price increases for medications, such as insulin, epinephrine autoinjectors, and naloxone,[3] persist. Although adult medicine, especially in the last year of life,[4] continues to consume most health care spending, newborn care comprises a major portion of health care costs in pediatrics.[5] It is estimated that in 2013, out of $233.5 billion spent on children's personal health

---

Financial Disclosure: Drs T. Ho, J.A.F. Zupancic, D.W.M. Pursley, and D. Dukhovny have received honoraria for faculty participation from Vermont Oxford Network.
Conflict of Interest: The authors have no commercial or financial conflicts of interest.
Funding Source: No funding was secured for this study.
Contributor's Statement: Dr T. Ho conceptualized and designed the work, drafted the initial article, and approved the final article as submitted. Dr J.A.F. Zupancic conceptualized and designed the work and approved the final article as submitted. Dr D.W.M. Pursley conceptualized and designed the work and approved the final article as submitted. Dr D. Dukhovny conceptualized and designed the work and approved the final article as submitted.
[a] Department of Neonatology, Beth Israel Deaconess Medical Center, Harvard Medical School, 330 Brookline Avenue, Boston, MA 02215, USA; [b] Department of Pediatrics, Oregon Health & Science University, Mail Code CRDC-P, 707 Southwest Gaines Street, Portland, OR 97239, USA
* Corresponding author. Department of Neonatology, Beth Israel Deaconess Medical Center, 330 Brookline Avenue, Boston, MA, 02215.
E-mail address: tho2@bidmc.harvard.edu

Clin Perinatol 44 (2017) 617–625
http://dx.doi.org/10.1016/j.clp.2017.05.009

care, the category of "well-newborn care," with $27.9 billion, was the single largest category of health care spending.[6]

Quality improvement in neonatal care has grown from its humble beginnings in single units to health care system–level quality collaboratives that improve care for thousands of infants.[7] Despite much effort to improve patient outcomes, however, there remain many opportunities to improve value in the care delivered to neonatal intensive care unit (NICU) patients. Quality improvement that focuses solely on clinical outcomes is no longer enough. Improvement efforts instead must reframe goals and aims to incorporate both outcomes and costs to add value to the care provided to infants and their families.

Many regulatory bodies now require some level of proficiency in quality improvement. In residency and fellowship training, the Accreditation Council for Graduate Medical Education requires programs to have a component of education around quality improvement.[8] In its Part 4 Maintenance of Certification requirements, Improving Professional Practice, the American Board of Pediatrics requires pediatricians to demonstrate competence in systematic measurement and improvement in patient care in a range of American Board of Pediatrics–approved quality improvement projects designed to assess and improve the quality of patient care.[9] Despite these recent training requirements, there are many clinicians who have never received any formal quality improvement training. Furthermore, lack of formal training in either quality improvement or basic health care economics make it intimidating for providers to achieve the challenge of practicing value-added care. Thus, for hospital-based care, leadership should be willing to properly invest in staff training and time to do the work, perhaps reinvesting some of the savings that result from quality improvement efforts back into quality programs.

In this review article, we start by defining value, introducing concepts described by Porter[10] and case examples of the use of the value equation in neonatology described by Dukhovny and colleagues.[11] We examine the integration of value in quality improvement and its relationship to the Institute of Healthcare Improvement Triple Aim.[12] We then present a review of the value literature in neonatology, with special emphasis on how quality improvement has led to change in value. Additionally, we discuss ways of adding value to quality improvement projects and then elaborate on the various perspectives (patient, NICU, and health care system–level) of quality improvement work and the relevant value-based measures for each of those viewpoints. Lastly, we break down the steps of adding value-based quality improvement components (charters, aims, and measures) to new or existing quality work.

DEFINITION OF VALUE

In a 2010 Porter[10] described a landscape in health care where conflicting goals and competing interests have resulted in lack of a shared vision and in an inability to improve performance. He defines value as "the health outcomes achieved per dollar spent" and argues that value ought to be the common goal in performance improvement. In the value equation, health outcomes achieved would thus be the numerator, and dollars spent the denominator.

Both Porter[10] and Dukhovny and colleagues[11] elaborate on the numerator, and the denominator within the value equation, but diverge with regard to specifics. With regards to the numerator, after acknowledging that value is difficult to measure and often misunderstood, Porter[10] argues that health outcomes should not be measured in terms of processes of care, that process measures are not substitutes for measuring actual clinical outcomes specific to particular diseases and conditions.

This view can make the inclusion of value-based measures within quality improvement difficult, because successful quality improvement initiatives often operate in the short term and focus on process measures as clinical outcome measures change more slowly. Dukhovny and colleagues[11] recognize this balance, and allow for several sources of outcomes, including "clinical stud[ies], process and outcome measures reported in ... institutions over time or in interinstitutional comparisons, [and] other markers of quality and safety." This broader view of outcomes allows for more practical inclusions of value-based measures in quality improvement work.

The denominator in the value equation in neonatology may go beyond direct medical costs, which include the dollar costs of equipment, procedures, medications, and health care provider time in person-hours. It also includes direct nonmedical costs not directly related to health care, such as travel to and from the hospital and additional child care necessary for other kids in the family, and loss of present and future productivity from missed work, for the family and eventually the patient.[11] More efficient use of resources, and thus waste reduction, increases value by directly decreasing the denominator.

THE ROLE OF VALUE IN QUALITY IMPROVEMENT

Even before Porter[10] explored value as it exists with respect to health care, one could already see glimpses of value objectives in performance improvement. Two years prior, in 2008, researchers at the Institute of Healthcare Improvement first introduced the Triple Aim, the idea that improvement initiatives must "pursue a broader system of linked goals... [called] the Triple Aim: improving the individual experience of care, improving the health of populations, and reducing the per capita costs of care for populations." All three arms of the Triple Aim should sound familiar to the reader, because the first two comprise the numerator, and the last represents the denominator of the value equation.[12]

Quality improvement remains one of the key methods for individual providers or units to improve the health outcomes and decrease care costs for their patients and families in a scientifically rigorous manner. Quality improvement may directly address outcomes through the application of evidence-based medicine. Similarly, quality goals may focus on cost reduction. Although these approaches may increase value, it is critical to consider outcomes and cost simultaneously because changes may result in unintended consequences and therefore require consideration of balancing measures.

Despite considerable evidence that quality improvement adds value by either improving outcomes or decreasing costs, a common misconception among health care providers is that adding value requires cost reduction. Borrowing ideas from comparative effectiveness research, adding value comes not only from reducing costs, but also from a more efficient allocation of resources for the best possible outcome, that is, the "biggest bang for the buck." Improving outcomes may, in fact, require additional expenditure, where those fiscal resources may have previously been spent in a less efficient manner.[11]

REVIEW OF THE LITERATURE ON VALUE IN NEONATOLOGY

Researchers in newborn medicine have been examining elements of outcomes, costs, and value since well before either the Triple Aim or value were described in the literature. Beginning nearly 20 years ago, Rogowski[13] described costs in neonatal medicine among a nationally representative sample of 25 hospitals with NICUs, including more than 3000 very low birth weight infants. Even then, the author concluded that "neonatal intensive care costs are high... [but] quality improvement efforts may increase or decrease costs... [and]... given the high cost of these stays, improvements in patient outcomes that [result in less] time spent in the NICU have the potential for significant cost savings."

Over the subsequent 5 years, Rogowski and Horbar compiled a compendium of publications that described value in one form or another. In 2001, a pair of publications shows that "multidisciplinary collaborative quality improvement has the potential to improve the outcomes of neonatal intensive care" within the Vermont Oxford Network (VON), a large, international network of NICUs,[14] and that cost savings were achievable and sustainable through collaborative quality improvement efforts when compared with controls.[15] Since then, VON has continued to use collaborative quality improvement to increase value. Through the use of intensive "home-rooms" targeting specific neonatal outcomes (eg, necrotizing enterocolitis, bronchopulmonary dysplasia, interventricular hemorrhage) and broader, Internet-based Neonatal Intensive Care Quality Collaborative (iNICQ) programs, VON has helped guide multidisciplinary teams of physicians, nurse practitioners, nurses, and parent advocates in their work together to improve outcomes and decrease costs across multiple domains in neonatal care.[11,16] The past focus of iNICQ topics has included respiratory management of the infant, neonatal abstinence syndrome (NAS),[17] alarm safety, and antibiotic stewardship. Other health care organizations, including the MEDNAX group, formerly Pediatrix, have also sought to define and increase value through quality improvement.[18]

An additional area of focus in health care has been in incorporating the patient as an educated consumer. Using this approach, the Choosing Wisely campaign arose from the American Board of Internal Medicine foundation, prompting professional organizations to develop top five lists of tests and treatments that physicians and patients should question. The American Academy of Pediatrics Section on Neonatal Perinatal Medicine developed its own top five list that addressed routine use of anti-reflux medications, antibiotic therapy beyond 48 hours without evidence of bacterial infection, pneumograms, daily chest radiographs for intubated patients, and term-equivalent brain MRIs.[19] The impact of this work on health care costs is still under investigation. However, the second item on the list, routine continuation of antibiotic therapy beyond 48 hours for asymptomatic infants without evidence of bacterial infection, has led to a unique partnership between the Centers for Disease Control and Prevention and VON to provide education in antibiotic stewardship. That collaboration has led to the most recent VON iNICQ, Choosing Antibiotics Wisely, in which more than 140 teams are participating to improve antibiotic stewardship.[20]

EXAMPLES OF VALUE-BASED MEASURES IN PUBLISHED QUALITY IMPROVEMENT

Since 2012 when *Pediatrics* first started publishing quality reports under a dedicated section, more than 20% (28 out of 136) of these articles describe improvement work in newborn care. Only 8 out of 136 reports incorporate value-based measures, with examples including total medical cost[21,22] and length of stay.[23–25] Hall and colleagues[21] published the first value-based quality report in *Pediatrics* that discussed cost savings with improvement efforts aimed at reducing the blood culture contamination rate. They found that the introduction of a standardized sterile collection process resulted in a greater than 50% reduction in blood culture contamination and an annual reduction in hospital charges of approximately $250,000. More recently, Holmes and colleagues[26] described a standardized approach to patients with NAS that resulted in less pharmacologic management, and a reduction of costs and length of stay. A separate quality report from a pediatric cardiovascular intensive care unit incorporated the use of a daily rounding checklist and computer order entry, resulting in decreased laboratory use and cost without a change in mortality or length of stay.[22]

Length of stay is a unique value measure because it represents costs that are incurred directly. Unnecessarily long hospitalizations (ie, prolonged length of stay) may also divert attention, resources, and care from other patients with greater needs. Such a measure has been considered part of a composite index of neonatal quality of care, but it was not selected as one of the final nine components in an expert consensus process.[27] Other attempts at systematically including value as an aggregate measure of quality have been undertaken but have been methodologically challenging.[28] One must be cautious in using the length of stay as a sole metric without appropriate balancing measures (eg, readmission rate), especially in health systems where the NICU and the postdischarge health care environment are distinct, and there are no repercussions for gaining through early discharge without considering readmission. Additionally, the length of stay measure is complicated by its relationship to revenue for some hospitals and providers. Nonetheless, the value of decreasing length of stay is substantial, especially when the impact on the family from prolonged hospitalization is considered.

THREE QUALITY IMPROVEMENT PERSPECTIVES

Quality improvement may be evaluated from different perspectives within a health care system. Analyses can reflect the viewpoint of the patient population (eg, very low birthweight infants, infants with NAS, infants at risk for chronic lung disease), the clinical unit (eg, mother-baby unit [MBU], NICU, hospital), or an entire system (eg, managed care organizations, regional or state quality collaboratives, accountable care organizations). For example, let us examine a quality improvement project seeking to decrease antibiotic overuse from three different perspectives. From the patient perspective, adherence to guidelines about antibiotic use ensures that only at-risk infants receive antibiotics. From the unit perspective, adherence to those same guidelines may lead to more consistent care between ordering providers and higher satisfaction rates among nurses, whereas from the system perspective, decreased antibiotic overuse reduces the incidence of antibiotic-resistant organisms in the community.

Sometimes, goals at different perspectives can work against each other, especially when incentives are misaligned. For example, consider the clinical practice of admitting infants undergoing sepsis rule outs on antibiotics to the NICU and a potential practice change of keeping those well-appearing infants in the MBU. From the patient perspective, keeping those infants in the MBU with their parents decreases separation time, increases bonding time, and facilitates successful breastfeeding.[29] From the unit perspective, cost savings may be seen from fewer person-hours spent admitting and caring for well-appearing infants. However, from both the system and the unit perspectives, fewer NICU admissions may result in less reimbursement, and this may conflict with the other two goals, potentially decreasing the operating margin necessary to achieve important objectives including optimal patient care. Awareness of such conflicts should prompt the incorporation of balancing measures for costs and outcomes, and proactive conversation with senior leadership regarding budget objectives, and help build a business case for additional resources needed for improvement.[30] The idea of misalignment of operating margin and optimal care is not unique to neonatology and should be acknowledged explicitly. Pairing clinical outcome measures with value-based balancing measures starts the process of addressing these types of differences. Incentive misalignment is further complicated by the payor environment; for example, longer lengths of stay may be rewarded with fee-for-service reimbursement, and penalized with bundled or population-based payments. Ultimately, even with fee-for-service reimbursement models, improving outcomes while decreasing lengths of stay may yet be beneficial from multiple perspectives. For example, decreasing the length of stay for one diagnosis may allow for more efficient use of fixed resources, such as NICU beds and staffing.

ADDING VALUE TO QUALITY IMPROVEMENT

Using the Model for Improvement,[31] every quality improvement project should start by answering the following question: "What are we trying to accomplish?" Because most quality improvement teams are composed of health care providers, the natural inclination of team members is to address a particular clinical outcome and focus only on the numerator of the value equation. If the quality improvement team expands its focus to improving value by either improving outcomes or reducing costs (or both), the entire aim of the project takes on a different flavor, leading to different change ideas and the incorporation of value-based measures.

When developing aims, we recommend using aims that are specific, measureable, attainable, relevant, and time-bound (SMART).[32] For example, a quality improvement team might hope to decrease the rate of chronic lung disease in its unit by 10% in a 6-month period. Change ideas might include development of clinical practice guidelines around criteria for initial respiratory support with continuous positive airway pressure, whereas a relevant process measure might be the percent of infants managed on continuous positive airway pressure in accordance with those guidelines. However, if the same improvement team thinks about the aim from a value-based perspective, alternative process measures may include chest radiographs of intubated infants, number of doses of surfactant used, hours of nursing care, or length of stay. Taking the time to consider costs and outcomes in the design of a quality improvement initiative, whether in the SMART aim or in the development of appropriate metrics (**Table 1**), can help improvement teams become aware of value as a shared goal. Alternatively, focusing solely on the denominator of the value equation and having a SMART aim that addresses cost alone also improves value. For example, a clinical unit in which facility costs for infants suffering from NAS are significantly greater than the national average might seek to decrease resource use for this population. Holmes and colleagues[26] showed that standardized protocols for scoring and weaning medication decreased hospital costs and increased value. Here, rather than introducing changes directed

Table 1
Value metrics in the NICU

General Categories	Specific Examples
Aggregate measures	Length of stay Ventilator days
Laboratory and radiology tallies	Number of radiographs, head ultrasounds, or MRIs Number of laboratory studies (all vs complete blood count)
Medication tallies	Antibiotic days per month Days of parenteral nutrition
People	Nursing or physician hours Parents (missed work, additional costs)
Material resources	Oxygen probes Endotracheal tubes

specifically toward outcome measures, changes to reduce costs may add value to the care of infants with NAS by shortening their length of stay. In this example, a shorter hospitalization may also impact outcomes by improving the parent-patient experience. However, caution must be taken to monitor clinical outcomes with balancing measures to ensure that any impact is in the positive direction.

Careful evaluation of stakeholder viewpoints in a practice change can reveal unique opportunities or potential pitfalls when addressing value. Other than nurses, nurse practitioners, respiratory therapists, and physicians, who else does a potential change or improvement impact? How are other hospital services, such as pharmacy, nutrition, or housekeeping, affected? How does the SMART aim change the workflow for these essential services, and is there an opportunity to save time, resources, or materials among other groups involved or will they be adversely affected? Answering these questions and others like them can prompt improvement teams to include important value-based measures not otherwise considered. Use of quality improvement tools, such as value stream mapping, can help assess the current state of a process inclusive of the various perspectives.[33]

Similarly, a complete understanding of the perspectives of people involved in patient care can lead to other concepts, measures, or data sources for value-based improvement. Are other areas of the hospital leading improvement efforts that interact with or impact value in the NICU? Does the pharmacy measure costs associated with medication ordering, delivery, or administration? Are the operating rooms measuring the time it takes to complete particular procedures relevant to patients in the NICU? How can these other sources of data help increase value in the NICU?

Finally, and perhaps most importantly, thinking about value-based aims and how they fit into the larger organizational goals of the institution or health care system allows improvement teams to frame quality improvement work in terms that reflect the multiple agendas of hospital and health care system leaders. Some data sources may not be accessible without senior leader involvement. Accessing an institution's fiscal experts can help disentangle the mysteries of health care financing and convert measures of resource use efficiency into relevant cost saving estimates. Moreover, the demonstration of responsible leadership and awareness of shared institutional goals through value aims presents an opportunity for building stronger relationships with senior leaders. These same leaders spend significant amounts of time and energy guiding organization-wide mission. One way to do this is to have a project charter or a systematic approach that defines the project, relates it to organizational goals, and helps build consensus and clarity among improvement team members and with senior leaders.[34]

In summary, it is becoming increasingly important to attach value to improvement work. Value should not be considered equivalent to cost reduction. Instead, improving value can occur through the simultaneous consideration of outcomes and the resources necessary to achieve a result. In doing so, core concepts of quality improvement remain applicable, including SMART aims, balancing measures, and inclusion of different perspectives. As with traditional quality improvement, value projects in neonatology benefit from early involvement with hospital administration.

SUMMARY

Ever-rising health care costs may seem like an insurmountable problem, especially for front-line providers in pediatrics and neonatal medicine. However, it is essential that every provider, no matter their specialty, strive not only to improve outcomes for populations of patients, but also to reduce costs of care and increase efficiency in the health care delivery system.[12] Making quality improvement commonplace in health care provides opportunities for everyone to participate in process improvement and value-added care.

REFERENCES

1. Moses H 3rd, Matheson DH, Dorsey ER, et al. The anatomy of health care in the United States. JAMA 2013;310(18):1947–63.
2. Liu Y, Jin GZ. Employer contribution and premium growth in health insurance. J Health Econ 2015;39:228–47.
3. Gupta R, Shah ND, Ross JS. The rising price of naloxone: risks to efforts to stem overdose deaths. N Engl J Med 2016;375(23):2213–5.
4. Hogan C, Lunney J, Gabel J, et al. Medicare beneficiaries' costs of care in the last year of life. Health Aff 2001;20(4):188–95.
5. Russell RB, Green NS, Steiner CA, et al. Cost of hospitalization for preterm and low birth weight infants in the United States. Pediatrics 2007;120(1):e1–9.
6. Bui AL, Dieleman JL, Hamavid H, et al. Spending on children's personal health care in the United States, 1996-2013. JAMA Pediatr 2017;171(2):181–9.
7. Ellsbury DL, Clark RH, Ursprung R, et al. A multifaceted approach to improving outcomes in the NICU: the Pediatrix 100,000 babies campaign. Pediatrics 2016;137(4) [pii:e20150389].
8. ACGME Program Requirements for Graduate Medical Education in Internal Medicine. 2016. Available at: http://www.acgme.org/portals/0/pfassets/programrequirements/140_internal_medicine_2016.pdf. Accessed January 2, 2017.
9. Improving Professional Practice (Part 4). Available at: https://www.abp.org/content/improving-professional-practice-part-4. Accessed December 16, 2016.
10. Porter ME. What is value in health care? N Engl J Med 2010;363(26):2477–81.
11. Dukhovny D, Pursley DM, Kirpalani HM, et al. Evidence, quality, and waste: solving the value equation in neonatology. Pediatrics 2016;137(3):e20150312.
12. Berwick DM, Nolan TW, Whittington J. The triple aim: care, health, and cost. Health Aff 2008;27(3):759–69.
13. Rogowski J. Measuring the cost of neonatal and perinatal care. Pediatrics 1999; 103(1 Suppl E):329–35.
14. Horbar JD, Rogowski J, Plsek PE, et al. Collaborative quality improvement for neonatal intensive care. NIC/Q Project Investigators of the Vermont Oxford Network. Pediatrics 2001;107(1):14–22.
15. Rogowski JA, Horbar JD, Plsek PE, et al. Economic implications of neonatal intensive care unit collaborative quality improvement. Pediatrics 2001;107(1):23–9.
16. Horbar JD. The Vermont Oxford Network: evidence-based quality improvement for neonatology. Pediatrics 1999;103(1 Suppl E):350–9.
17. Patrick SW, Schumacher RE, Horbar JD, et al. Improving care for neonatal abstinence syndrome. Pediatrics 2016;137(5) [pii:e20153835].
18. Clark RH, Spitzer AR. Understanding outliers and defining value in neonatal healthcare. J Pediatr 2016;173:15–6.
19. Ho T, Dukhovny D, Zupancic JA, et al. Choosing wisely in newborn medicine: five opportunities to increase value. Pediatrics 2015;136(2):e482–9.
20. Ho T, Dukhovny D, Zupancic JA, et al. Antibiotic stewardship in 143 neonatal intensive care units (NICUs). Paper presented at: Pediatric Academic Societies Meeting. San Francisco, CA, May 9, 2017.

21. Hall RT, Domenico HJ, Self WH, et al. Reducing the blood culture contamination rate in a pediatric emergency department and subsequent cost savings. Pediatrics 2013;131(1):e292–7.
22. Algaze CA, Wood M, Pageler NM, et al. Use of a checklist and clinical decision support tool reduces laboratory use and improves cost. Pediatrics 2016;137(1): e20143019.
23. Deindl P, Unterasinger L, Kappler G, et al. Successful implementation of a neonatal pain and sedation protocol at 2 NICUs. Pediatrics 2013;132(1):e211–8.
24. DeMauro SB, Douglas E, Karp K, et al. Improving delivery room management for very preterm infants. Pediatrics 2013;132(4):e1018–25.
25. Asti L, Magers JS, Keels E, et al. A quality improvement project to reduce length of stay for neonatal abstinence syndrome. Pediatrics 2015;135(6):e1494–500.
26. Holmes AV, Atwood EC, Whalen B, et al. Rooming-in to treat neonatal abstinence syndrome: improved family-centered care at lower cost. Pediatrics 2016;137(6) [pii:e20152929].
27. Profit J, Gould JB, Zupancic JA, et al. Formal selection of measures for a composite index of NICU quality of care: baby-MONITOR. J Perinatol 2011;31(11): 702–10.
28. Kaempf JW, Zupancic JA, Wang L, et al. A risk-adjusted, composite outcomes score and resource utilization metrics for very low-birth-weight infants. JAMA Pediatr 2015;169(5):459–65.
29. Moore ER, Bergman N, Anderson GC, et al. Early skin-to-skin contact for mothers and their healthy newborn infants. Cochrane Database Syst Rev 2016;(11):CD003519.
30. Bartlett Ellis RJ, Embree JL, Ellis KG. A business case framework for planning clinical nurse specialist-led interventions. Clin Nurse Spec 2015;29(6):338–47.
31. Langley GJ. The improvement guide : a practical approach to enhancing organizational performance. 2nd edition. San Francisco (CA): Jossey-Bass; 2009.
32. Doran GT. There's a S.M.A.R.T. way to write management's goals and objectives. Management Rev (AMA Forum) 1981;70(11):35–6.
33. Graban M. Lean hospitals : improving quality, patient safety, and employee engagement. 2nd edition. New York: Productivity Press/Taylor & Francis; 2012.
34. Kaplan HC, Provost LP, Froehle CM, et al. The model for understanding success in quality (MUSIQ): building a theory of context in healthcare quality improvement. BMJ Qual Saf 2012;21(1):13–20.

Using Statistical Process Control to Drive Improvement in Neonatal Care

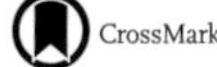

A Practical Introduction to Control Charts

Munish Gupta, MD, MMSc[a,*], Heather C. Kaplan, MD, MSCE[b]

KEYWORDS

• Control chart • Statistical process control • Quality improvement
• Special cause variation • Common cause variation

KEY POINTS

- Quality improvement requires the analysis of data measured over time and the ability to understand variation in that data in order to evaluate processes and guide change.
- Common cause variation is natural variation inherent to any process; special cause variation is unnatural variation owing to external factors.
- Control charts are tools within statistical process control (SPC) that provide a robust method for understanding data over time and identifying common and special cause variation.
- Health care providers engaging in quality improvement should use SPC methods and control charts to help guide their efforts.

INTRODUCTION

Data measurement is critical for quality improvement (QI). Although health care practices are often designed or changed based on the knowledge and expertise of the clinical care team, only by measuring processes or outcomes can practices truly be assessed and evaluated.

Data for QI, however, differ fundamentally from data measured for other purposes in health care. Typically, health care outcomes are measured statically, meaning that any given outcome is measured for a specific population over a fixed period of time.

The authors have nothing to disclose.

[a] Department of Neonatology, Beth Israel Deaconess Medical Center, 330 Brookline Avenue, Boston, MA 02215, USA; [b] Perinatal Institute and James M. Anderson Center for Health Systems Excellence, Cincinnati Children's Hospital Medical Center, University of Cincinnati School of Medicine, 3333 Burnet Avenue, MLC 7009, Cincinnati, OH 45229, USA

* Corresponding author.

E-mail address: mgupta@bidmc.harvard.edu

Clin Perinatol 44 (2017) 627–644
http://dx.doi.org/10.1016/j.clp.2017.05.011
perinatology.theclinics.com

Examples include population-level public health measures (ie, rates of preterm birth for a state for a particular period), metrics reported to regulatory agencies by hospitals (ie, central line infection rates for an intensive care unit for a particular year), and outcomes measured by research trials (ie, the rate of chronic lung disease in preterm infants who received a medication as compared with the rate in preterm infants who did not). These types of static measures can be analyzed using traditional statistics familiar to most in health care, including descriptive statistics such as mean values and standard deviations, and comparative statistics such as χ^2 tests, *t* tests, analyses of variance, and regression models.

Conversely, QI requires that data be measured dynamically over time, to allow for the ability to evaluate the reliability of current processes and to measure adequately the impact of changes in practice on desired outcomes. Over the past several decades, the quality and safety movement in health care has made clear the need to be able to understand dynamic rather than static data.[1,2] Analyzing data over time to understand and address the performance of the underlying system or process requires a different set of tools than traditional statistics, and statistical process control (SPC) methods are the most commonly used tools for this type of analysis.

In this review, we provide a practical overview of SPC and its most powerful tool, the Shewhart control chart, with an emphasis on the use of these methods in neonatology. Of note, the focus of this article is the analysis of data over time; we do not address other essential aspects of QI, including defining the improvement goal, setting specific aims, choosing and defining appropriate measures, understanding processes and current states, developing a theory of change, and using structured plan–do–study–act cycles to test and then implement changes. Also, this article is not meant to be a complete guide to the use of SPC. This review focuses on control charts, and does not address other important SPC tools such as run charts. In addition, although the intent of this review is to encourage clinicians to adopt control charts in their QI efforts, more comprehensive resources and textbooks should be consulted to understand important considerations of control chart use that are beyond the scope of this article.[3–6]

THE IMPORTANCE OF DATA OVER TIME

There is a natural tendency for those engaged in QI in health care to use more familiar traditional statistics. This practice often translates into the use of comparative tests to compare outcomes before and after an intervention, with the *P* value determining the impact of that intervention. Before–after comparisons do not adequately describe trends and patterns that may be essential to understanding the impact of changes in QI. A hypothetical example is provided in **Figs. 1** and **2**. In **Fig. 1**, a certain outcome is measured before and after an intervention, with the average score in each group shown. This before–after comparison suggests the intervention reduced the average score from 8 to 3, and if the improvement goal was to lower this measure, the obvious conclusion would be that the intervention was successful. **Fig. 2** shows 3 potential patterns of the same measure plotted over time. In each, the average score of the points before and after the intervention are 8 and 3, respectively, and would produce identical before–after bar graphs. However, the 3 patterns lead to very different conclusions regarding the impact of the intervention. In **Fig. 2**A, the pattern suggests the intervention did have a meaningful impact, with the score consistently higher before the intervention and then consistently lower after. In **Fig. 2**B, the pattern suggests the intervention had no impact at all, with the measure naturally declining over time. In **Fig. 2**C, the pattern suggests

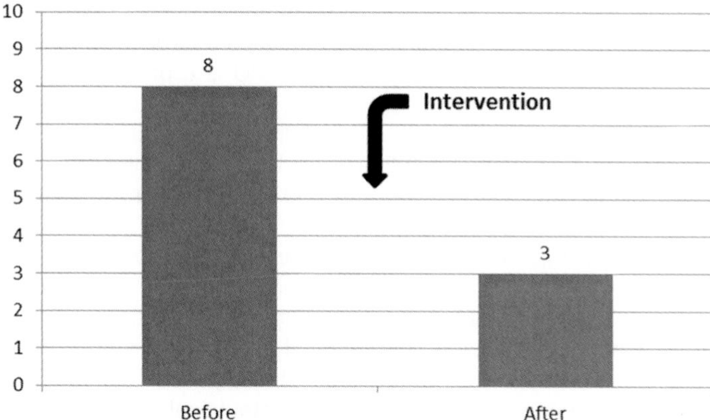

Fig. 1. Outcome measured before and after an intervention, with the average score in each group shown.

the intervention may have had a significant impact initially, but that this impact has not been sustained with the measure score increasing again over time. Although these examples are designed to be illustrative, the lessons are important: visualizing measures over time will provide a much more robust understanding of trends and patterns than before and after comparisons.

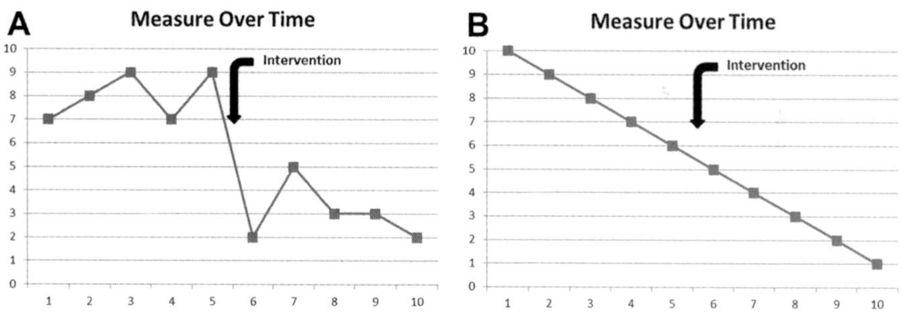

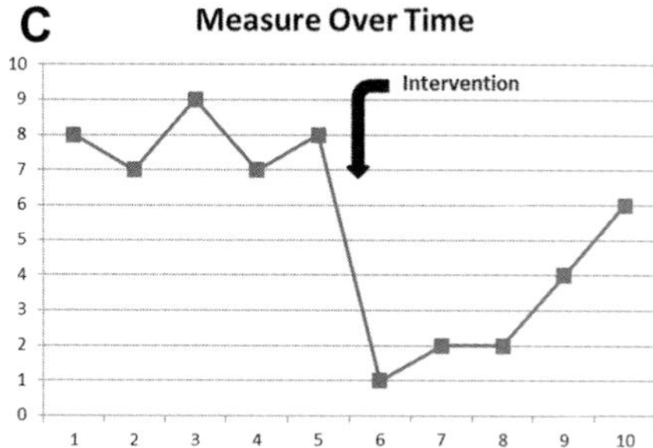

Fig. 2. Example of 3 potential patterns of change after an intervention. (*A*) The pattern suggests the intervention did have a meaningful impact, with the score consistently higher before the intervention and then consistently lower after. (*B*) The pattern suggests the intervention had no impact at all, with the measure naturally declining over time. (*C*) The pattern suggests the intervention may have had a significant impact initially, but that this impact has not been sustained, with the measure increasing again over time.

STATISTICAL PROCESS CONTROL AND VARIATION

Simple visualization of data over time can provide important context to evaluate and guide improvement efforts, but optimal understanding of data patterns requires more rigorous analysis. SPC is a field of analytical statistics that provides the robust tools necessary for this type of analysis. At its core, SPC is a philosophy that supports learning through data, incorporating process thinking, analytical study, prediction, and the analysis of process stability and capability.[7] The theories that underpin this approach were developed in the late 1920s by Dr. Walter Shewhart while he was working at Western Electric and Bell Laboratories and were popularized internationally by W.E. Deming.[8,9]

SPC is built on tools that help to understand variations in data measured over time. All processes measured over time will vary, and understanding this variation is critical to understanding that process and evaluating improvement efforts. Shewhart observed that, although all processes will vary, if a process is stable, the variation is predictable and can be described by a known statistical distribution. This statistical distribution was the foundation of control charts—statistical tools developed by Shewhart to help individuals working on the frontlines of manufacturing systems to understand variation in their processes. Shewhart realized the importance of reducing variation and that continual process adjustment in reaction to natural variation actually increased variation and worsened quality. The control chart combines the graphical display of data over time with statistical testing in a way that makes it easy for nonstatisticians to detect process changes. Shewhart believed the control chart could help individuals on the frontlines react appropriately to variation and it is one of the core tools of SPC.

Shewhart identified 2 types of variation that can be seen in data measured over time (**Table 1**). Common cause variation is natural variation that is inherent in a particular process, occurring on a regular basis. Repeated measures of the same factor or process, even without changes to that system, often produce slightly different values. For example, repeated measures of a patient's P_{CO_2} on blood gas, time to first skin-to-skin hold in the neonatal intensive care unit (NICU), or measures of parent satisfaction may differ over time even if there is no change in the patient's status or NICU processes. The differences in these measurements in these situations are due to normal fluctuations in the patient's physiology, small differences in unit workflow among staff, or even discrepancies in how the measures themselves are captured and recorded, and reflect natural or common cause variation within that system. A process that has only common cause variation is considered a stable process, with predictable variation. Special cause variation, in contrast, refers to unnatural variation that is due to events, changes, or circumstances that have not been characteristic of the

Table 1
Definitions

Term	Definition
Common cause variation	Natural variation, inherent as part of usual process
Special cause variation	Unnatural variation, owing to causes not part of usual process, either intended or unintended
Stable process	Process with only common cause variation, with variation predictable within natural common cause bounds
Unstable process	Process with special and common cause variation, with unpredictable variation

regular process. For example, an extremely elevated P_{CO_2} on a patient's blood gas owing to a plugged endotracheal tube, a significant decrease in the NICU's average time to first skin-to-skin hold after educating staff to encourage skin-to-skin care with umbilical lines in place, or low parent satisfaction scores after a flood in the NICU would all reflect variation not inherent in the system, but rather variation owing to some external special cause introduced into the system. Importantly, special cause variation can be the result of an external event over which we have little control (eg, plugged endotracheal tube, flood in the NICU) or the results of a planned intervention (eg, education of staff on skin-to-skin care with umbilical lines). Furthermore, special cause variation can be transient or maintained permanently as part of the system. A process with special cause variation is considered an unstable process, with unpredictable variation.

Graphical displays of data over time can aid in distinguishing common cause and special cause variation. An illustrative example is given in **Fig. 3**, which graphs time to get to work measured daily by an individual for 1 month. It is clear from the graph that the natural process results in getting to work in approximately 30 minutes, but that on days 21 and 22, a different process impacted the commute, resulting in a time to get to work of 54 and 56 minutes, clearly different than the usual time. This special cause, perhaps construction, was not persistent, because the time to get to work then returned to its typical values. In this example, the variation seen on days 1 to 20 and 23 to 30, where time to work ranged from 25 to 34 minutes, would be considered common cause variation. The variation seen on days 21 and 22 would be special cause variation.

In this example, identifying common cause and special cause variation was clear; in most displays of data over time, characterizing the type of variation will not be as evident, and simple visualization will not reliably distinguish natural variation from

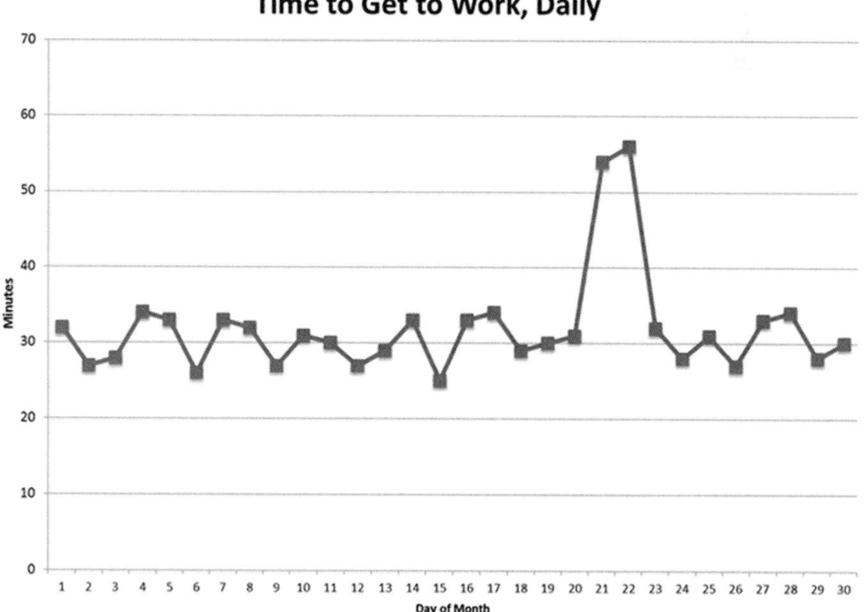

Fig. 3. Graph example of data over time. Time to get to work (in minutes) measured daily by an individual for 1 month.

unnatural. SPC control charts are meant to identify common cause and special cause variation. Furthermore, although built on rigorous statistical methods, control charts are designed to be used by frontline staff, to allow for improvement teams to rapidly and continuously understand their data and appropriately respond.

THE CONTROL CHART

Anatomy of a Control Chart

Classic statistical methods are based on examining data collected over time in aggregate without attention paid to the time order.[3] The first step in any statistical testing is to examine and describe the distribution of the data, often by creating a histogram of the data. The distribution can be described by its mean, median, and standard deviation. A control chart, instead, takes the same series of measurements and plots them in time order (**Fig. 4**). The *x*-axis is a unit of time, which may be daily, weekly, monthly, or a grouping of consecutive units. The *y*-axis plots the variable or measure of interest. In a control chart, the distribution of the data is still described by its mean and standard deviation, but graphically, with the mean plotted as the center line and the standard deviation plotted as upper and lower control limits, placed at ±3 standard deviations from the mean (see **Fig. 4**). The graphical display of the mean and control limits allow for visual assessment of whether data follows an expected distribution (common cause variation) or unexpected (special cause variation). If the parameters of the process have not changed, common cause variation will be predictable based on the underlying statistical distribution. For example, a stable process with data that follows a normal distribution will have 99.73% of measurements falling within ±3 standard deviations around the mean. Control limits reflect the inherent variability in the data.

Different Types of Control Charts

The theory underlying SPC, and control charts, is based on the observation that measurements coming from a stable process exhibit variation that is predictable and can be described by a known statistical distribution. Measurements may come from a normal (or Gaussian), Poisson, binomial, or geometric distribution. There are examples of measures in health care coming from each of these distributions (**Table 2**)

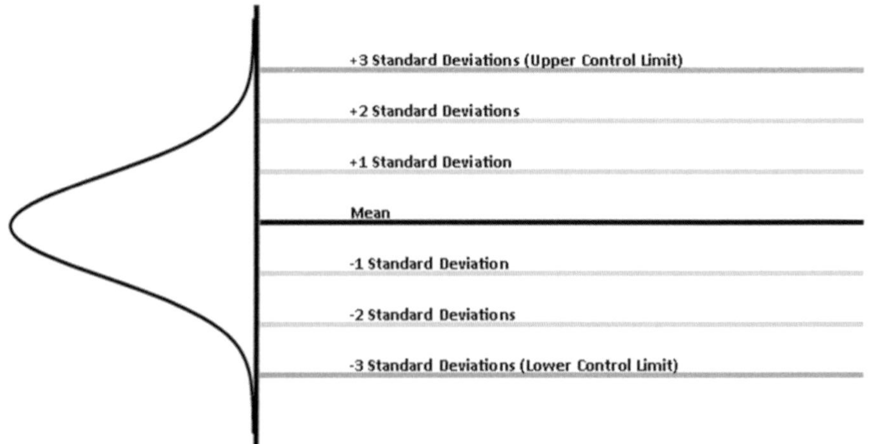

Fig. 4. Control chart showing mean plotted as the center line and the standard deviation plotted as upper and lower control limits, placed at ±3 standard deviations from the mean.

Table 2
Control charts based on type of data and distribution

Type of Data	Distribution	Examples	Type of Control Chart
Continuous	Continuous (Gaussian)	Time to first skin to skin Admission temperature Birth weight Duration of stay[a]	X-bar and S charts
Discrete dichotomous	Binomial	Patient develops BPD (Y/N) Patient develops severe IVH (Y/N) Patient develops NEC (Y/N) Patient receives breast milk (Y/N)	P chart
Discrete count	Poisson	Number of CLABSIs Number of unplanned extubations Number of alarms Number of medication errors	U chart

Abbreviations: BPD, bronchopulmonary dysplasia; CLABSIs, central line–associated bloodstream infections; IVH, intraventricular hemorrhage; NEC, necrotizing enterocolitis.
[a] Often skewed distribution.

It is important to understand which distribution your data come from to select the appropriate control chart. Depending on the type of control chart used and the specific statistical distribution associated with that chart, a different formula will be used for calculating the standard deviation, and therefore the upper and lower control limits (see **Table 2**). For example, if we are monitoring the proportion of very low birthweight infants who develop bronchopulmonary dysplasia at 36 weeks, the appropriate formula for calculating the upper and lower control limits on the p-chart will use the standard deviation from the binomial distribution. In contrast, if we are monitoring our NICU's central line–associated bloodstream infection rate per 1000 line-days, the appropriate formula for calculating the upper and lower control limits on the u-chart will use the standard deviation from the Poisson distribution. For any given QI (or process monitoring) effort, one needs to first clearly identify the measure of interest, then determine what type of data populate that measure (continuous, discrete count data, or discrete dichotomous data). This information will help to determine which type of control chart to use based on the type of data (**Fig. 5**). Although multiple different control charts exist, 3 types are the most common used in health care: the X-bar and S chart for continuous data, the P chart for discrete dichotomous data, and the U chart for discrete count data.

For discrete data (P chart and U chart), only 1 chart is needed to understand the performance of the process metric over time. With continuous data, 2 charts are needed because there can be 2 types of special cause variation or process changes; the mean or standard deviation could change, and either could change without the other. The X-bar chart looks at variation across the subgroups, whereas the S chart (as in standard deviation chart) looks at variation within each subgroup. For example, with X-bar and S charts examining average monthly time to first skin-to-skin hold in a NICU, the X-bar chart would show variation from month to month, and the S chart would show the variation within each month. Typically, if the S chart shows significant variation within each subgroup (eg, special cause variation), then it becomes more difficult to interpret variation seen on the X-bar chart.

Control charts can be constructed manually, although this is fairy labor intensive. Instead, specific control chart software (eg, Chartrunner, PQ Systems), add-ins to

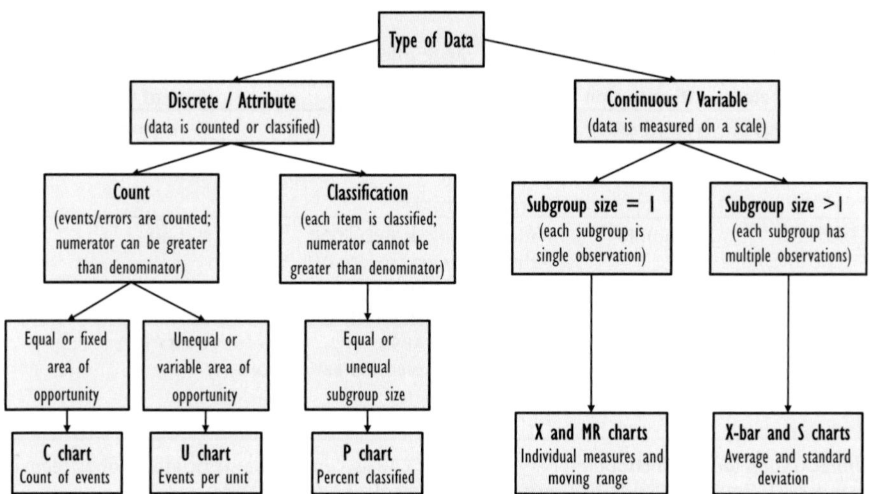

Fig. 5. How to choose a control chart based on type of data. (*Adapted from* Provost LP, Murray SK. The health care data guide: learning from data for improvement. 1st edition. San Francisco, CA: Jossey-Bass; 2011. p. xxviii 445; and Carey RG. Improving healthcare with control charts: basic and advanced SPC methods and case studies. Milwaukee, WI: ASQ Quality Press; 2003.)

Microsoft Excel (eg, QI Macros for Excel, SPC for Excel, QI Charts), and general statistical software (eg, SAS, STATA, SPSS, Minitab) can be purchased to construct control charts from data.

Rules for Special Cause

Control charts can help to assess whether a given process is stable as well as the impact of process changes by looking for evidence of special cause variation. If a process produces data that deviates from the random distribution models predicted by a given distribution, special cause variation is likely present. Data that fall outside the control limits or display nonrandom patterns are signs of special cause variation, meaning that is highly probable that something inherently different in the process led to these data.

Having an appropriate threshold for distinguishing special versus common cause variation is important because the type of variation present dictates your improvement actions. Originally, Shewhart suggested that points outside of the upper and lower control limits likely indicated special cause variation. Since then, additional rule-based conventions have been developed that also identify special cause variation based on other patterns of control chart data. Placement of the upper and lower control limits at ± 3 standard deviations and the selection of rules to identify nonrandom patterns in the data are designed to balance the risk of falsely detecting special cause variation when the data suggest a predictable (but extreme) value resulting from common cause variation (type I error) and failing to detect special cause variation when it is present (type II error). Placing the upper and lower control limits at ± 3 standard deviations on a control chart with 25 data points has a tolerable false positive probability of $1 - (0.9973)^{25} = 6.5\%$.[3]

The various conventions for identifying special cause variation in a control chart are based on patterns of data around control limits. In addition to points outside of control limits at ±3 standard deviations, some of these conventions use 'inner control limits' at ±1 and ±2 standard deviations. At least 8 such rule-based conventions have been developed (**Table 3**). Although all of these rules are used in some industries, in health care, only a subset of the rules are typically used. Although applying more rules to detect special cause increases the power of control charts to detect true process changes, they also increase the likelihood of a false-positive finding and, as shown in **Table 3**, authors and organizations vary in the rules recommended for routine use. To a great extent, the choice of rules should be made based on the relative importance of missing true positives versus identifying false positives. If it is highly important to identify all potential positives and any false positives can be managed easily, then using more rules to increase detection power may be appropriate. This may apply when monitoring for adverse events. If it is important to identify special cause variation only when true change has happened, then using fewer rules may be appropriate. This may apply when responding to special cause variation would require major system changes. Given the number of conventions and rules available, when beginning an improvement initiative, it is important to decide a priori which set of rules will be used to identify special cause variation.

CONTROL CHART EXAMPLES

Admission Hypothermia

A NICU has an ongoing initiative to reduce admission hypothermia in very low birth weight (VLBW) infants through improvements in delivery room management. Through structured use of the plan–do–study–act cycle, they have tested and implemented multiple changes over several years. They track first temperature on admission to the NICU, and an infant is categorized as having admission hypothermia if that first temperature is less than 36°C. Their goal is to reduce the percent of VLBW infants with admission hypothermia to less than 25%.

Table 3
Rule-based conventions for special cause variation in control charts and author recommendations

	Provost & Murray,[5] 2011	Benneyan et al,[3] 2003	Carey,[4] 2003	Montgomery,[10] 2013
One or more points more than 3 SD from mean	✔	✔	✔	✔
2 of 3 consecutive points more than 2 SD from the mean	✔	✔	✔	✔
4 of 5 consecutive points more than 1 SD from the mean		✔		✔
8 consecutive points on 1 side of the mean	✔	✔	✔	✔
6 consecutive points increasing or decreasing	✔	✔	✔	✔
15 consecutive points within 1 SD of the mean	✔			✔
14 consecutive points alternating up and down		✔		✔
8 points in a row more than 1 SD from the mean				✔

Abbreviation: SD, standard deviation.

They are using a control chart to help assess the impact of their improvement efforts. As they are plotting the percent of VLBW infants with admission hypothermia, they consider this discrete dichotomous data, and use a P chart. They are using quarterly subgroups. Their control chart showing their data after 4 years is shown in **Fig. 6**.

Improvement in their outcome is readily evident, with a progressive decrease in the percent of VLBW infants with admission hypothermia. Using control chart rules, evidence of special cause variation is seen in 2009, with 2 out of 3 points outside of 2 SDs and 1 point outside of 3 SDs, after 2011 with more than 8 points in a row below the mean, and again in 2013 with 2 out of 3 points outside of 2 SDs. Their overall admission hypothermia rate for the entire time period is 31.7%.

Skin-To-Skin Events

As part of an improvement initiative focused on increasing the use of human milk, a NICU team would like to understand their performance around encouraging skin-to-skin contact between NICU infants and their mothers. They are tracking the number of skin-to-skin events in their NICU, and measure this as a rate per patient day in weekly subgroups. They consider this discrete count data, and use a U chart, shown in **Fig. 7**.

Numerous signals of special cause variation are present, with multiple points outside of outer control limits, and multiple instances of clusters of points near the outer control limits. In addition, the patterns of special cause variation do not seem to be consistent. The team concludes that this is an unstable process, and focuses on determining the reasons for the special cause variation and removing those variations in practice before seeking fundamental process improvements.

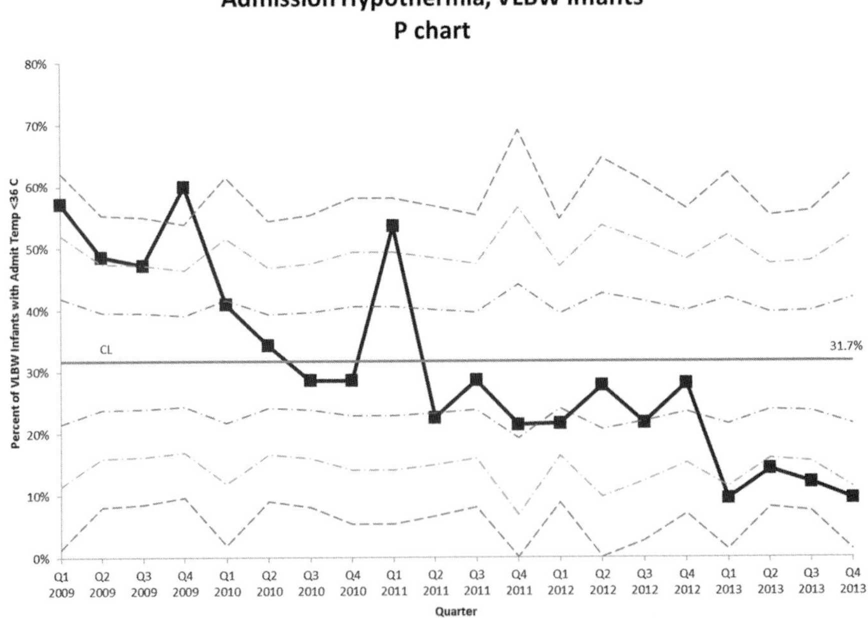

Fig. 6. P chart for admission hypothermia in very low birthweight (VLBW) infants.

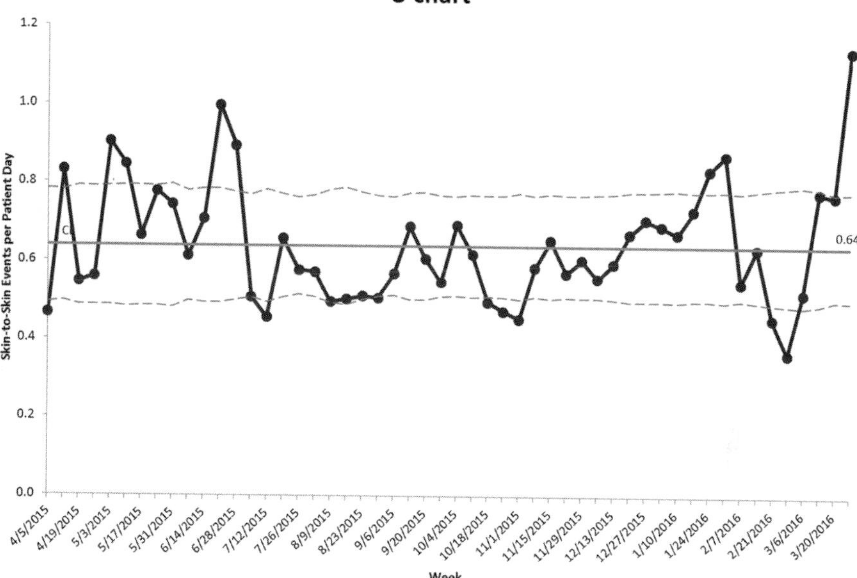

Fig. 7. U chart showing to skin event rates in infants in the neonatal intensive care unit (NICU).

Time to First Administration of Colostrum

As part of an improvement effort to increase the use of human milk, a NICU team is tracking the time to first administration or feeding of breast milk as a process measure reflecting early initiation of breast feeding, pumping, or hand expression. They are measuring time to first breast milk use by the infant.

To examine their performance using a control chart, the team plots the average time to first use by month. Because these are continuous data with a sample size each month that is greater than 1, they use an X-bar–S chart. Their chart is shown in **Fig. 8**.

The team can see significant improvements in this process measure. They first examine the S chart, and note that the standard deviation of time to first breast milk use has decreased substantially, with special cause variation noted in early 2011 and again after April 2012. This suggests that their process has become more consistent, with less variability between infants each month. They then examine the X-bar chart, and note that the average time to first breast milk use has also decreased substantially, with special cause variation noted in early 2011 and again in 2012. This suggests infants are receiving their first breast milk earlier. Thus, the team concludes they have made their process more reliable by reducing variation between infants, and made their process better by reducing the overall time to first breast milk use.

SPECIAL CONSIDERATIONS WHEN USING CONTROL CHARTS

Number of Data Subgroups

As discussed, control charts are particularly powerful tools for guiding QI efforts because of their ability to identify common and special cause variation. However, an adequate number of data subgroups is necessary for control charts to determine

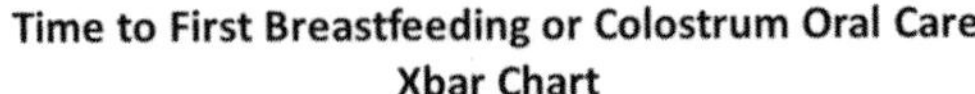

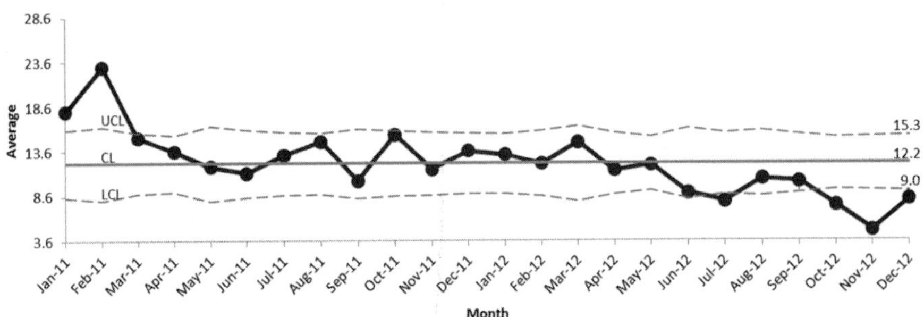

Time to First Breast Feeding or Colostrum Oral Care
S chart

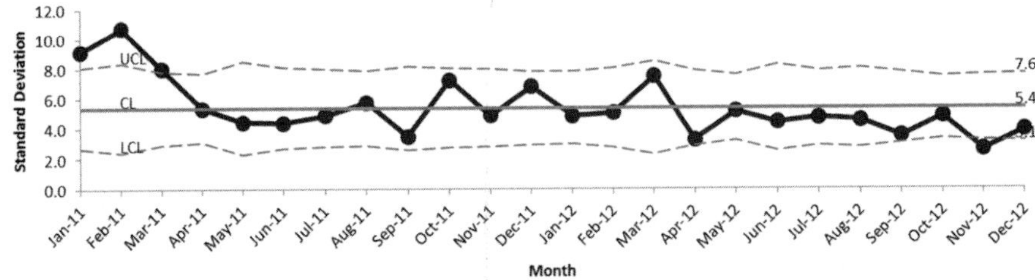

Fig. 8. X-bar-S chart measuring time to first breast milk use by infant.

reliably whether a process is in statistical control; with too few data points, typical special cause rules do not adequately indicate that only common cause variation is present. Most experts agree that a minimum of 20 to 25 data points are needed to be able to calculate robust upper and lower control limits and, thereby, distinguish common cause from special cause variation.[3–6]

This has obvious implications for data collection and definition of subgroups. Most control charts plot data over time. For data measured daily, nearly 1 month of data will be needed to produce an adequate number of subgroups for a robust control chart. For data measured weekly, this will be nearly 6 months of data, and for data measured monthly, this will be 2 years of data. When developing control charts, there is a constant tension between having frequent subgroups of a small sample size that enable rapid detection of change versus less frequent subgroups of larger size that create more robust control limits.

Of note, it is possible to have too many subgroups in a control chart. Too many data points will increase the likelihood of detecting inconsequential special cause variation in a process that would otherwise be considered stable for practical purposes. Some authors recommend limiting control charts to 35 to 40 subgroups, whereas others suggest control charts can have up to 80 subgroups.[4,5]

Ideally, retrospective data abstraction can provide adequate baseline data to create an appropriate control chart for a new improvement initiative. If data are being newly collected and baseline data are not available, then trial limits can be calculated with as few as 12 data points for the most commonly used control charts in health care, including P, U, and X-bar and S charts.[5] Trial limits can provide important information regarding common or special cause variation, but must be interpreted with caution. Special cause variation seen with trial limits likely reflects an unstable process, and should be responded to accordingly. It is more difficult to use trial limits to conclude a process is stable with only common cause variation if special cause variation is not seen. Trial limits should be recalculated as data are obtained from additional subgroups. In addition, run charts can be a powerful tool to examine processes before having adequate data for construction of a control chart. Although not discussed here, other references review run charts in detail.[11]

Fixing Limits

When a process is being newly measured, and it is uncertain whether the process is stable or unstable, then all of the data available can be used to calculate the center line and control limits and then assess for common or special cause variation. For a process that has been shown to be stable with only common cause variation, if the goal is to detect improvement or change, then the center line and limits should be fixed, and future data points should then be compared with these existing limits. Special cause variation will be detected in new subgroups more quickly then if the center line and limits were recalculated to include the additional data points. An example of this is given in **Fig. 9**A–C, in which any mother's milk at discharge for NICU infants is being monitored by a NICU interested in increasing their human milk use. Review of their data over a 24-month period through December 2014 with a P chart (**Fig. 9**A) reveals a stable process with only common cause variation around a mean of 77.0%. If 12 additional monthly subgroups are added and the mean and control limits are recalculated with each subgroup, review of 36 months of data again reveals only common cause variation around a mean of 78.8% (see **Fig. 9**B). If the center line had been fixed at 77.0% after the initial control chart had demonstrated a stable process over a 24-month period, then adding the 12 subsequent subgroups would have revealed special cause variation, with more than 8 data points in a row in 2015 above the mean (see **Fig. 9**C).

Importantly, as described, at least 20 to 25 data points will be necessary to determine whether a process is in control with only common cause variation, and thus allow for fixing of limits. Also, in general, limits should not be fixed if a process is not stable; if a process has special cause variation, then this variation should be understood and addressed before limits are fixed.

Updating or Changing Limits

If a control chart shows special cause variation suggesting a sustained change in the process, then the center line and control limits can be revised to describe more accurately the new process. This is commonly seen in successful improvement initiatives, in which changes made to a process result in sustained special cause variation as compared with the baseline data. In these situations, limits can be calculated for the baseline data, and new limits for the data obtained after the process change.

Updating limits to reflect a new process requires an understanding of the process as well as evidence of special cause variation. In general, new limits can be calculated when all of the following are true: the data show a clear change from previous (special cause variation); the change in the data can be explained by a change in the process; and the change in the process is expected to be sustained.[6] In the mother's milk at discharge example, if the NICU team had made changes to their process that they felt contributed to the special cause variation seen in 2015, and they expected those changes to be sustained, they could revise their central line and control limits to reflect this new process. **Fig. 10** shows their control chart with the revised limits, showing that

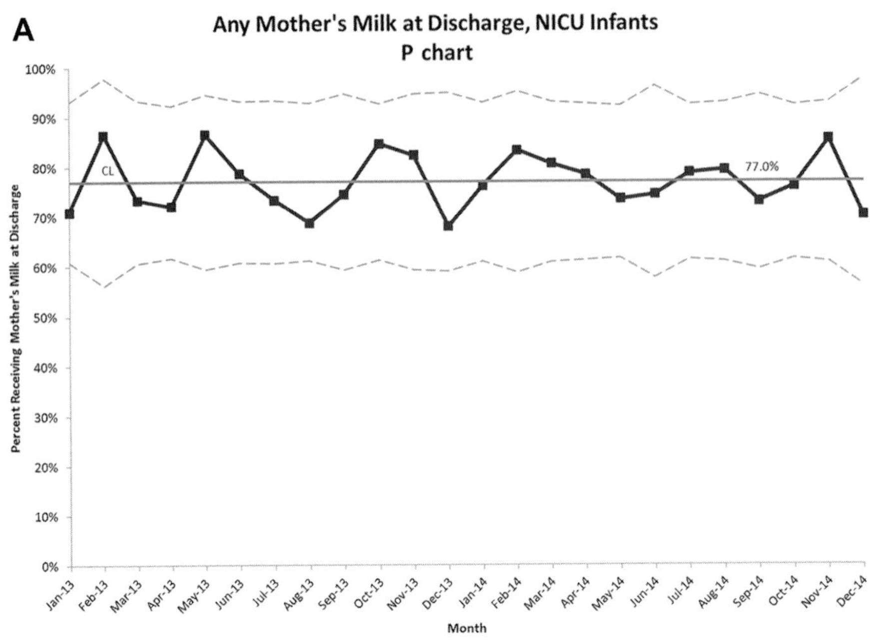

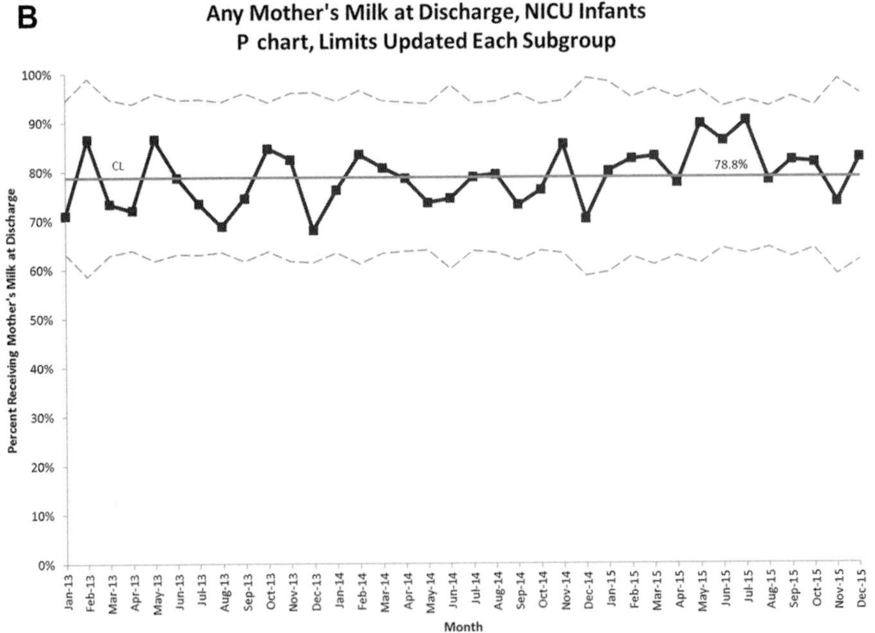

Fig. 9. P charts of any mother's milk at discharge, illustrating value of fixing limits appropriately. (*A*) 24 months of data showing only common cause variation around a mean of 77%. (*B*) 12 additional months of data added with mean recalculated with each additional subgroup, showing only common cause variation around mean of 78.8%. (*C*) 12 additional months of data added with mean fixed at original value of 77%, showing special cause variation in 2015 with 8 points in a row above the mean.

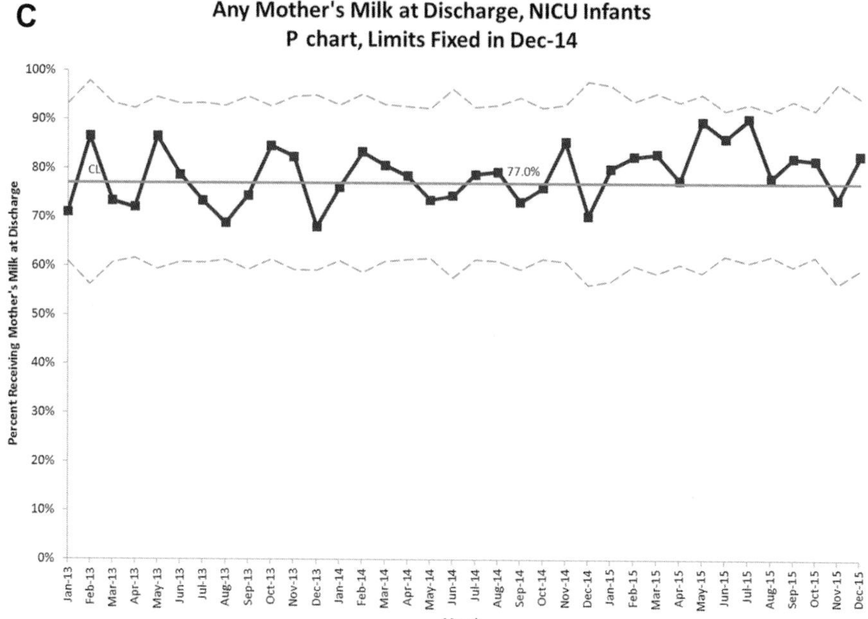

Fig. 9. (*continued*).

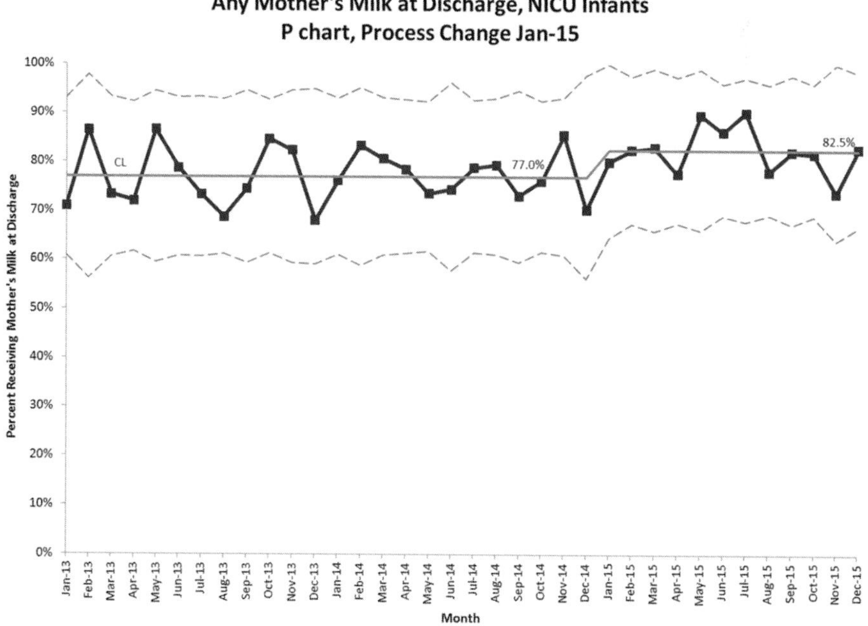

Fig. 10. P chart of any mother's milk at discharge with revised limits after January 2015, showing increase in overall rate from 77.0% to 82.5%.

their overall rate of any mother's milk at discharge in NICU infants increased from 77.0% in 2013 and 2014 to 82.5% in 2015.

Subgroup Sample Size

Although more frequent measurement of data over time generally provides greater ability to evaluate processes and detect change in a control chart, it can also result in small subgroup sample sizes that lessen the chart's usefulness. Larger subgroup sizes provide greater power to detect process changes, but require less frequent subgroup sampling. These considerations are particularly true for control charts of attribute data, where small subgroup sizes can result in many measure values of zero or 100%, or a lack of upper or lower control limits. In general, subgroup sizes should be adequate to allow for reasonably symmetric distribution of the sampled data, adequate sensitivity to detect process changes, and detectable outer control limits.[12] Several simplified approaches to determining minimum subgroup size are discussed here, although control chart users are encouraged to consult other references for more detailed mathematical explanations of sample size calculations.[12,13]

For P charts, a common guideline is for the minimum subgroup size to be greater than 3 divided by the overall average proportion of the outcome of interest [$n>(3/p)$], where n is the minimum sample size and p is the overall population proportion). If the proportion of the outcome is greater than 50%, the minimum sample size would be 3 divided by 1 minus the overall proportion [$n>3/(1-p)$].[5,12,13] Although 3 divided by the overall proportion is the minimum subgroup size needed, P charts will have more power when the subgroup size is greater than 5 divided the by overall proportion.[12] For example, if a certain measure has an overall occurrence rate of 20% (0.2), the minimum sample size for each subgroup would be 3 divided by 0.2, or 15, whereas a more powerful control chart would have a subgroup size greater than 5 divided by 0.2, or 25. If the occurrence rate was 90% (0.9), the minimum sample size would be 3 divided by 1 – 0.9, or 30, and the optimal chart subgroup size would be greater than 5 divided by 1 – 0.9, or 50. Measures with occurrence rates closer to zero or 100% will require larger sample sizes than measures with occurrence rates that are less extreme.

For u-charts, common guidelines are for the minimum subgroup size to be greater than 1.4 to 3 divided by the overall occurrence rate, with optimal subgroup size being 5 to 9 divided by the overall occurrence rate.[5,12] For example, if a U chart were being used to monitor hospital-acquired infections with a rate of 3 per 1000 patient-days (0.003 per day), then the subgroup size would need to be at a minimum 466 to 1000, and optimally 1666 to 3000.

Although similar sample size considerations do apply to control charts for continuous data (X-bar and S charts), in general, these charts tend to be more robust and can allow for reasonable sensitivity to detect process change even with small subgroup sizes. In fact, control charts for continuous data exist that can plot individual measures over time (the I or XmR chart); these tend to be less powerful than X-bar and S charts, however, and are not commonly used. References are available that provide detailed calculations for sample sizes for X-bar and S charts.[12]

A reasonable, practical approach to subgroup sizes for control charts in general is to seek to develop charts with outer control limits >0% and <100%, and with most data points not at zero or 100%. For example, if the goal of an improvement initiative is to lower a certain measure, then the control chart should have a measurable lower control limit and most data points should not be zero. If the goal of an improvement initiative is to increase performance on a certain measure to 100%, then the control chart should have a measurable upper control limit and most data points should not be 100%.

Measures of rare events that approach zero or measures that are near 100% would likely require subgroup sizes that prohibit timely data evaluation. For example, this circumstance commonly occurs in NICUs monitoring central line–associated bloodstream infection rates, after improvement efforts have led to enough improvements that CLABSIs become rare events. A U chart of central line–associated bloodstream infection rates in many NICUs, even if the NICU is quite large, would require subgroups measured at most yearly, and a U chart plotted monthly or even quarterly would be uninformative. Yearly data have limited usefulness in guiding clinical improvement efforts. In these situations, special control charts designed for rare events such as G charts and T charts would likely be more useful.[5,14]

HOW SPECIAL CAUSE VARIATION TRANSLATES TO IMPROVEMENT ACTION

Although control charts are powerful tools for identifying common cause and special cause variation, their true usefulness comes from health care providers using control charts to drive improvement based on expert knowledge of their systems. There are 2 general approaches to improving processes using SPC. First, because processes that exhibit a lot of special cause variation are unstable, they should be improved by eliminating special cause variation. If something has affected the process negatively, it should be identified and removed. If it had a positive effect, in contrast, it should be understood and incorporated into the ongoing process. However, once a process has only common cause variation, it will continue to produce the same results (within statistical limits) unless the process is fundamentally changed or revamped. If the process average (center line) is higher or lower than goal, then a formal improvement project should be undertaken to alter the process. Even if the process average is at goal, the process could likely be improved by reducing variation (narrowing the control limits by reducing the standard deviation) through efforts directed at standardizing work. **Fig. 11** provides an approach for thinking about how the type of variation (common vs special cause) leads to a given type of improvement action.

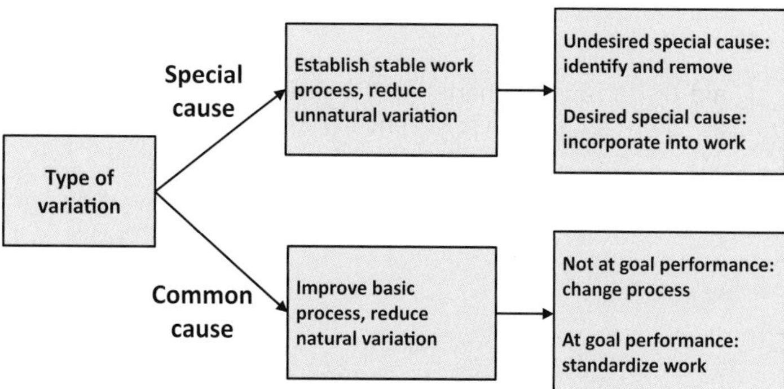

Fig. 11. How type of variation can help determine type of improvement action.

SUMMARY

Understanding variation is the core of SPC and is essential to ultimately improving quality of care. Control charts provide graphical and statistical tools that are easily used by those on the frontlines to distinguish common from special cause variation and direct improvement efforts.

ACKNOWLEDGMENTS

Among many others, we gratefully acknowledge Lloyd Provost and Jim Benneyan for providing countless hours of education and guidance regarding statistical process control, control charts, and quality improvement.

REFERENCES

1. Berwick DM. Controlling variation in health care: a consultation from Walter Shewhart. Med Care 1991;29(12):1212–25.
2. Blumenthal D. Total quality management and physicians' clinical decisions. JAMA 1993;269(21):2775–8.
3. Benneyan JC, Lloyd RC, Plsek PE. Statistical process control as a tool for research and healthcare improvement. Qual Saf Health Care 2003;12(6):458–64.
4. Carey RG. Improving healthcare with control charts: basic and advanced SPC methods and case studies. Milwaukee, WI: ASQ Quality Press; 2003.
5. Provost LP, Murray SK. The health care data guide: learning from data for improvement. 1st edition. San Francisco: Jossey-Bass; 2011.
6. Wheeler DJ, Chambers DS. Understanding statistical process control. 3rd edition. Knoxville, TN: SPC Press; 2010.
7. Thor J, Lundberg J, Ask J, et al. Application of statistical process control in healthcare improvement: systematic review. Qual Saf Health Care 2007;16(5):387–99.
8. Shewhart WA. Economic control of quality of manufactured product. New York: D. Van Nostrand Company, Inc; 1931.
9. Deming WE. The new economics: for industry, government, education. 2nd edition. Cambridge, MA: MIT Press; 2000.
10. Montgomery DC. Introduction to statistical quality control. 7th edition. Hoboken, NJ: Wiley; 2013.
11. Perla RJ, Provost LP, Murray SK. The run chart: a simple analytical tool for learning from variation in healthcare processes. BMJ Qual Saf 2011;20(1):46–51.
12. Benneyan JC. The design, selection, and performance of statistical control charts for healthcare process improvement. International Journal of Six Sigma and Competitive Advantage 2008;4(3):209–39.
13. Benneyan JC. Statistical quality control methods in infection control and hospital epidemiology, part II: chart use, statistical properties, and research issues. Infect Control Hosp Epidemiol 1998;19(4):265–83.
14. Benneyan JC. Number-between g-type statistical quality control charts for monitoring adverse events. Health Care Management Sci 2001;4(4):305–18.

Creating a Highly Reliable Neonatal Intensive Care Unit Through Safer Systems of Care

Patoula G. Panagos, MD[a,b,c], Stephen A. Pearlman, MD, MSHQS[c,d,*]

KEYWORDS

- Patient safety • Neonatal • Culture of safety • Communication tools
- Unplanned extubation

KEY POINTS

- Creating a culture of safety is the key to making the neonatal intensive care unit (NICU) safer.
- Incident reporting and analysis are critical to improving patient safety.
- A nonpunitive approach promotes staff engagement in safety activities.
- An interdisciplinary approach is fundamental to NICU safety efforts.
- Unplanned extubation is a NICU safety concern that can be addressed using quality improvement methodology.

INTRODUCTION

Infants in the neonatal intensive care unit (NICU) are at high risk for serious medical errors.[1–5] Studies estimate that about 80% of medical errors are system derived.[6] The key to designing a safe system of care is to reduce the overall frequency of errors and when they do occur ensure that harm does not reach patients.[7]

Quality improvement (QI) and patient safety are interrelated but also distinct entities. Although each focuses on the system and processes of patient care, QI strives to improve patient outcomes, whereas safety attends to avoiding errors

The authors have nothing to disclose.

[a] Division of Neonatology, Nemours Alfred I. duPont Hospital for Children, 1600 Rockland Road, Wilmington, DE 19803, USA; [b] Nemours Neonatology, Thomas Jefferson University Hospital, Philadelphia, PA, USA; [c] Sidney Kimmel School of Medicine, Thomas Jefferson University, Philadelphia, PA, USA; [d] Division of Neonatology, Women and Children's Services, Christiana Care Health System, MAP I Suite 217, Newark, DE 19713, USA

* Corresponding author. Division of Neonatology, Women and Children's Services, Christiana Care Health System, MAP I Suite 217, Newark, DE 19713.

E-mail address: SPearlman@christianacare.org

Clin Perinatol 44 (2017) 645–662
http://dx.doi.org/10.1016/j.clp.2017.05.006
perinatology.theclinics.com

and patient harm. QI uses methodology to apply well-established approaches often as a bundle of care in order to improve patient outcomes. The methods used include the Institute of Healthcare Improvement (IHI) Model for Improvement, Plan-Do-Study-Act method, or Lean Six Sigma. Patient safety focuses on developing safe systems of care. This process starts with greater transparency and, hence, reporting of medical errors. Many tools for improving patient safety focus on better communication.

The focus of this article is on patient safety. Numerous tools for developing a safety framework that can be applied in neonatal care are reviewed. Unplanned extubation (UE) is then used as an example of a major safety concern for NICU patients to illustrate how a systematic approach to improving patient safety can lead to reduction in patient harm.

DESIGNING A SAFE WORK SYSTEM

The IHI has established a framework for patient safety that integrates 2 broad areas with a common focus on patient and family engagement[1]: establishing a safety culture and[2] developing a learning system (**Fig. 1**). A safety culture must incorporate psychological safety, accountability, teamwork, communication, and negotiation. The continuous learning system relies on transparency, reliability, improvement, and measurement. Engagement of leadership at the highest levels is essential to the success of both domains.

There are several other models describing patient safety efforts that bear mentioning. Reason's[8] Swiss Cheese Model describes how the holes in different parts of a process must line up in order for an error to be propagated. Vincent and colleagues[9] expanded on Reason's model by organizing the factors that affect clinical practice into distinct categories, such as team factors, patient characteristics, and

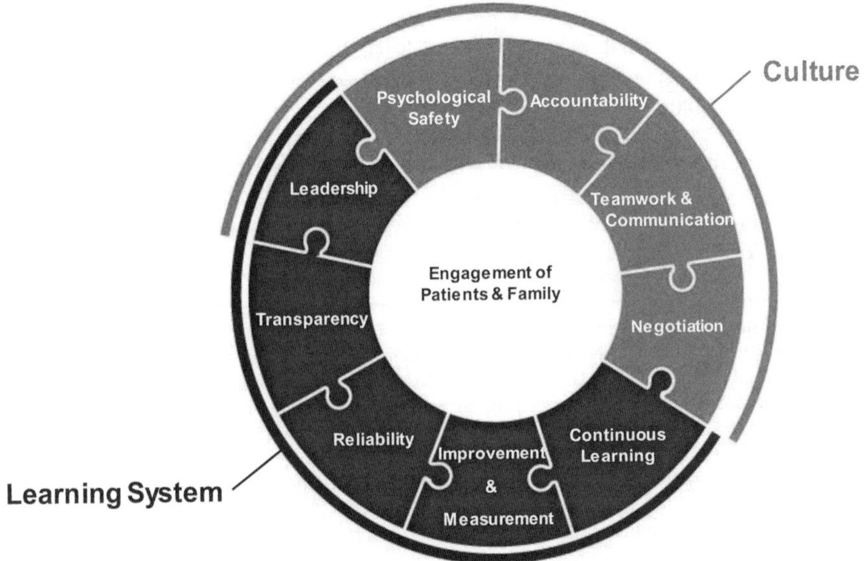

Fig. 1. Patient safety framework. (*Reprinted from* www.IHI.org with permission of the Institute for Healthcare Improvement (IHI), © 2016.)

work environment. The Donabedian[10] model is a framework that subdivides the work system into structure, process, and outcomes.

Building on Donabedian's work, a group at the University of Wisconsin has developed the more advanced System Engineering Initiative for Patient Safety (SEIPS) model.[11] SEIPS is based on the human factors specialty of industrial engineering and stresses the importance of interaction between people and the environment in which they work. Using this approach, the model makes observations and predictions about performance, the quality of work life, and the services delivered. A safety system is built for each health care process and is broken down into (1) people, (2) tasks, (3) tools and technologies, (4) physical environment, and (5) organizational conditions. This model has been applied in various health care settings but requires the expertise of individuals knowledgeable in human factors science and the systems approach to building safer systems of care. Undoubtedly, the NICU with its complex care processes and high acuity could benefit from the SEIPS approach.

Returning to the IHI approach, in the following sections, the authors describe specific patient safety tools that can be used in the NICU to address the major components of their model. The authors address both safety culture and the learning system by exploring approaches to each domain's underlying principles.

SAFETY CULTURE

Culture is defined as the shared ways of thinking, acting, and interacting among a group of individuals.[12,13] Medicine has learned about safety from highly reliable industries, such as aviation and nuclear energy, that define a culture of safety as enhancing organizational learning capacity and reducing mistakes.[12,14–16] A strong culture promotes improvements in the quality of health care.[12,17–19] IHI describes a culture of safety as one with high situational awareness throughout an organization and leadership that encourages reporting safety concerns. Developing a strong safety culture leads to a system with high reliability. The authors describe several specific tools that are essential to a safety culture. Following that, the authors characterize safety approaches that contribute to the learning system.

Psychological Safety

Incident reporting is a critical first step in defining a safety culture and must be done with psychological safety measures that ensure no retribution against those who report. Reporting must be integral to the daily work routine. Staff members should be encouraged to report adverse events, medical errors, and near misses.[20] The Harvard Medical Practice Study defined an adverse event as "an injury that was caused by medical management (rather than the underlying disease) and that prolonged the hospitalization, produced a disability at the time of discharge, or both."[21] Whereas a medical error is "an act of commission (doing something wrong) or omission (failing to do the right thing) leading to an undesirable outcome or significant potential for such an outcome."[21] The definition of a near miss is "any event that could have had adverse consequences but did not and was indistinguishable from fully fledged adverse events in all but outcome."[22] Quantifying both adverse events and errors has value because studies have shown that errors may not always be linked to patient harm.[23,24]

Having a standardized system for reporting and review of medical errors, adverse events, and near misses is a critical component to a safety culture. Incident reporting is important because trending event reports has the added value of early identification of those issues that need a rapid response. Reports of frequently occurring events often lead to QI initiatives contributing to the learning system. Reporting also allows for common cause analysis across the continuum of care to address the underlying causes of safety events that are similar in nature.

Studies show that only a small percentage of adverse events and even fewer near misses are detected by incident reporting.[25] In order to improve the effectiveness of event reporting it (1) must be quick and user friendly so that providers can easily incorporate it into their work flow; (2) must be nonpunitive; (3) should not emphasize individual performance but rather the system of care during event analysis; (4) should be integrated into staff performance assessments; (5) should provide rapid feedback about the response to an event to improve reporter validation; and (6) should display the value in reporting and increase the likelihood of reporting future events.[25]

Accountability

Creating a safety culture requires that everyone involved focuses on making the system of care more reliable. This focus may, at times, conflict with the desire of health care providers and even leadership to assign individual responsibility. Although individual accountability sometimes plays a role in safety issues, this is commonly dealt with through the peer review process. A just culture must be used to ensure fairness in the peer review process with a stepwise approach that ranges from consoling initially to discipline for recurrent episodes.[26] A just culture enables open discussion to develop strategies to prevent the next potential error.[7,27] Management is responsible for establishing reliable processes that provide feedback regarding event reports. Systems that engage in these learning practices identify deviations from safe practices early, enable analysis of the underlying causes, and reduce the probability of recurrence. Human error should never be considered the cause of an adverse event but rather the underlying conditions that allowed a human error to propagate and reach patients. A just culture encourages staff to become problem solvers as opposed to the defenders of the status quo.

Teamwork

Many safety tools are available that develop a safety culture through improvements in teamwork and communication. Some of these tools focus on developing a shared mental model so that ad hoc teams can function effectively. The tools that will be discussed include safety briefings and team training. Closely tied to these are safety tools that seek to improve communication including identifying safety leaders, leadership rounds, huddles, standardized communication, checklists, read backs, and debriefing.

Safety briefings are a tool that frontline staff can use to communicate information about potential concerns on a daily basis.[28] These briefings are often led by the NICU manager to facilitate situational awareness of specific patient safety issues within the unit. Successful safety briefings must be nonpunitive, brief, open, easy to use, and applicable to all patient safety issues. Briefings ensure that the entire team is aware of safety concerns.

Good teamwork is essential to effective neonatal care. Simulation is one tool that enhances situational awareness and improves communication in a nonthreatening environment. Joint simulation exercises between the obstetric and neonatal team may lead to a more seamless delivery of care. Simulation emphasizes the importance of role assignments and teaches communication skills. Video recording of resuscitations helps identify gaps in care and potential areas for improvement.[29] There are programs, such as Team Strategies and Tools to Enhance Performance and Patient Safety, that create a common mental model for those involved in high-acuity care.[30]

Communication

One of the more useful approaches to improving communication is ensuring that front-line staff knows who to contact with their safety concerns. This objective can be achieved through several different approaches. One potential solution is designating a patient safety officer (PSO) who has knowledge of safety tools and improvement methodologies.[7] The individual in this role imports and reinforces best practices and develops organizational policies to advance patient safety. The PSO can function within the context of the NICU alone but should report through the safety infrastructure of the organization to ensure alignment with the system-level safety goals. Ideally, the PSO helps to integrate risk management, quality assurance, QI, and other focused resources that share a common strategic aim. QI and data measurement experts support the PSO to measure and reduce gaps in patient safety.

Another option to build a communication network from the grassroots level is to identify safety champions within the neonatal unit. These individuals should receive basic training in patient safety so that when staff raises concerns they know when to escalate these up the chain of command.[31]

Organizations can demonstrate commitment to building a safety culture with patient safety leadership walk rounds.[32] There is great value in having executive leadership together with unit-specific leadership make safety rounds throughout the institution. NICU and executive leaders can have informal and confidential interactions with front-line staff about safety issues and encourage reporting errors. Leadership safety rounds can serve as a catalyst for improvement by establishing communication between executive leadership, management, and staff.

Huddles identify high-risk situations and alert staff to impending problems. These huddles are often held at the start of each shift and have been shown to decrease the likelihood of medical errors and adverse events.[20] Because neonatology and obstetrics are so interdependent, it is useful to huddle together to maximize the benefit. Huddles are another safety tool that leads to better communication by aligning thought processes among staff.

Structured communication within an organization facilitates patient safety. The communication tool Situation-Background-Assessment-Recommendation provides the framework for communication between 2 members of a health care team about a patient's condition.[7,33] Standardized communication between members of the NICU team removes ambiguity and improves care. This approach to communication was developed in highly reliable organizations.

The use of timeouts in the NICU is an important component to enhance communication for procedures. This activity, done before the procedure, properly identifies the patient, the procedure being done, and the laterality. Although more widely used in the operating room, use of a time-out before a NICU procedure improves safety by ensuring that the right patient gets the right procedure on the right side.[34]

Checklists are integral to health care safety and remind the care team of all necessary steps in the process and facilitate communication when a component is either omitted or done out of sequence.[35] Checklists are particularly useful in the NICU to improve communication for rare procedures, such as exchange transfusion.

Read backs optimize communication in a high-risk setting like the NICU. These read backs may be particularly useful during resuscitation when verbal orders are used. This closed-loop communication reduces the risk of medication and other errors in any critical care environment.[36]

Debriefing, borrowed from the aviation and aerospace industries, is a communication tool that is becoming more pervasive in health care.[37] After an event, such as a delivery, surgery, or resuscitation, the staff reviews what happened in a critical but nonjudgmental manner. A debrief should have structure, be brief, and occur proximal to the event. Ideally, a debrief should follow all events not only those during which a problem occurred.

Negotiation

Negotiation is one of the tenets of a safety culture. It involves having the health care providers of different disciplines come to general agreement on important matters. This negotiation can be challenging because historically, physicians have been trained to practice with autonomy. Physicians are likely to resist standardization and adherence to clinical practice guidelines.[7,38,39] One effective strategy is for senior leaders to identify physician safety champions who are effective at removing the hierarchy thereby promoting communication and collaboration among team members of various disciplines.

THE LEARNING SYSTEM

In 2004 at the World Alliance for Patient Safety, Sir Liam Donaldson stated "To err is human, to cover up is unforgivable, and to fail to learn is inexcusable."[40] Developing a learning system is integral to the IHI Framework for Patient Safety and equally important to the safety culture. The foundations for the learning system are transparency, reliability, continuous learning, and improvement/measurement. Specific tools for each of these fundamental concepts are shared in this next section.

Transparency

Keeping families well informed about their baby's condition and plan of care is an essential component of family centered neonatal care. Maintaining transparency and open lines of communication can be challenging but also rewarding. In the NICU setting, parents can participate in multidisciplinary daily rounds as a model for shared decision-making. Improving health literacy and reducing ethnic disparities are key drivers in delivering high-quality patient-centered care.[7] The use of interpreters in medical settings enhances communication for families with limited English proficiency and improves safety.[41] Transparency can be especially difficult when our patients are subjects of a medical error or when end-of-life discussions are necessary. Disclosure and palliative care programs promote open, honest communication and assist the health care team to care for the family under challenging circumstances.[42]

By engaging the family, they become integrated into the NICU safety program. Family members can provide another layer of defense against adverse events by observing things that others may miss.[7,20] Some institutions have gone so far as to incorporate family members into the root cause analysis (RCA) process, QI initiatives, and other patient safety activities.[43] Engaging families creates a learning environment for the entire health care team.

Reliability

Reliability is defined as failure-free operation over time that improves patient safety. A reliable system is designed to compensate for the limits of human ability. The principles of reliability can be applied to a health care system using the 3-step model proposed by the IHI[44]:

1. Prevent failure in an operation by the standardization of care with best practices.
2. Identify and mitigate failure.
3. Redesign the process based on the critical failure identified.

Leadership that follows these steps will be nimbler to reduce variation and maintain safety.

One simple tool that can enhance reliability of a specific process is the double check verification. Double checks improve patient safety in the NICU by having 2 providers verify a medication order or breastmilk feeding. Having a second person confirm reduces the likelihood of an error occurring during these processes. Many NICUs now use electronic scanners for medications and breastmilk feedings, but when this technology is not available the double check is a reasonable alternative.

Continuous Learning

Advances in information technology (IT) have afforded health care providers substantial benefits to make care safer. One advantage is the ability to categorize and monitor different types of medical errors and perform common cause analysis to ascertain how often a certain type of error is occurring, whether it is occurring in the same type of patient or if the same providers are involved.[45] These data allow a unit to benchmark their results against other similar units and focus safety efforts. These IT tools are the key to learning from past errors and using that knowledge to prevent future adverse events.

IT also promotes learning through the use of clinical decision support (CDS).[46] These reminders alert providers about possible drug interactions, correct dosages, and the correct time to order certain treatments. CDS works well in the NICU environment with its high acuity, frequent handoffs, and multiple providers. Hard stops, another IT safety tool, work by preventing providers from entering incorrect orders or discharging patients without completing certain tasks. IT is a critical aspect of the learning system that will continue to flourish as new tools are developed.

Improvement/Measurement

W. Edwards Deming, one of the early leaders of the QI movement said, “In God we trust, all others bring data.”[47] Fundamental to the learning system is to measure our errors before we can begin to improve them. There are different ways to capture the data and compare our results to those of others. A trigger tool is defined as an occurrence or flag found on review of the medical record that triggers further investigation to determine the presence of an adverse event.[48] The initial use of trigger tools was to identify medication safety events.[49] Triggers identify up to 10 times as many adverse events than random chart review or event reporting by narrowing the field to patients likely to have experienced an adverse event.[48,50,51] An example in the NICU would be a blood glucose level of greater than 150 to identify patients who potentially received too high a glucose infusion rate. This trigger narrows the scope of your investigation but will also capture some patients who are hyperglycemic for other reasons.

A study of 15 North American NICUs yielded a list of 17 NICU-specific trigger tools to identify adverse events.[48] The study found that early gestation infants were at the highest risk for adverse events, the most common being nosocomial infections, catheter infiltrates, abnormal cranial imaging, and unplanned extubation. Fifty-six percent were deemed preventable, and only 8% had a safety report associated with the event. Trigger tools improve the rate of the identification of adverse events, provide a consistent methodology that promotes tracking over time, and allow benchmarking.

ERROR ANALYSIS

Once errors have been measured they must be carefully analyzed before moving forward with improvements. RCA, failure modes and effects analysis (FMEA), and random safety auditing (RSA) are 3 methods that can contribute to the learning system by effectively analyzing errors and improving safety in the complex NICU workflow.[1]

RCA identifies factors that influence variation in system performance in a retrospective approach. This method serves to identify and correct weaknesses that propagate errors. There are 5 steps to completion of an RCA:

1. Identify events that require an RCA.
2. Assemble a team including frontline staff.
3. Diagram the process.
4. Determine why an event happened with a thorough investigation.
5. Develop and implement a functional action plan.

Fig. 2 is an example of one approach to the organization of an RCA. The Joint Commission has an evidence-based model for RCA.[52]

FMEA is a prospective tool that can be used to evaluate high-risk processes by identifying possible system failures before they occur.[53] Failures are unintended deviations that affect a system. Modes are the pathways in which a system can fail. Effects are the consequences that result from an error. Analysis examines the way that individual processes might interact. The process is diagrammed, potential failure modes identified, and the effects determined. The root causes of these failure modes are prioritized to permit redesigning the process. Continued measurement of the new process is imperative.

RSA can be used to monitor a subset of processes within a system that are prone to error. This method requires a designated audit team and a finite number of audit questions pertinent to the unit. RSA can provide blameless feedback to frontline staff and promote behavioral changes.[3,54] The questions asked can be revised to reflect changing safety priorities. Auditing prevents errors and identifies system failures before they become ingrained in daily practice.

We now have in our armamentarium specific safety tools that address each of the essential components of a safety culture and a learning system. These tools can be applied to a multitude of adverse events and medical errors. UE is one of the more common adverse events in the NICU population with the potential for serious patient harm. The authors applied these tools to mitigate harm from UE in their NICU and characterize their approach in the next section.

A NEONATAL SAFETY ISSUE: UNPLANNED EXTUBATION

UE is generally defined as the unintended removal of an endotracheal tube (ET) in intubated patients. However, there is variation in the neonatal literature as to how UE is defined.[55] Neonates are particularly vulnerable to UE because of longer periods of invasive mechanical ventilation, shorter tracheal anatomy, use of uncuffed ETs, movement due to parents holding their intubated babies, and infrequent use of sedation and paralytic medications. UE may be associated with acute cardiorespiratory compromise and the risks associated with reintubation, such as airway trauma, subglottic stenosis, and ventilator-associated pneumonia, making it a serious safety concern.[56–59]

Data from the Vermont-Oxford Network show that UE requiring reintubation is the fourth most common adverse event in North American NICUs.[48] The incidence of UE in neonates varies from 0.14 to 6.6 UE per 100 ventilator days.[60] The literature from pediatric intensive care units recommends a benchmark of less than 1 UE per 100 ventilator days, whereas no such quality metric exists for the NICU population.[61]

Sentinel Event (SE): Root Cause Analysis Process

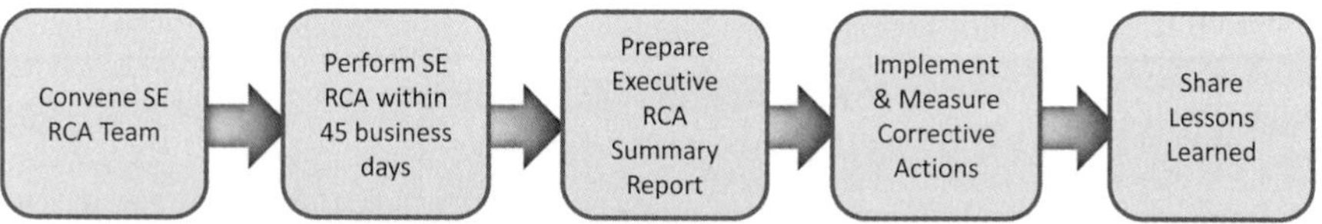

Root Cause Analysis (RCA)

A process for identifying the basic or causal factor(s) that underlie system variation in performance when a sentinel event occurs by examining what happened, why did it happen, what can be done differently to prevent it from happening again and did the actions taken make a difference.

Plan: RCA Planning Process

- Gather clinical facts via post-event debrief, interviews, event simulation, event site visit(s), and pertinent documentation
- Identify current state of processes
- Compile data, policies and evidence-based literature related to the event
- Draft Team Charter with potential system opportunities
- Identify process owners, subject matter experts and ad hoc members
- Develop timeline and appropriate analysis tool(s)

RCA Ground Rules

- Everyone has been invited to this process analysis for their ability to be objective and unbiased
- This process is meant to identify system issues and not point fingers nor assign blame
- We will examine existing processes and systems not individuals
- We will maintain non-judgmental and open discussions
- We will work together to identify opportunities in our system
- We will think creatively to improve care and services

Do: RCA Team Analysis

GOAL: Promote systems thinking and evaluation of human factors

Review Charter with team:

- System opportunities
- Date for completion: The Joint Commission requirement for completion is within 45 business days from sentinel event determination date
- Team member role and responsibility: Each member identified has a specific role and responsibility in the team process

Review Event Timeline with team

Share pertinent literature and data

Utilize analysis tools (see legend) and triggering questions:

- Discuss what happened, what normally happens and what should happen
- Identify key causal factors

Determine potential root cause(s) and significant contributing factors

Develop cause and effect statements

Fig. 2. RCA tool.

Although no widely accepted NICU benchmark exists, recent QI efforts with defined neonatal preventive strategies have led to a reduction in this complication to less than 1 UE per 100 ventilator days.[55,57,60] Recently the *US News & World Report* ranking includes evaluation of the NICU UE rate.[62] As medicine moves toward measuring quality of care through outcome metrics, there is already evidence that UE is becoming one way to evaluate NICU quality.

Factors Affecting Endotracheal Tube Safety

Published reports about neonatal UE place much emphasis on defining the risk factors that contribute to UE in order to develop effective risk reduction strategies. The length

Sentinel Event: Root Cause Analysis Process

Do: RCA Action Plan Reporting

GOAL: Develop and design mistake proofing strategies to promote change and prevent future harm

- Utilize the hierarchy of action matrix to develop and implement mistake proofing strategies and corresponding action plans for each causal factor identified
- Identify the process owner for accountability of each action plan
- Finalize with the process owner a target date for implementation of each action plan

Do: RCA Feedback

GOAL: Feedback to organization of team analysis findings and recommendations for actions

- Prepare and disseminate final RCA reports

Check: RCA Control Plan

GOAL: Develop a plan for measurement and control of action plans to achieve new performance

Develop control plans to:

- Identify and track specific metrics to assess effectiveness of strategies
- Identify mode and frequency of measurement
- Identify who collects the data and a mechanism for reporting
- Develop a response plan, including criteria for taking action

Act: RCA Followup

GOAL: Promote accountability, benchmarking and organizational sharing

- Monitor strategy completion
- Display results of actions
- Identify and address barriers to success with appropriate senior leadership involvement
- Share Lessons Learned for application in all areas of the organization

Fig. 2. (*continued*).

of neonatal intubation, correlation to birth weight, methods for securing the ET tube, kangaroo care, and staff models and competency have all been defined in the literature as risk factors for neonatal UE.[57,63–66]

Length of intubation was characterized in a retrospective study that showed that infants who experienced UE had both longer length of stay and days of ventilation.[63] Additionally, a multivariate analysis of the risk for UE in 222 neonates showed that the duration of the mechanical ventilation was the only statistically significant independent predictor of UE.[64] What remains unclear is if UE leads to longer periods of ventilation or if being intubated for more time increases the risk of UE. There is variation in the reported rates of reintubation following UE from 30% to 50% in 2 studies, which raises questions about different levels of tolerance for extubation based on experience, local practices, and the willingness to use noninvasive forms of ventilation.[57,63] An effective strategy to prevent many UEs is to have clinical practice guidelines that select which patients require intubation and promote a daily assessment for weaning ventilator support to facilitate planned extubation.[67]

With regard to the correlation of UE and birth weight (BW), a study over a 5.5-year period showed that there was an inverse relationship between the rate of UE and birth weight with a degree of variation from 3.6 UE per100 ventilator days in infants born less than 1000 g compared with 1 UE per 100 ventilator days in infants greater than

2500 g.[57] Understanding that this relationship may not be causal, it can still help target QI efforts to the highest-risk patients.

Even though a recent Cochrane library review was unable to conclude the optimal method for securing an ET,[65] Loughead and colleagues[57] were able to show a decreased UE rate after standardization of securing the ET tube and no other practice change. Standardization has been shown to be a founding principle of continuous QI.[68] Furthermore, biases against ventilated neonates receiving kangaroo care were challenged when a study demonstrated that intubated neonates could safely complete kangaroo care without UE if they were ventilated for greater than 24 hours, on low ventilator settings, had stable vital signs, and no vasopressor administration.[69] Lastly, research has not demonstrated a correlation between UE and nurse to patient ratios or years of nursing experience.[63,66]

Using Safety and Quality Improvement Tools to Address Unplanned Extubation

Prospective data collection tools provide an objective investigation of the UE and can be used to characterize the causes in a specific unit.[57] A data collection sheet, which describes the UE event, is completed by the frontline staff at the time of the UE, after stabilization of the infant. Use of a data collection tool promotes a structured approach for an immediate interdisciplinary team debrief that encourages shared responsibility without placing blame. A sample of a data collection sheet is provided in **Fig. 3**.[70] One critical factor to the authors' success is conducting a local RCA within 72 hours of each UE event.

In the authors' unit, the RCA was conducted by an interdisciplinary team, which includes the QI champions consisting of physician lead, nurse champion, and respiratory therapy champion, in addition to the clinical nurse educator, nurse manager, and medical director. The RCA began with review of the UE event data collection sheet by the physician QI leader. Then the entire team reviewed the summary of the event and added information from interviews with the involved frontline staff. After identifying the circumstances surrounding the UE event, the RCA team determined systemic causes and vulnerabilities that answer the question of why the event happened. The focus of the event analysis is never on individual performance, and effort is made to make the determination of causes that are systems based and blameless.[71] The RCA team then formulated casual statements that led to recommendations for action and implementation. This process promotes further team collaboration and improvement of their outcome measure. Using a NICU huddle board allowed safety information to be shared about UE. Recommendations from the RCA were distributed to each discipline's leadership and frontline staff electronically, at staff meetings, and displayed on the unit huddle board. In addition, the number of days since the last UE was posted to further highlight the NICU's team effort surrounding UE prevention and promote motivation for interdisciplinary collaboration.

A Pareto chart is a simple tool to focus improvement efforts on the aspects of process that will have the greatest impact by listing contributing factors in order of descending frequency.[59] The QI team focuses their improvement efforts on those factors that account for the top 80% of the problem also known as the "vital few."[68] The prospective data analysis provided reliable information from which a Pareto chart could be made to narrow the focus of the proposed QI interventions.

A key driver diagram is helpful as a road map for QI efforts. **Table 1** shows an example developed in the authors' tertiary care level IV NICU. The changes can then be refined with repeated cycles of improvement. It is useful for staff engagement to develop risk reduction strategies around one primary driver first to

Patient identifier information: Date and Time of UE event:	Birth gestation age: Birth weight:	Corrected gestation age: Current weight:

Review below questions with the interdisciplinary team after stabilization of infant.
Check box where applicable.

Infant is in:
☐ Isolette ☐ Radiant warmer ☐ Open crib

ET Tube secured with tube holder per unit guideline:
☐ YES ☐ NO (if no, please state reason for exception)
Was adhesive secured to face?
☐ YES ☐ NO
Was ET tube secured at the correct position?
☐ YES ☐ NO

Ventilator tubing secured in 2 places per unit guideline?
☐ YES ☐ NO (if no, please state reason for exception)

Is infant receiving sedation medication?
☐ YES, Continuous infusion: ______ ☐ YES, last PRN given:_____ ☐ NO
Was sedation adequate for the activity of the infant?
☐ YES ☐ NO

What were the events surrounding the UE? (check all that apply)
☐ Infant was moving ☐ Infant was sleeping ☐ Radiograph performed ☐ Nurse care hands on
☐ Infant kangarooing ☐ Infant being weighed ☐ Infant repositioned ☐ ET tube re-secured
☐ Infant given bath ☐ Other: ___________

Nurse to patient ratio at time of UE: (check one)
☐ 1:1 ☐ 1:2 ☐ 1:3
Number of infants with ET tube in the NICU at the time of UE:
Provide number 1-18: ______
NICU census:
Provide number 1-18: ______

Was the infant re-intubated?
☐ YES ☐ NO
If yes:
# of attempts: ________
Medications used: ________
Complications: __________

Describe the events surrounding this UE?
Are there any factors that may have prevented this UE?
Providers present for this event review (circle): RN RT Charge nurse NP Resident Fellow Attending
Incident report completed by (write nurse name): ___________

Fig. 3. Unplanned extubation event data collection tool is completed and reviewed by the multidisciplinary team after each Unplanned extubation. NP, nurse practitioner; RN, registered nurse; RT, respiratory therapist.

establish small gains and then build on them. The authors' interventions incorporated the use of checklists: (1) a checklist for standardized ventilator setup by respiratory therapy, (2) a checklist for a standardized bed space setup by nursing staff, and (3) a checklist to assess the security of the ET used by the interdisciplinary team.

The process control chart (U chart) in **Fig. 4** shows the progression of the implementation of the key drivers in the authors' level IV NICU. The authors' unit was able to reduce the UE rate from 3.3 to 0.98 UE per 100 ventilator days from 2014 to 2016.

Table 1
Key driver diagram for UE: Four primary drivers were identified to reduce UE in the NICU

Aim	Primary Drivers	Secondary Drivers (Interventions)
Reduce UE in the NICU from 3.6 UE per 100 ventilator days to <1.0 UE per 100 ventilator days	Standardize ET tube securing method	Guideline for preparing skin, securing and resecuring ET tube holder Staff checks for competency Establish special population that may deviate from guideline
	Standardize ventilator setup	Guideline for conventional vent setup Guideline for high-frequency oscillator vent setup Guideline for high-frequency jet ventilator
	Standardize care of ventilated infant	2 Clinicians required to move intubated infant Standardize documentation of ET tube location checks Chest radiographs with head midline Rounding tool checklist
	Increase communication, awareness, and spreading safety culture	Team debriefing immediately after UE Clinicians document event: RN incident report and progress note, RT event form, MD notify project leader for review Display run chart and days since last UE on central huddle board

These primary drivers include interventions (secondary drivers) that underwent multiple PDSA (Plan-Do-Study-Act) cycles.

Abbreviations: MD, doctor of medicine; RN, registered nurse; RT, respiratory therapist.

Data from Boc J, Muller J, Gilroy P, et al. Reducing unplanned extubation in a level IV neonatal intensive care unit. Abstract presented at the Pediatric Academic (PAS) 2016 Meeting. Baltimore (MD), April 30-May 3, 2016.

The success of this project was that they were able to identify and mitigate the contributing factors unique to their unit.

With the prevalence of intubation decreasing due to increased use of noninvasive ventilation, there is an even greater need to standardize the authors' processes around neonatal ET care. The QI efforts were able to overcome a plateau in improvement during 2015 (see **Fig. 4**) by shifting the focus to interdisciplinary collaboration and empowering staff to take responsibility for each UE. Teamwork and an interdisciplinary approach are tantamount for the successful implementation of improvement strategies.

UE is a safety issue that demonstrates how reporting and monitoring adverse events supports the development of continuous QI. A well-designed safety infrastructure and the use of selective safety and QI tools enables a health system to be more facile at recognizing and managing deviations from the desired standard of care. The authors used a data collection tool to develop a shared mental model and perform a focused RCA on each event. Checklists were used to standardize processes and reduce variation. Pareto analysis enabled the authors to determine which factors contributed the

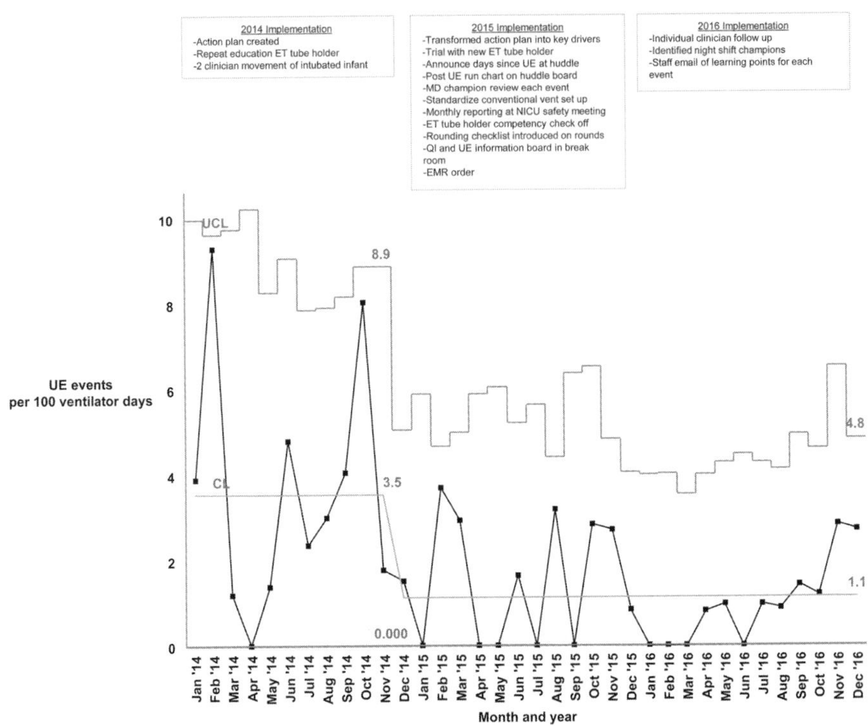

Fig. 4. Process control chart (U chart) UE count per intubated day displayed monthly from 2014 to 2016. The solid gray line represents the mean during measurement period, 2 UE per 100 ventilator days. After multiple PDSA (Plan-Do-Study-Act) cycles, special cause variation achieved by December 2015. CL, control limit; EMR, electronic medical record; UCL, upper control limit. (*Data from* Boc J, Muller J, Gilroy P, et al. Reducing unplanned extubation in a level IV neonatal intensive care unit. Abstract presented at the Pediatric Academic (PAS) 2016 Meeting. Baltimore (MD), April 30-May 3, 2016.)

most to UE in their unit. A driver diagram was helpful in deciding how to facilitate improvement in a stepwise fashion.

Engaging staff and changing the culture in your unit is the key to successful QI initiatives. This engagement was done by displaying data in a visually apparent way, such as showing days from last UE on the authors' huddle board. Celebrating success helps to keep everyone involved and focused on the same goal. Maintaining change can be challenging, which is why it behooves the QI team to continue monitoring the outcome measures even after the project has reached its completion.

SUMMARY

The NICU population is more vulnerable to adverse events because of inherent characteristics and the high-intensity environment of the NICU. There is a growing importance of establishing a high-level safety infrastructure as neonatal outcomes are being measured to determine the quality of care. A patient safety framework must include a work system that is designed for safety, a strong culture of safety that is nonpunitive yet balances systems improvement with individual accountability, and improved teamwork and communication. Equally important is a learning system based on transparency, reliability, improvement, and measurement. In order to create a highly reliable NICU, it requires constant system evaluation and measurement of quality metrics. Adverse events must be analyzed and communicated back to frontline staff in order to propagate a true safety culture. None of this is possible without leadership support throughout the organization.

UE is an example of a safety and quality metric that affects the long-term outcome of ventilated neonates. Improvement in the rate of UE rate is clearly possible and demonstrates specific metrics can be assessed to achieve a higher level of performance.

Patient safety in the NICU is an obligation and a challenge. Learning from adverse events and near misses is essential to the process of improvement. Working together as an interdisciplinary team and using the correct tools, we can create a safer environment of care for high-risk neonates and improve their outcomes.

ACKNOWLEDGMENTS

The authors wish to thank Ann Principe MBA, MSM, RN, CPHQ, Senior Patient Safety Project Manager in the Department of Patient Safety and Accreditation at Christiana Care Health System for developing **Fig. 2**.

REFERENCES

1. Ursprung R, Gray J. Random safety auditing, root cause analysis, failure mode effects analysis. Clin Perinatol 2010;37:141–65.
2. Kaushal R, Bates DW, Landrigan C, et al. Medication errors and adverse drug events in pediatric inpatients. JAMA 2001;285(16):2114–20.
3. Ursprung R, Gray JE, Edwards WH, et al. Real time patient safety audits: improving safety every day. Qual Saf Health Care 2005;14(4):284–9.
4. Gray JE, Suresh G, Ursprung R, et al. Patient misidentification in the neonatal intensive care unit: quantification of risk. Pediatrics 2006;117(1):e43–7.
5. Simpson JH, Lynch R, Grant J, et al. Reducing medication errors in the neonatal intensive care unit. Arch Dis Child Fetal Neonatal Ed 2004;89(6):F480–2.
6. Leonard M, Graham S, Bonacum D. The human factor: the critical importance of effective teamwork and communication in providing safe care. Qual Saf Health Care 2004;13:i85–90.
7. Botwinick L, Bisognano M, Haraden C. Leadership guide to patient safety. IHI innovation series white paper. Cambridge, (MA): Institute for Healthcare Improvement; 2006. Available at: www.IHI.org.
8. Reason J. Human error. Cambridge (England): Cambridge University Press; 1990.
9. Vincent C, Taylor Adams S, Stanhope N. Framework for analyzing risk and safety in clinical medicine. Br Med J 1998;316:1154–7.
10. Donabedian A. The quality of medical care. Science 1978;200:856–64.
11. Calayon P, Schoofs Hundt A, Karsh BT, et al. Work system design for patient safety: the SEIPS model. Qual Saf Health Care 2006;15(Suppl 1):i50–8.
12. Hoff TJ, Pohl H, Bartfield J. Implementing safety cultures in medicine: what we learn by watching physicians. In: Henriksen K, Battles JB, Marks ES, et al, editors. Advances in patient safety: from research to implementation (volume 1: research findings). Rockville (MD): Agency for Healthcare Research and Quality (US); 2005.

13. Schein E. The learning culture: managing the contradictions of stability, learning and change. In: organizational culture and leadership. San Francisco (CA): Jossey-Bass Inc; 1992. p. 363–73.
14. Gaba DM. Structural and organizational issues in patient safety. Calif Manage Rev 2000;43(1):83–101.
15. Helmreich RL, Merritt AC, Wilhelm JA. The evolution of crew resource management in commercial aviation. Int J Aviat Psychol 1999;9(1):19–32.
16. Weick KE, Roberts KH. Collective mind in organizations: heedful interrelating on flight decks. Admin Sci Quart 1993;38(September):357–81.
17. Argyris C. On organizational learning. Boston: Blackwell Publishers, Inc; 1999.
18. Senge PM. The fifth discipline: the art and practice of the learning organization. New York: Currency and Doubleday; 1990.
19. Schön D. The reflective practitioner: how professionals think in action. New York: Basic Books, Inc; 1983.
20. Institute for Healthcare Improvement. Develop a culture of safety. Available at www.ihi.org. Accessed November 3, 2016.
21. Brennan TA, Leape LL, Laird NM, et al. Incidence of adverse events and negligence in hospitalized patients – results of the Harvard medical practice study I. N Engl J Med 1991;324:370–6.
22. Barach P, Small SD. Reporting and preventing medical mishaps: lessons from non- medical near miss reporting systems. Br Med J 2000;320:759–63.
23. Griffin FA, Resar RK. IHI global trigger tool for measuring adverse events. (second edition). IHI innovation series white paper. Cambridge, (MA): Institute for Healthcare Improvement; 2009. Available at: www.IHI.org.
24. Layde PM, Maas LA, Teret SP, et al. Patient safety efforts should focus on medical injuries. JAMA 2002;287(15):1993–7.
25. Kaldjian LC, Jones EW, Wu BJ, et al. Reporting medical errors to improve patient safety. Arch Intern Med 2008;168(1):40–6.
26. Dekker S. Just culture: balancing safety and accountability. 3rd edition. Boca Raton (FL): CRC Press; 2012.
27. Reason J. Managing the risks of organizational accidents. Hampshire (England): Ashgate Publishing Limited; 1997.
28. Institute for Healthcare Improvement. Safety briefings. Available at: www.ihi.org. Accessed November 3, 2016.
29. Carbine DN, Finer NN, Knodel E, et al. Video recording as a means of evaluating neonatal resuscitation performance. Pediatrics 2000;106(4):654–8.
30. Clancy CM, Tornberg DN. Team STEPPS: assuring optimal teamwork in clinical settings. Am J Med Qual 2007;22(3):214–7.
31. Shekelle PG, Pronovost PJ, Wachter RM, et al. Advancing the science of patient safety. Ann Intern Med 2011;154(10):693–6.
32. Campbell DA, Thompson M. Patient safety rounds: description of an inexpensive but important strategy to improve the safety culture. Am J Med Qual 2007;22(1): 26–33.
33. Kaiser Permanente of Colorado. SBAR technique for communication: a situational briefing model. Available at: www.ihi.org. Accessed November 3, 2016.
34. Samner CE, Lykens K, Singh K, et al. What is a patient safety culture? A review of the literature. J Nurs Scholarsh 2010;42(2):156–65.
35. Hales B, Terblanche M, Fowler R, et al. Development of medical checklists for improved quality of patient care. Int J Qual Health Care 2008;20(1):22–30.

36. Hargestam M, Lindkvist M, Brolin C, et al. Communication in interdisciplinary teams: exploring closed-loop communication during in situ trauma team training. BMJ Open 2013;3:e003525.
37. Edelson DP, Litzinger B, Arora V, et al. Improving in-hospital cardiac arrest process and outcomes with performance debriefing. Arch Intern Med 2008; 168(10):1063–9.
38. Wachter R, Shojania K. Internal bleeding: the truth behind America's terrifying epidemic of medical mistakes. New York: Rugged Land Press; 2004.
39. Pronovost PJ. Enhancing physicians' use of clinical guidelines. JAMA 2013; 310(23):2501–2.
40. Available at: http://www.who.int/patientsafety/launch/en/index1.html Accessed February 24, 2017.
41. Flores G. The impact of medical interpreters on the quality of healthcare: a systematic review. Med Care Res Rev 2005;65(3):255–99.
42. Boss R, Kavanaugh K, Kobler K. Prenatal and neonatal palliative care in textbook of interdisciplinary pediatric palliative care. Philadelphia: Elsevier; 2011.
43. Zimmerman TM, Amori G. Including patients in root cause and system failure analysis. J Healthc Manag 2007;27(2):27–34.
44. Nolan T, Esar R, Haraden C, et al. Improving the reliability of healthcare. IHI innovation series white paper. Cambridge, (MA): Institute for Healthcare Improvement; 2004. Available at: www.IHI.org.
45. Clapper C, Crea K. Common cause analysis. 2010. Available at: http://www.psqh.com/analysis/common-cause-analysis/. Accessed January 9, 2017.
46. Garg AX, Adhikari NKJ, McDonald H, et al. Effects of computerized clinical decision support systems on practitioner performance and patient outcomes. JAMA 2005;293(10):1223–38.
47. Available at: http://www.goodreads.com/quotes/34849-in-god-we-trust-all-others-bring-data. Accessed February 27, 2017.
48. Institute for Healthcare Improvement. Trigger tool for measuring adverse drug events. Available at: www.ihi.org. Accessed November 3, 2016.
49. Sharek PJ, Horbar JD, Mason W, et al. Adverse events in the neonatal intensive care unit: development, testing, and findings of a NICU focused trigger tool to identify harm in North American NICUs. Pediatrics 2006;118(4):1332–40.
50. Rozich JD, Haraden CR, Resar RK. Adverse drug event trigger tool: a practical methodology for measuring medication related harm. Qual Saf Health Care 2003;12:194–200.
51. Resar RK, Rozich JD, Classen DC. Methodology and rationale for the measurement of harm with trigger tools. Qual Saf Health Care 2003;12:39–45.
52. Root cause analysis and action plan framework template. 2013. Available at: https://www.jointcommission.org/framework_for_conducting_a_root_cause_analysis_and_action_plan/. Accessed February 22, 2017.
53. Reiling JG, Knutzen BL, Stoecklein M. FMEA – the cure for medical errors. Qual Prog 2003;67–71.
54. United States Agency for Healthcare Research and Quality, University of California San Francisco-Stanford Evidence-Based Practice Center. Making health care safer: a critical analysis of patient safety practices. Rockville (MD): Agency for Healthcare Research and Quality, U.S. Dept. of Health and Human Services; 2001.
55. Meyers JM, Pinheiro J, Nelson MU. Unplanned extubation in NICU patients: are we speaking the same language? J Perinatol 2015;35:676–7.

56. Brown MS. Prevention of accidental extubation in newborns. Am J Dis Child 1988; 142(11):1240–3.
57. Loughead JL, Brennan RA, DeJulio P, et al. Reducing accidental extubation in neonates. Jt Comm J Qual Patient Saf 2008;34(3):164–70.
58. Elward AM, Warren DK, Fraser VJ. Ventilator-associated pneumonia in pediatric intensive care unit patients: risk factors and outcomes. Pediatrics 2002;109(5): 758–64.
59. Lucas da Silva PS, Reis ME, Aguilar VE, et al. Unplanned extubation in the neonatal ICU: a systematic review, critical appraisal, and evidence-based recommendations. Respir Care 2013;58(7):1237–45.
60. Merkel L, Beers K, Lewis MM, et al. Reducing unplanned extubations in the NICU. Pediatrics 2014;133(5):e1367–72.
61. Rachman BR, Watson R, Woods N, et al. Reducing unplanned extubations in a pediatric intensive care unit: a systematic approach. Int J Pediatr 2009;2009: 820495.
62. Available at: www.usnews.com/best hospitals/pediatric-rankings/neonatal-care. Accessed January 8, 2017.
63. Veldman A, Trautschold T, Weib K, et al. Characteristics and outcomes of unplanned extubation in ventilated preterm and term newborns on a neonatal intensive care unit. Paediatr Anaesth 2006;16(9):968–73.
64. Carvalho FL, Mezzacappa MA, Calil R, et al. Incidence and risk factors of accidental extubation in a neonatal intensive care unit. J Pediatr (Rio J) 2010;86(3): 189–95.
65. Kamlin CO, Davis PG, Morley CJ. Predicting successful extubation of very low birthweight infants. Arch Dis Child Fetal Neonatal Ed 2006;91:F180–3.
66. Lai M, Inglis GDT, Hose K, et al. Methods for securing endotracheal tubes in newborn infants (review). Cochrane Database Syst Rev 2014;(7):CD007805.
67. Barber JA. Unplanned extubation in the NICU. J Obstet Gynecol Neonatal Nurs 2013;42:233–8.
68. Ellsbury DL, Ursprung R. A primer on quality improvement methodology in neonatology. Clin Perinat 2010;37:87–99.
69. Ludington-Hoe SM, Ferreira C, Swinth J, et al. Safe criteria and procedure for Kangaroo care with intubated preterm infants. J Obstet Gynecol Neonatal Nurs 2003;32(5):579–88.
70. Boc J, Muller J, Gilroy P, et al. Reducing unplanned extubation in a level IV neonatal intensive care unit. Abstract presented at: Pediatric academic (PAS) 2016 meeting. Baltimore, MD, April 30–May 3, 2016.
71. Institute for healthcare improvement open school. Root cause and systems analysis. Available at: http://www.ihi.org/education/ihiopenschool. Accessed February 17, 2017.

Tackling Quality Improvement in the Delivery Room

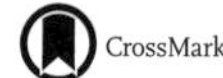

Wannasiri Lapcharoensap, MD[a], Henry C. Lee, MD, MS[b,*]

KEYWORDS

- Quality improvement • Neonatal resuscitation • Very-low-birth-weight infant
- Delivery room • Labor and delivery

KEY POINTS

- Quality improvement (QI) in the delivery room requires a multidisciplinary approach and careful consideration of the unique aspects of the delivery room setting.
- Delivery room attendants may refine their technical and behavioral skills through simulation sessions and use those skills to meet delivery room QI objectives.
- QI projects may be further enhanced by participation in collaborative projects with other neonatal ICUs (NICUs) to promote a culture of information sharing and improvement.
- Improvements in discrete areas of delivery room management of the neonate have the potential to have an impact on neonatal outcomes.

INTRODUCTION

The initial cry of a newborn baby is part of a sequence of events marking a successful transition from intrauterine to neonatal life. With that first cry, the infant pushes fetal lung fluid out and fills the alveoli with air to oxygenate. The pulmonary vasculature relaxes, pulmonary blood flow increases, and oxygenated blood returns to the heart, allowing the infant to achieve independence from placental blood supply. Although this process occurs smoothly in most deliveries, an estimated 5% to 10% of all newborn deliveries require active assistance at birth (stimulation, suction, and so forth) and 1% of births require intensive resuscitation measures.[1] The incidence of intensive

Conflicts of Interest: None.
Funding source for this article: This project was supported by grant number P30HS023506 from the Agency for Healthcare Research and Quality. The content is solely the responsibility of the authors and does not necessarily represent the official views of the Agency for Healthcare Research and Quality.
[a] Department of Pediatrics, CDRCP, Oregon Health & Science University, 707 Southwest Gaines Street, Portland, OR 97239, USA; [b] Department of Pediatrics, California Perinatal Quality Care Collaborative, Stanford University, 1265 Welch Road, Stanford, CA 94305, USA
* Corresponding author.
E-mail address: hclee@stanford.edu

Clin Perinatol 44 (2017) 663–681
http://dx.doi.org/10.1016/j.clp.2017.05.003

measures, such as cardiopulmonary resuscitation, is inversely correlated with gestational age and independently associated with increased morbidity and mortality.[2–5] Furthermore, in each delivery room, the safety of both mother and infant are paramount and the sheer number of equipment and personnel required can contribute to a seemingly chaotic environment. Given the unpredictable nature of the delivery room, there is a need to establish standardized practices and optimize workflow among labor and delivery units to ensure effective care in a timely manner.

The International Liaison Committee on Resuscitation (ILCOR) and the Neonatal Resuscitation Program (NRP) guidelines help provide a framework for the workflow of a delivery room.[6–8] Skilled personnel present at the delivery must possess the technical and behavioral skills for resuscitation, while also ensuring that equipment is readily available. Implementation of these guidelines and training of personnel are often carried out and improved on by institutional QI projects. Delivery room QI is aimed at identifying and improving quantifiable processes to ensure that teams are prepared for all resuscitations. This article discusses what makes the delivery room a unique environment for QI, the various facets of delivery room QI, and specific examples on how to approach delivery room QI.

THE CONTEXT OF THE DELIVERY ROOM FOR QUALITY IMPROVEMENT

The conceptual frameworks for quality of care in the health care setting share a common theme of developing a work environment in which providers work as a team to reliably execute processes of care that are known to work and to avoid care that may be harmful.[9] When considering the environment, team, and processes that are relevant to delivery room care, several distinguishing features may differ from other health care settings (**Box 1**).

Unique Physical Environment

First, the environment of the delivery room can be challenging due to the sheer number of people involved. For example, in the operating room before an infant is born by emergency cesarean section, there can be more than 10 people encompassing 3 different medical teams (obstetrics, pediatrics, and anesthesia) who must work together to ensure safety of both the mother and the fetus/newborn in a discrete amount of time and often in a small amount of space. Each medical specialty plays an important role to improve neonatal outcomes.

Box 1
Unique considerations for delivery room quality improvement

Unique physical environment

- Two patients simultaneously receiving care
- Multidisciplinary personnel and equipment
- Can be chaotic and noisy
- Inadequate space

Unpredictable nature

- Emergency preparedness for every delivery
- Equipment readily available at all times
- Varying personnel

Quality data acquisition

- Efficient and accurate delivery room documentation
- Data collection and reporting for mother and neonate

One Point in a Continuum of Care

Delivering optimal care in the delivery room requires specific preparation and a team's actions in the delivery room can have immediate consequences. The delivery and birth of an infant, however, are but parts of the overall care of the mother and fetus/neonate. When considering QI to improve processes and outcomes for neonatal resuscitation, care of the mother and fetus/neonate can be closely examined prenatally and postnatally. The goal to improve neonatal outcomes through QI in the delivery room may be hindered by suboptimal care that happens prior to or after delivery. For example, administration of antenatal steroids prior to preterm birth is an evidence-based practice; therefore, QI to facilitate consistent practice may complement ongoing delivery room QI for respiratory management.[10] Similarly, a lack of standardization in the NICU for postextubation management could negate gains made in the delivery room.

Unpredictable Nature of Deliveries

Although perinatal risk factors may assist with risk stratification and subsequent preparation for deliveries, a newborn infant may require emergency resuscitation without the presence of any warning signs. Thus any delivery room QI should also consider the unpredictable nature of the delivery room to consistently apply processes to infants most at risk and in need of delivery room assistance. Providers and staff caring for mothers and infants should be familiar with their own institutional processes on how to call for assistance initially and for further help when there is a need to escalate care.

Quality Data Acquisition

A crucial component of QI is standardized data collection to track performance. In considering Donabedian's[11] framework of contextual, process, and outcome measures (including balancing measures), delivery room QI includes those outcomes that are measured immediately but also may include longer-term outcomes. Data collection in the delivery room can be more challenging than in other health care settings. During and after a neonatal resuscitation, the clinicians involved may not have time to document in real time or even immediately after the resuscitation, because they may be busy with postresuscitation care in the NICU. Therefore, working on data quality may be an important aspect of a delivery room QI project.

STRATEGIES FOR IMPLEMENTATION

The unique context of the delivery room translates to aspects of implementation that also may be different from traditional QI strategies (**Box 2**).

Data Collection: Standardized Forms

Acquiring appropriate data from the delivery room for review and QI activities may be challenging. Data may be present in the medical records of mother, infant, or both, and there may be inconsistencies across multiple data sources. The activities surrounding the delivery and resuscitation may not be recorded immediately and subject to errors in recall. Often, there is a circulating nurse assigned to the obstetric team to record times and other actions that are called out as they occur. Such record keeping for neonatal resuscitation, however, is often less consistent.

An aid in data collection for neonatal resuscitation activities can be a standardized form that contains all the pertinent variables considered important for the medical record and for assessment of quality. In the current environment of electronic medical records, most systems facilitate a customized form that contains both standard items

Box 2
Strategies for implementation

Standardized forms for data collection

Video recording and review

Development and utilization of checklists

Simulation training

CRM

Briefings and debriefings

Utilizing technology/telemedicine

required at every delivery (time of birth and Apgar scores), additional variables if resuscitation is required, and free text. An electronic medical record system that automatically fills preselected fields with data from the maternal record can also reduce errors in manual transfer of data. In the process of pursuing a QI project, there may be additional variables that can be standardized for data collection. For example, in 2015, the California Perinatal Quality Care Collaborative (CPQCC) implemented an optional data collection for delayed cord clamping (DCC) to facilitate QI in this area.[12] For this purpose, participating centers have collected data on the following 4 questions:

1. Was delayed umbilical cord clamping performed?
2. (If yes to 1) How long was DCC?
3. Was umbilical cord milking performed?
4. Did breathing begin before umbilical cord clamping?

By standardizing the data collection for DCC, the electronic medical record can be used to keep track of process measures that are relevant to the QI project.

Video Review for Data Collection and Quality Improvement

Video recording and review in the delivery room is one solution to improving data collection and facilitating QI activities.[13,14] Investigators at the University of California, San Diego (UCSD), have had extensive experience in the implementation of video recording of neonatal resuscitations to facilitate QI.[15] Video review can be used to evaluate the performance of teams in providing neonatal resuscitation in regard to following the NRP guidelines, which can be used to develop specific QI goals to address deficiencies.[16] Performance in following NRP guidelines may include excessive action, or errors of commission, such as giving oxygen unnecessarily, as well as errors of omission, such as missing corrective steps to address ineffective positive pressure ventilation (PPV).[16,17]

The UCSD team has used audio and video recordings of neonatal resuscitations since 1999 for quality assurance.[15] Their experience has shown that the medical record is not always consistent with actual practice and can facilitate areas for improvement in communication, systems issues, and team performance. In addition to video recordings, the team at UCSD can also use simultaneous physiologic recordings to align team actions with clinical data.[15]

When considering the start of a video recording program, each center needs to research local regulations and resources available to support the program. A recording system and procedures that can ensure confidentiality for both patients' families and personnel are crucial. In the UCSD program, video recordings are erased at most 14 days after the event.[15] Centers like UCSD have determined that video recording in the delivery room for QI does not require family consent, because it is for the purpose of QI and adequate protections for privacy have been established. If videos are saved for teaching purposes, an explicit consent can be obtained. Similar to UCSD, a center in Germany video records resuscitations as a part of routine patient care and is approved to do so without consent.[18] Other centers, however, may determine that consent is required, which may be obtained as either part of a general consent form completed on admission, as a specific consent for recording in the delivery room, or by signs posted noting the potential recording.

For particularly salient video and audio recordings that could inform future educational efforts, there may be procedures to save recordings for that purpose with consent obtained from patients' families and any personnel who may have been involved in the resuscitation. State regulations may protect recordings that are for the purpose of quality assurance from medicolegal use. Such regulations should be reviewed by local risk management and quality assurance teams prior to program implementation.

Incorporation of the Checklist

The delivery of a newborn and the potential neonatal resuscitation that follows is a quick process. Resuscitation equipment and supplies should be readily available for every delivery. Therefore, preparation prior to delivery is a crucial element to consider in QI. Utilization of checklists can help ensure consistent and accurate set-up of equipment and supplies for each delivery room. Checklists in health care improve safety, reduce human error, and ensure that safety standards are met.[19,20] In a survey of the most optimal elements in a delivery room checklist, participants of a yearlong collaborative QI project noted the broad category of checking and preparing all equipment as the most important content of a checklist.[19] For those clinicians who attended more than 20 deliveries annually, introducing the team and assigning roles were also considered important. The NRP textbook provides a quick equipment checklist and encourages users to tailor the list to their own institutions (**Box 3**).[7] Checklists may be categorized according to specific NRP steps or tasks, and often a supplemental checklist is required for very premature infants. Incorporation of the checklist is consistent across multiple successful QI initiatives in different areas of the delivery room, including equipment checks, predelivery and postdelivery briefings, communication techniques, and specialized care for the extremely premature infant.[19,21–26] In addition to facilitating resuscitations, checklists are a tool for identifying areas for improvement in future QI projects.

Enhancing Skills with Simulation-Based Learning

Institutions have different requirements for who is required to attend deliveries, often depending on known risk factors.[27] Ensuring that these are standardized to best care for mother and infant is important. The skills of any person attending a delivery can be divided into content knowledge, technical skills, and behavioral skills. These skills are often acquired via NRP course completion, which is renewed once every 2 years. Studies have demonstrated waning knowledge retention by 6 months after completion of an NRP course,[28,29] thus supporting the argument that more frequent skill sessions are required. Simulation is a powerful methodology of adult learning with the benefit of allowing mistakes to occur without harm to a real patient.[30,31] For technical skills, such as proper mask positioning or intubation, performing short, brief skill sessions may be beneficial. This allows providers to familiarize themselves with the delivery room environment and equipment. Behavioral skills can be enhanced with a more multidisciplinary approach, complex simulation sessions, and debriefing of the session to

Box 3
Neonatal Resuscitation Program quick equipment checklist

Warm
- Preheated warmer
- Warm towels or blankets
- Temperature sensor and sensor cover for prolonged resuscitation
- Hat
- Plastic bag or plastic wrap (<32 weeks' gestation)
- Thermal mattress (<32 weeks' gestation)

Clear airway
- Bulb syringe
- 10F or 12F suction catheter attached to wall suction, set at 80 mm Hg to 100 mm Hg
- Meconium aspirator

Auscultate
- Stethoscope

Ventilate
- Flowmeter set to 10 L/min
- Oxygen blender set to 21% (21%–30% if <35 weeks' gestation)
- PPV device
- Term-sized and preterm-sized masks
- 8F feeding tube and 20-mL syringe

Oxygenate
- Equipment to give free-flow oxygen
- Pulse oximeter with sensor and cover
- Target oxygen saturation table

Intubate
- Laryngoscope with size 0 and size 1 straight blades (size 00, optional)
- Stylet (optional)
- Endotracheal tubes (sizes 2.5, 3.0, and 3.5)
- CO_2 detector
- Measuring tape and/or endotracheal tube insertion depth table
- Waterproof tape or tube-securing device
- Scissors
- Laryngeal mask (size 1) and 5-mL syringe

Medicate
- Access to
  - 1:10,000 (0.1 mg/mL) epinephrine
  - Normal saline
  - Supplies for placing emergency umbilical venous catheter and administering medications
  - ECG monitor leads and ECG monitor

This checklist includes only the most essential supplies and equipment needed at the radiant warmer for most neonatal resuscitations. Tailor this list to meet unit-specific needs. Ensure that an equipment check has been done prior to every birth.

Reprinted from the Textbook of Neonatal Resuscitation. American Academy of Pediatrics and American Heart Association. 2015; with permission.

provide real-time feedback. In particular, simulation training is a unique opportunity to improve communication skills across multidisciplinary teams.[32,33] Moreover, simulation-based training can be incorporated into QI initiatives—such as improving time to continuous positive airway pressure (CPAP) application, using new equipment to reduce hypothermia, and implementing new communication techniques—allowing delivery room attendants to practice new skills, familiarize themselves with new equipment, and identify system errors in a safe environment.

Multidisciplinary Team Approach: Crew Resource Management

The multidisciplinary nature of the delivery room lends itself to QI methodology while also necessitating a multidisciplinary approach to QI. Labor and delivery room staff are often required to be trained to resuscitate infants and may be called on to assist in the event of a neonatal emergency. Furthermore, in the rare event that both mother and infant are in duress, the teams need to be prepared to work in close quarters to resuscitate 2 individual patients. Formal interdisciplinary simulation training of maternal emergencies with both obstetric and pediatric teams present has the potential to improve neonatal outcomes.[34–36]

The development of teamwork across disciplines may be enhanced by crew resource management (CRM)—a concept developed by the aviation industry. In particular, communication failures heavily contribute to medical errors and can be improved on by CRM training.[37] QI projects may incorporate CRM training as a tool to improve communication in specific arenas, such as ensuring closed-loop communication during assessment of an infant's heart rate during delivery room resuscitation. Simulation is the optimal environment to assess and teach components of CRM.

Briefings and Debriefings

Although ILCOR and NRP guidelines continue to suggest performing briefings and debriefings whenever possible,[38] briefings and debriefings are important components of the delivery room that are often neglected. In a study of 84 NICUs, briefings occurred 66% of the time and debriefings occurred only 19% of the time for very-low-birth-weight infants.[39] Regular use of briefs and debriefings has been demonstrated to improve overall team communication during resuscitations.[24] The brief prior to delivery creates a shared mental model for the resuscitation team and ensures team readiness, similar to a team pause prior to procedures and surgical cases. After a delivery, debriefing can be challenging because team members often disperse to continue care for the infant. Nonetheless, implementation of debriefing is crucial for identifying what went well, what did not go well, and what might be improved. Taking the time to debrief is a powerful tool for revealing systematic, technical, or behavioral errors.

Utilizing Technology for Resuscitation

Because a neonatal emergency may occur in any location, hospital staff should be aware of what resources are available at their own hospital. Many community hospitals now have the capability to use communication technology, such as telemedicine, to assist with resuscitation and care of the neonate.[40] The use of telemedicine in adult trauma and burn patients has been shown to improve adherence to guidelines and overall management of patients and to increase provider confidence in taking care of patients in a remote location.[41–44] In neonates, telemedicine is a proved health information technology used to screen for retinopathy of prematurity due to scarce availability of qualified ophthalmologists.[45,46] Although research in the neonatal resuscitation setting is limited, a high-fidelity simulation study concluded that video-assisted resuscitation significantly improved provider time to effective ventilation and adherence to the NRP guidelines.[47] If live video-assisted telemedicine is unavailable, another recent high-fidelity simulation study demonstrated that a tablet application turned on at the beginning of a resuscitation also allows staff to deliver resuscitation measures (PPV, intubation, and chest compressions) in a timely manner and improve performance.[48] The incorporation of new technology into the workflow requires appropriate training and familiarization but may have a positive impact on delivery room management of infants.

SPECIFIC QUALITY IMPROVEMENT OPPORTUNITIES/APPROACHES

Although neonatal resuscitation occurs in a short window of time, there are many unique aspects of neonatal care that can be used as focus points for improvement (**Box 4**). As QI efforts are undertaken, the various components that lead to successful implementation may include equipment, training in technical and behavioral skills (as discussed previously), and consideration of what outcome and balancing measures are available or feasible for collection during the project (**Table 1**). Although several areas of potential improvement are listed in **Box 4**, a few of those are discussed in more detail in this section. In particular, key components of delivery room QI are highlighted, for which there are examples where QI has successfully led to improved processes and outcomes.

Optimizing the Resuscitation Cart

Delivering effective and timely resuscitation also depends on the ability to readily access effective code carts (resuscitation cart and code cart). Standardization of the code cart is shown in the adult literature to affect patient safety by improving nursing familiarity, confidence, and performance.[49,50] Using the Lean methodology to improve resuscitation and emergency carts is a proved approach in not only neonatal emergencies but also pediatrics and adult care.[51–54] Human factors engineering principles can be used for QI projects to optimize the resuscitation cart as a tool to increase usability while reducing human error and wasteful actions. Further training to familiarize staff to the contents and location of the code cart is also paramount. Within each unit, establishing a culture of safety allows for appropriate use of the neonatal code cart during urgent and emergent situations.

Temperature Management

Admission hypothermia and hyperthermia of a newborn are associated with adverse effects, including increased risk of respiratory distress, intraventricular hemorrhage, and death.[55–57] Several published QI initiatives have successfully reduced admission

Box 4
Examples of quality improvement opportunities in the delivery room

Delivery room layout

Optimizing the neonatal code cart

Appropriate delivery room attendance

Activation of code/back-up team

Temperature management

Respiratory management

Communication among team members

Communication with family

Time to hold in the delivery room

DCC

Care of the very-low-birth-weight infant (golden hour)

hypothermia by using published recommendations by NRP and the World Health Organization, such as ensuring correct use of blankets, hats, radiant warmers, and chemical mattresses and polyethylene wraps when indicated.[25,58–61] Working to increase the ambient temperature of the delivery room or operating room is an effective method to prevent both maternal and neonatal hypothermia.[62] Many of the studies on delivery room QI focus on improving admission temperatures among very-low-birth-weight infants while using checklists and a multidisciplinary approach to ensure adherence to guidelines. In one such study, rates of moderate hypothermia (admission temperature <36°C) were reduced from 55% to approximately 6% without any increase in rates of admission hyperthermia (>37.5°C).[59] Given the known risks of hypothermia, QI focus on admission temperature has the potential to have an impact on clinical outcomes.

Respiratory Support in the Delivery Room

The most recent recommendations from the American Academy of Pediatrics Committee on Fetus and Newborn support the use of CPAP immediately after birth in the preterm infant.[63] The rationale for this approach is the recognition that early CPAP applied optimally is associated with less intubation and may reduce the potential for long-term respiratory morbidity in the form of bronchopulmonary dysplasia, which may translate into lower health care utilization and improved childhood respiratory function.[64–67] The efficient and optimal application of CPAP in the delivery room will benefit from applying many of the principles discussed previously, including appropriate equipment set-up; briefing, including assignment of roles; and communication skills.

Optimal respiratory management in the delivery room has multiple facets and steps (**Table 2**). Because the NRP algorithm relies on accurate measurements of heart rate and oxygen saturation, role assignment and equipment set-up are key factors for effective QI. Further team training in communication and technical skills for ongoing assessment and providing effective PPV are needed to delivery optimal respiratory care.

Delayed Cord Clamping

Recent evidence for DCC has changed the practice of immediate cord clamping over the past decade. DCC has been shown to decrease incidence of intraventricular hemorrhage, lower need for transfusion, and lower rates of necrotizing enterocolitis in premature infants and iron deficiency anemia in term infants.[68,69] Current recommendations from the American College of Obstetricians and Gynecologists, ILCOR, and NRP support DCC for 30 seconds to 60 seconds in infants not requiring resuscitation at birth.[70] Incorporation of DCC in the delivery room requires close coordination and clear communication between the neonatal and obstetrics teams to keep time as well as determine safety of the mother and infant during DCC. The briefing prior to delivery can serve as a reminder on whether the mother and infant are appropriate candidates for DCC. Policies and procedures can be developed by the obstetrics and neonatal teams to determine a list of patients (mothers or infants) to be excluded from DCC in addition to logistics of who will be the responsible team member for the infant while attached to the umbilical cord. Setting local guidelines and expectations as well as active communication during the delivery will help to avoid confusion that may potentially arise during DCC, such as who is holding the infant, who is assessing tone, and who is providing gentle stimulation. The CPQCC has developed a Web page with resources for improving quality of data collection and education surrounding DCC.[12]

Table 1
Examples of various aspects of specific delivery room quality improvement opportunities and what to measure

	Equipment	Systems Issues	Technical and Behavioral Skills	Measurable Outcomes	Balancing Measures
Optimizing the resuscitation cart	• Correct size and number of carts • Appropriate emergency supplies	• Space for placement of resuscitation carts in optimal locations	• Training staff to increase familiarity with resuscitation cart • Culture of safety to utilize cart as appropriate	• % times cart used during code situations	• Number of times equipment cannot be located
Appropriate delivery room attendance	• Communication devices • Institution-specific communication system during emergencies (button, phone, pager, overhead)	• Policies and procedures for calling appropriate team (standard/complex/back-up)	• Familiarity with policies and procedures • Communication between obstetrics and pediatrics team	• % appropriate delivery room notifications • % appropriate delivery room attendance	• Number of codes called per month that were false alarms
Temperature management	• Hat • Blankets • Plastic wrap • Temperature sensor • Warming mattress • Radiant warmer	• Appropriate operating/delivery room temperature	• Team member assigned to monitor temperature and apply equipment	• NICU admission temperature • % infants with hypothermia	• % infants with hyperthermia
Respiratory management	• T-piece resuscitator • Appropriate-sized mask • Oxygen blender • Monitors (O_2, ECG) • CO_2 detector	• Air, oxygen, and suction capabilities in all delivery rooms	• Familiarity with NRP algorithm including ventilation corrective steps (MR SOPA) • Accurately recognize whether ventilation is effective or ineffective	• % delivery room CPAP use • % delivery room intubation • Time to nasal CPAP	• % infants with air leak/pneumothorax

Time to hold in delivery room (for NICU admissions)	• Warm blankets • Hat • Stethoscope	• Availability to monitor infant during hold time • Policies for appropriate patient population and length of time	• Communication between obstetrics and pediatrics teams for appropriateness • Ability to wrap infant and/or place skin to skin on mother • Ability to monitor infant during hold	• % appropriate infants held by mother in the delivery room prior to NICU admission • Time until delivery room hold	• Number of cases requiring early interruption of hold time
DCC	• Sterile blankets, towels, or medical-grade plastic wrap	• Policies and procedures for DCC (who, how long) as determined by pediatric and obstetric teams	• Team member to monitor time until cord clamping • Identified team member to provide infant stimulation during DCC	• % appropriate infants receiving DCC • Length of DCC time	• % infants with hyperbilirubinemia requiring phototherapy • % mothers with hemorrhage complications • Number of times there is a break in sterile field

Table 2
Stepwise quality improvement goals and activities related to delivery room respiratory management

Progression	Quality Improvement Goals	Activities
↓ Time	Initial and continual evaluation of infant need for respiratory support	• Role assignment • Teamwork and communication • ECG placement and assessment • Pulse oximetry with appropriate F_{IO_2} titration
	Early and effective application of CPAP	• Equipment preparation and familiarization on how to deliver PEEP • Technical skills for appropriate equipment use (eg, mask size, orogastric tube placement) • Time to nasal CPAP, if indicated/available
	Safe, effective PPV	• Training in T-piece resuscitator/anesthesia bag/respiratory delivery systems • Assessment of effective PPV using CO_2 detectors and team communication • Technical skills on ventilation corrective steps (MR SOPA) • Equipment preparation for intubation
	Volume targeted ventilation	• Timely surfactant administration, if indicated • Obtaining physiologic measurements via respiratory monitors or ventilators • Ongoing feedback and reactive behavior

COLLABORATIVE QUALITY IMPROVEMENT

Aside from using local resources, institutions may elect to participate in collaborative QI groups. These groups may be national, such as the Vermont Oxford Network; statewide, such as the CPQCC; or institution–network specific. Collaboration allows for sharing of potentially better practices and creates a culture of information sharing. For example, a specific toolkit for delivery QI was published by CPQCC and is freely available online.[71] Furthermore, collaborative QI has been demonstrated effective in improving outcomes. In a CPQCC study on delivery room QI, those who participated in a collaborative QI had superior outcomes with decreased hypothermia and increased CPAP use compared with those hospitals that participated in stand-alone QI projects.[25] Furthermore, the collaborative QI group also had significantly reduced odds of developing bronchopulmonary dysplasia.[72]

In an analysis of focus groups of participants in collaborative QI for delivery room management, several factors were noted as key drivers for positive change: tracking of individual and comparative performance measurement, visible positive impacts on key components of the project, and initial and ongoing education on the evidence behind practices.[73] In regard to tracking data, both an institution's quality data over time and comparisons to similar institutions can be facilitated by belonging to a QI network. For example, if an institution noted that their rates of chest compression or epinephrine use for extremely preterm infants were significantly higher than those of other network hospitals, there may be benefit to evaluating the reasons for the higher rates.[5]

GOLDEN HOUR

The term, *golden hour*, has come to represent different concepts and protocols in various medical fields and in neonatology refers to the key procedures and tasks that should be performed in the first hour after delivery for very preterm infants.[74] Protocols should be tailored to each institution because there are differing personnel availability, policies, and procedures. The plan starts in the delivery room prior to the delivery, when providers are assigned specific tasks (**Table 3**). This may involve administrative tasks, such as entering orders, communication with the obstetric team and parents, and preparing umbilical lines. After an infant is born, the initial steps of clinical management of temperature and respiration are performed in the delivery room according to the NRP. The golden hour protocol then often continues into the NICU, with timed goals for vascular access, dextrose infusion, antibiotic and surfactant administration (as appropriate), and closure of the incubator. Team member tasks may include entering orders, securing vascular access, obtaining laboratory specimens, setting up the ventilator and giving surfactant, and providing a family update.[75] An example of a detailed plan for respiratory management is shown in **Fig. 1**.

Table 3
Golden hour Neonatal Resuscitation Program algorithm delineated by role

Time (seconds)	Provider Action	Respiratory Therapist Action	Nurse Action
0	• Wrap infant (already done) • Place hat on head • Position head • Hold mask (both hands)	• Set Apgar timer • Open mouth • Place mask • Begin mCPAP 5 cmH_2O, F_{IO_2} 0.3 with colorimeter detector	• Flatten wrap against skin • Place pulse oximetry probe on right wrist • Place temperature probe • Use stethoscope to listen for HR and tap HR out • Listen for breath sounds
30	• State HR out loud (<60, <100, or >100)	• Start PPV at 20/5, F_{IO_2} 0.3 with T-piece[a]	• Listen and tap heart rate • Listen for breath sounds • Look for chest rise
45	• State HR out loud • Reposition head[a] • May assist with MR SOPA measures	• Reapply mask[a] • Open mouth[a] • Increase PIP • Consider need for prolonged iTime	• Listen and tap heart rate • Suction mouth, if needed • Listen for breath sounds • Look for chest rise
60	• State HR out loud • Intubate within 30 s[a,b]	• Tape the ETT	• Listen for bilateral breath sounds • Look for chest rise • Listen and tap heart rate
90	• Start chest compressions[b] • Second provider to place emergent UVC[b]	• Provide breaths via ETT at 3:1 ratio • Ensure adequate chest rise with each breath	• Place ECG leads • Call neonatal code blue • Listen and tap heart rate (until monitoring is accurate)

Abbreviations: bpm, beats per minute; ETT, endotracheal tube; F_{IO_2}, fraction of inspired oxygen; HR, heart rate; mCPAP, mask CPAP; iTime, inspiratory time; MR SOPA, mask adjustment—ensure good seal, reposition—ensure head in sniffing position, suction mouth then nose if secretions present, open mouth—ventilate infant with mouth slightly open, pressure increase—increase pressure if no improvement, airway alternative—consider intubating if PPV by mask not effective; PIP, peak inspiratory pressure; UVC, umbilical venous catheter.

[a] HR <100 bpm and not rising.

[b] HR <60 bpm.

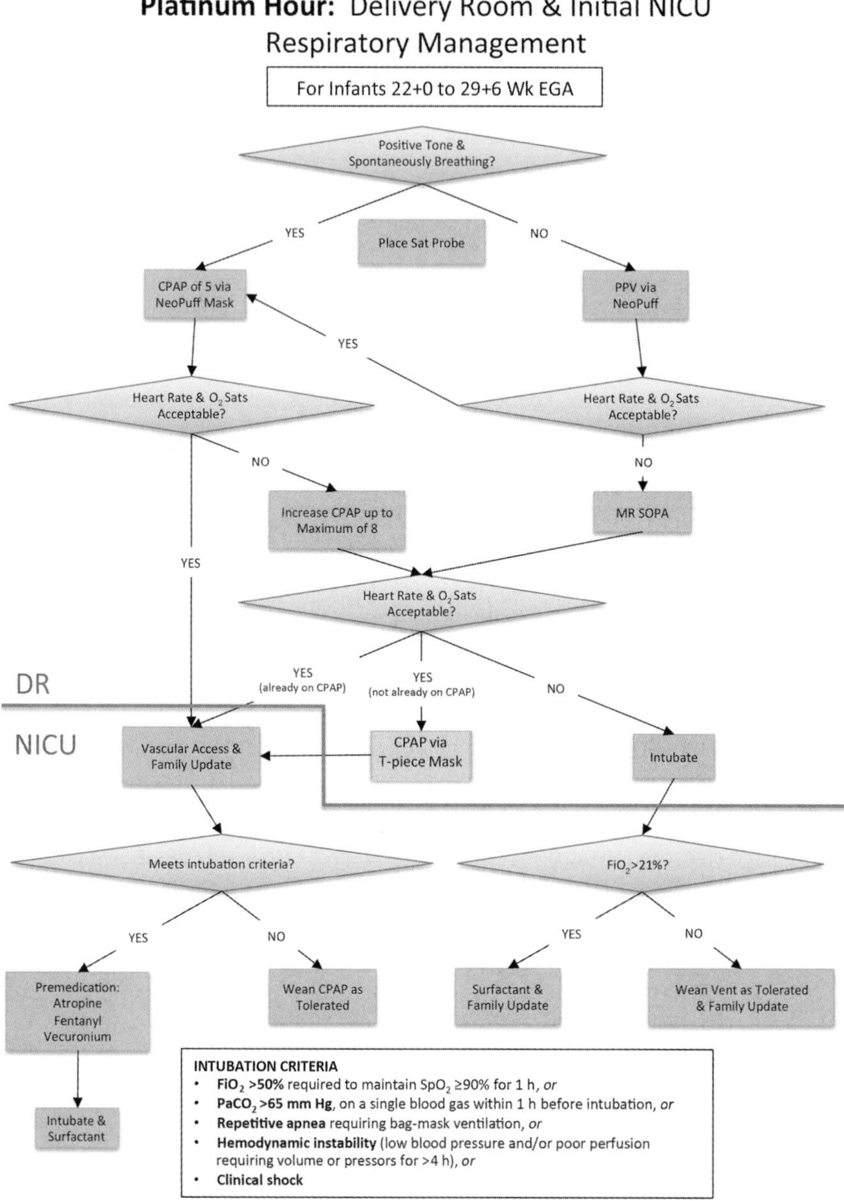

Fig. 1. Delivery room and initial NICU respiratory management. (*Reprinted from* Johnson C, Cohen R, McCallie K. NICU guide. Lucile Packard Children's Hospital. Stanford, CA; with permission.)

SUMMARY

The unique nature and complexity of the delivery room makes QI an excellent methodology for implementing positive changes in the delivery room. This article has given a broad overview of some of the unique aspects of QI in the delivery room and points to multiple resources that QI teams can use for this purpose. Ultimately, QI teams need to assess their own institutions' data, the context of their hospital, and corresponding networks to design the best approach for their local projects. Ongoing research on optimal methods to pursue delivery room QI and the short-term and long-term impacts of such activities will continue to inform best practices.

REFERENCES

1. Finer N, Rich W. Neonatal resuscitation for the preterm infant: evidence versus practice. J Perinatol 2010;30(Suppl):S57–66.
2. Soraisham AS, Lodha AK, Singhal N, et al. Neonatal outcomes following extensive cardiopulmonary resuscitation in the delivery room for infants born at less than 33 weeks gestational age. Resuscitation 2014;85(2):238–43.
3. Chamnanvanakij S, Perlman JM. Outcome following cardiopulmonary resuscitation in the neonate requiring ventilatory assistance. Resuscitation 2000;45(3): 173–80.
4. Finer NN, Horbar JD, Carpenter JH. Cardiopulmonary resuscitation in the very low birth weight infant: the Vermont Oxford Network experience. Pediatrics 1999;104(3 Pt 1):428–34.
5. Handley SC, Sun Y, Wyckoff MH, et al. Outcomes of extremely preterm infants after delivery room cardiopulmonary resuscitation in a population-based cohort. J Perinatol 2015;35(5):379–83.
6. Perlman JM, Wyllie J, Kattwinkel J, et al. Part 7: Neonatal Resuscitation: 2015 International Consensus on Cardiopulmonary Resuscitation and Emergency Cardiovascular Care Science With Treatment Recommendations (Reprint). Pediatrics 2015;136(Suppl 2):S120–66.
7. Weiner GM. Textbook of neonatal resuscitation. 7th edition. Elk Grove Village (IL): American Academy of Pediatrics and American Heart Association; 2016.
8. Wyckoff MH, Aziz K, Escobedo MB, et al. Part 13: Neonatal Resuscitation: 2015 American Heart Association Guidelines update for cardiopulmonary resuscitation and emergency Cardiovascular care (Reprint). Pediatrics 2015;136(Suppl 2): S196–218.
9. Profit J, Lee HC, Gould JB, et al. Evaluating and improving the safety and quality of neonatal intensive care. In: Martin R, Fanaroff A, Walsh M, editors. Fanaroff and Martin's neonatal-perinatal medicine. Philadelphia: Elsevier; 2014. p. 59–88.
10. Lee HC, Lyndon A, Blumenfeld YJ, et al. Antenatal steroid administration for premature neonates in California. Obstet Gynecol 2011;117(3):603–9.
11. Donabedian A. Evaluating the quality of medical care. Milbank Mem Fund Q 1966;44(3:Suppl):166–206.
12. California Perinatal Quality Care Collaborative. Available at: https://www.cpqcc.org/perinatal-programs/cpqcc-data-center/2016-delayed-cord-clamping-pilot-project-dccpp.
13. Finer NN, Rich W. Neonatal resuscitation: toward improved performance. Resuscitation 2002;53(1):47–51.
14. Gelbart B, Hiscock R, Barfield C. Assessment of neonatal resuscitation performance using video recording in a perinatal centre. J Paediatr Child Health 2010;46(7–8):378–83.
15. Rich WD, Leone T, Finer NN. Delivery room intervention: improving the outcome. Clin Perinatol 2010;37(1):189–202.
16. Carbine DN, Finer NN, Knodel E, et al. Video recording as a means of evaluating neonatal resuscitation performance. Pediatrics 2000;106(4):654–8.

17. Chitkara R, Rajani AK, Oehlert JW, et al. The accuracy of human senses in the detection of neonatal heart rate during standardized simulated resuscitation: implications for delivery of care, training and technology design. Resuscitation 2013;84(3):369–72.
18. Konstantelos D, Gurth H, Bergert R, et al. Positioning of term infants during delivery room routine handling - analysis of videos. BMC Pediatr 2014;14:33.
19. Brown T, Tu J, Profit J, et al. Optimal Criteria survey for preresuscitation delivery room checklists. Am J Perinatol 2016;33(2):203–7.
20. Hales BM, Pronovost PJ. The checklist–a tool for error management and performance improvement. J Crit Care 2006;21(3):231–5.
21. Bennett SC, Finer N, Halamek LP, et al. Implementing delivery room checklists and communication standards in a multi-neonatal ICU quality improvement collaborative. Jt Comm J Qual Patient Saf 2016;42(8):369–76.
22. Castrodale V, Rinehart S. The golden hour: improving the stabilization of the very low birth-weight infant. Adv Neonatal Care 2014;14(1):9–14 [quiz: 15–6].
23. DeMauro SB, Douglas E, Karp K, et al. Improving delivery room management for very preterm infants. Pediatrics 2013;132(4):e1018–25.
24. Katheria A, Rich W, Finer N. Development of a strategic process using checklists to facilitate team preparation and improve communication during neonatal resuscitation. Resuscitation 2013;84(11):1552–7.
25. Lee HC, Powers RJ, Bennett MV, et al. Implementation methods for delivery room management: a quality improvement comparison study. Pediatrics 2014;134(5): e1378–86.
26. Vergales BD, Dwyer EJ, Wilson SM, et al. NASCAR pit-stop model improves delivery room and admission efficiency and outcomes for infants <27 weeks' gestation. Resuscitation 2015;92:7–13.
27. Aziz K, Chadwick M, Baker M, et al. Ante- and intra-partum factors that predict increased need for neonatal resuscitation. Resuscitation 2008;79(3):444–52.
28. Patel J, Posencheg M, Ades A. Proficiency and retention of neonatal resuscitation skills by pediatric residents. Pediatrics 2012;130(3):515–21.
29. Kaczorowski J, Levitt C, Hammond M, et al. Retention of neonatal resuscitation skills and knowledge: a randomized controlled trial. Fam Med 1998;30(10): 705–11.
30. Halamek LP. Simulation as a methodology for assessing the performance of healthcare professionals working in the delivery room. Semin Fetal Neonatal Med 2013;18(6):369–72.
31. Ades A, Lee HC. Update on simulation for the neonatal resuscitation program. Semin Perinatol 2016;40(7):447–54.
32. Dadiz R, Weinschreider J, Schriefer J, et al. Interdisciplinary simulation-based training to improve delivery room communication. Simul Healthc 2013;8(5): 279–91.
33. Yamada NK, Fuerch JH, Halamek LP. Impact of standardized communication techniques on errors during simulated neonatal resuscitation. Am J Perinatol 2016;33(4):385–92.
34. Lipman SS, Daniels KI, Arafeh J, et al. The case for OBLS: a simulation-based obstetric life support program. Semin Perinatol 2011;35(2):74–9.
35. Draycott T, Sibanda T, Owen L, et al. Does training in obstetric emergencies improve neonatal outcome? BJOG 2006;113(2):177–82.
36. Zabari M, Suresh G, Tomlinson M, et al. Implementation and case-study results of potentially better practices for collaboration between obstetrics and neonatology to achieve improved perinatal outcomes. Pediatrics 2006;118(Suppl 2):S153–8.

37. Grogan EL, Stiles RA, France DJ, et al. The impact of aviation-based teamwork training on the attitudes of health-care professionals. J Am Coll Surg 2004; 199(6):843–8.
38. Wyckoff MH, Aziz K, Escobedo MB, et al. Part 13: neonatal resuscitation: 2015 American Heart Association Guidelines Update for Cardiopulmonary Resuscitation and Emergency Cardiovascular Care. Circulation 2015;132(18 Suppl 2): S543–60.
39. Edwards EM, Soll RF, Ferrelli K, et al. Identifying improvements for delivery room resuscitation management: results from a multicenter safety audit. Matern Health Neonatol Perinatol 2015;1:2.
40. Fang JL, Collura CA, Johnson RV, et al. Emergency video telemedicine Consultation for newborn resuscitations: the Mayo Clinic experience. Mayo Clin Proc 2016;91(12):1735–43.
41. Duchesne JC, Kyle A, Simmons J, et al. Impact of telemedicine upon rural trauma care. J Trauma 2008;64(1):92–7 [discussion: 97–8].
42. Wibbenmeyer L, Kluesner K, Wu H, et al. Video-enhanced telemedicine improves the care of Acutely Injured burn patients in a rural state. J Burn Care Res 2015; 37(6):e531–8.
43. Agarwal AK, Gaieski DF, Perman SM, et al. Telemedicine REsuscitation and Arrest Trial (TREAT): a feasibility study of real-time provider-to-provider telemedicine for the care of critically ill patients. Heliyon 2016;2(4):e00099.
44. Ajami S, Arzani-Birgani A. Fast resuscitation and care of the burn patients by telemedicine: a review. J Res Med Sci 2014;19(6):562–6.
45. Fierson WM, Capone A Jr. American Academy of Pediatrics Section on Ophthalmology, American Academy of Ophthalmology, American Association of Certified Orthoptists. Telemedicine for evaluation of retinopathy of prematurity. Pediatrics 2015;135(1):e238–54.
46. Quinn GE, Ying GS, Repka MX, et al. Timely implementation of a retinopathy of prematurity telemedicine system. J AAPOS 2016;20(5):425–30.e421.
47. Fang JL, Carey WA, Lang TR, et al. Real-time video communication improves provider performance in a simulated neonatal resuscitation. Resuscitation 2014; 85(11):1518–22.
48. Fuerch JH, Yamada NK, Coelho PR, et al. Impact of a novel decision support tool on adherence to Neonatal Resuscitation Program algorithm. Resuscitation 2015; 88:52–6.
49. Rousek JB, Hallbeck MS. Improving medication management through the redesign of the hospital code cart medication drawer. Hum Factors 2011;53(6): 626–36.
50. Shultz J, Davies JM, Caird J, et al. Standardizing anesthesia medication drawers using human factors and quality assurance methods. Can J Anaesth 2010;57(5): 490–9.
51. Agarwal S, Swanson S, Murphy A, et al. Comparing the utility of a standard pediatric resuscitation cart with a pediatric resuscitation cart based on the Broselow tape: a randomized, controlled, crossover trial involving simulated resuscitation scenarios. Pediatrics 2005;116(3):e326–33.
52. Chan J, Chan B, Ho HL, et al. The neonatal resuscitation algorithm organized cart is more efficient than the airway-breathing-circulation organized drawer: a crossover randomized control trial. Eur J Emerg Med 2016;23(4):258–62.
53. Chitkara R, Rajani AK, Lee HC, et al. Comparing the utility of a novel neonatal resuscitation cart with a generic code cart using simulation: a randomised, controlled, crossover trial. BMJ Qual Saf 2013;22(2):124–9.

54. Weigel WA. Redesigning an airway cart using lean methodology. J Clin Anesth 2016;33:273–82.
55. Lapcharoensap W, Lee HC. Temperature management in the delivery room and during neonatal resuscitation. NeoReviews 2016;17(8):e454–62.
56. Laptook AR, Watkinson M. Temperature management in the delivery room. Semin Fetal Neonatal Med 2008;13(6):383–91.
57. Miller SS, Lee HC, Gould JB. Hypothermia in very low birth weight infants: distribution, risk factors and outcomes. J Perinatol 2011;31(Suppl 1):S49–56.
58. Lee HC, Ho QT, Rhine WD. A quality improvement project to improve admission temperatures in very low birth weight infants. J Perinatol 2008;28(11):754–8.
59. Russo A, McCready M, Torres L, et al. Reducing hypothermia in preterm infants following delivery. Pediatrics 2014;133(4):e1055–62.
60. Manani M, Jegatheesan P, DeSandre G, et al. Elimination of admission hypothermia in preterm very low-birth-weight infants by standardization of delivery room management. Perm J 2013;17(3):8–13.
61. Billimoria Z, Chawla S, Bajaj M, et al. Improving admission temperature in extremely low birth weight infants: a hospital-based multi-intervention quality improvement project. J Perinat Med 2013;41(4):455–60.
62. Duryea EL, Nelson DB, Wyckoff MH, et al. The impact of ambient operating room temperature on neonatal and maternal hypothermia and associated morbidities: a randomized controlled trial. Am J Obstet Gynecol 2016;214(4):505.e1-7.
63. Committee on Fetus and Newborn, American Academy of Pediatrics. Respiratory support in preterm infants at birth. Pediatrics 2014;133(1):171–4.
64. Finer NN, Carlo WA, Walsh MC, et al. Early CPAP versus surfactant in extremely preterm infants. N Engl J Med 2010;362(21):1970–9.
65. Stevens TP, Finer NN, Carlo WA, et al. Respiratory outcomes of the surfactant positive pressure and oximetry randomized trial (SUPPORT). J Pediatr 2014; 165(2):240–9.e244.
66. Morley CJ, Davis PG, Doyle LW, et al. Nasal CPAP or intubation at birth for very preterm infants. N Engl J Med 2008;358(7):700–8.
67. Dunn MS, Kaempf J, de Klerk A, et al. Randomized trial comparing 3 approaches to the initial respiratory management of preterm neonates. Pediatrics 2011; 128(5):e1069–76.
68. Perlman JM, Wyllie J, Kattwinkel J, et al. Part 7: Neonatal Resuscitation: 2015 International Consensus on Cardiopulmonary Resuscitation and Emergency Cardiovascular Care Science with treatment recommendations. Circulation 2015; 132(16 Suppl 1):S204–41.
69. Raju TN. Timing of umbilical cord clamping after birth for optimizing placental transfusion. Curr Opin Pediatr 2013;25(2):180–7.
70. Committee on Obstetric Practice, American College of Obstetricians & Gynecologists. Committee Opinion No.543: timing of umbilical cord clamping after birth. Obstet Gynecol 2012;120(6):1522–6.
71. Bell R, Finer N, Halamek L, et al. on behalf of the Perinatal Quality Improvement Panel, California Perinatal Quality Care Collaborative. Delivery Room Management Quality Improvement Toolkit. California Perinatal Quality Care Collaborative. 2011. Available at: http://cpqcc.org/quality_improvement/qi_toolkits/delivery_room_management_toolkit_revised_july_2011. Accessed July 2, 2012.
72. Lapcharoensap W, Bennett MV, Powers RJ, et al. Effects of delivery room quality improvement on premature infant outcomes. J Perinatol 2016;37(4):349–54.

73. Lee HC, Arora V, Brown T, et al. Thematic analysis of barriers and facilitators to implementation of neonatal resuscitation guideline changes. J Perinatol 2016; 37(3):249–53.
74. Wyckoff MH. Initial resuscitation and stabilization of the periviable neonate: the Golden-Hour approach. Semin Perinatol 2014;38(1):12–6.
75. Doyle KJ, Bradshaw WT. Sixty golden minutes. Neonatal Netw 2012;31(5): 289–94.

Reducing Incidence of Necrotizing Enterocolitis

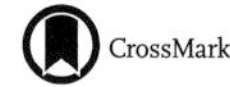

Aloka L. Patel, MD[a,*], Patoula G. Panagos, MD[b], Jean M. Silvestri, MD[c]

KEYWORDS

- Necrotizing enterocolitis • Quality improvement • Feeding guidelines • Antibiotics • Probiotics • Transfusion • Anemia • Human milk

KEY POINTS

- Own mother's milk (OMM) is associated with reduced odds of necrotizing enterocolitis (NEC) in observational studies, and quality improvement (QI) efforts to increase OMM have been successful at decreasing NEC.
- Donor milk (DM) has also been associated with NEC reduction when OMM is unavailable, although DM has not been associated with other health benefits as seen with OMM feedings in preterm infants.
- Institution of standardized feeding guidelines has been associated with reduced NEC rates, although the optimal rates of advancement and fortification are uncertain. Prolonged periods of nothing by mouth are associated with increased rates and severity of NEC and thus enteral feedings should be instituted soon after birth.
- Acid antagonists and prolonged empiric antibiotics in the setting of negative cultures are associated with increased odds of NEC, and both should be minimized or avoided if possible.
- Probiotics have been associated with reduced NEC in some, but not all, studies. Meta-analyses demonstrate reduction in NEC. At present, however, there remains controversy about probiotics due to concerns regarding quality and reliability of available products.
- Anemia and blood transfusions have been linked to NEC. Controversy remains regarding these relationships and best practices regarding enteral feeding during blood transfusions.

INTRODUCTION

Despite the many years of investigation into NEC,[1] the pathophysiology remains uncertain. This uncertainty poses several challenges to QI efforts to prevent this significant complication. The current consensus is that NEC is a multifactorial disease that occurs when multiple risk factors and/or stressors overlap, leading to profound inflammation

Disclosure Statement: The authors have nothing to disclose.
[a] Department of Pediatrics, Rush University Children's Hospital, 1653 West Congress Parkway, Pavilion 353, Chicago, IL 60612, USA; [b] Department of Pediatrics, Rush University Children's Hospital, 1653 West Congress Parkway, Pavilion 361, Chicago, IL 60612, USA; [c] Department of Pediatrics, Rush University Children's Hospital, 1653 West Congress Parkway, Pavilion 357, Chicago, IL 60612, USA
* Corresponding author.
E-mail address: Aloka_Patel@rush.edu

Clin Perinatol 44 (2017) 683–700
http://dx.doi.org/10.1016/j.clp.2017.05.004
perinatology.theclinics.com

and intestinal injury (**Fig. 1**).[2–4] Diagnosis of this multifactorial disease remains primarily dependent on clinical features that vary significantly due to the multiple predisposing conditions. This heterogeneity complicates efforts to identify broad strategies for NEC prevention as a part of QI efforts. A clinically based classification system (**Table 1**) has been proposed as one strategy to increase understanding of the multiple etiologies underlying NEC, which could potentially lead to novel insights and/or interventions for NEC prevention.[4] In addition to the challenge provided by differences in clinical features and predisposing factors, another difficulty in identifying strategies to reduce NEC relates to the timing of presentation varying with gestational age (GA). NEC has a later onset in the most immature infants with a central peak at approximately 29 weeks' to 32 weeks' postmenstrual age (PMA).[5] Furthermore, the low incidence of NEC (approximately 5% in very-low-birth-weight [VLBW] infants)[6] has led to difficulty in identifying those infants at the highest risk who might benefit from targeted prevention strategies.

Even with these limitations and obstacles, the incidence of NEC has gradually been decreasing over the past 10 years, in part due to QI initiatives directed at preventing

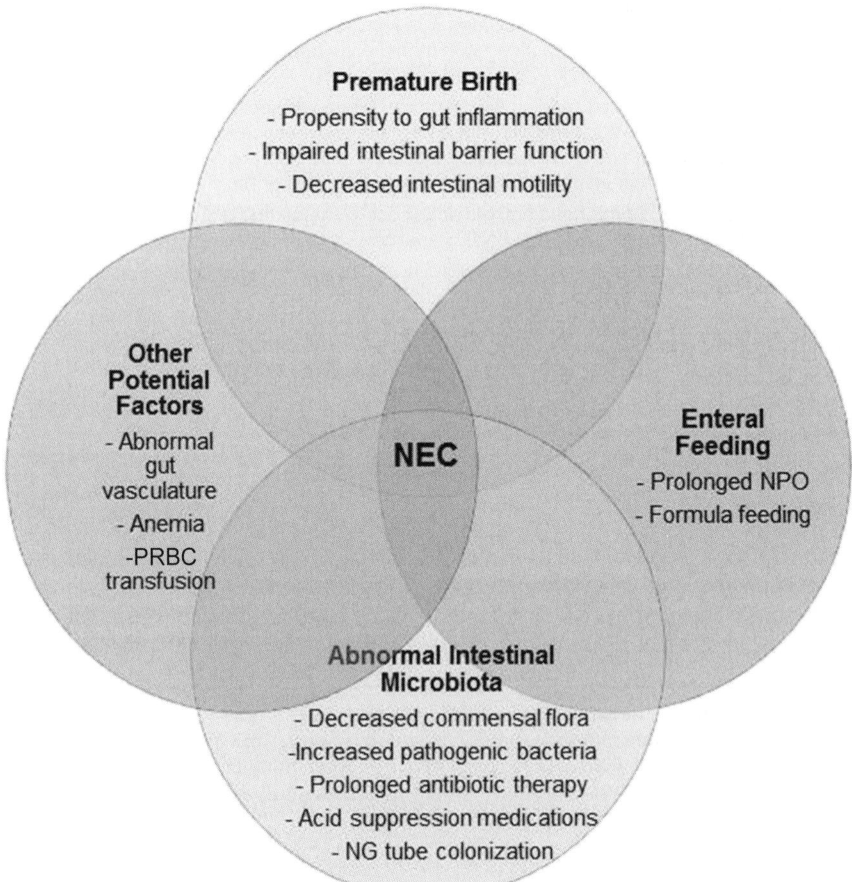

Fig. 1. Multifactorial nature of NEC. (*Adapted from* Patel RM, Denning PW. Intestinal microbiot and its relationship with necrotizing enterocolitis. Pediatr Res 2015;78(3):233; with permission from Macmillan Publishers Ltd.)

Table 1
Proposed catalog of necrotizing enterocolitis subsets

Category	Criteria—Necrotizing Enterocolitis Associated with...
Transfusion-associated NEC (TANEC)	Within 48 h after a PRBC transfusion
NEC associated with neonatal cow's milk allergy (MOONEC)	Bloody stools, history of feeding intolerance/ severe reflux, any absolute eosinophil count >2000/mL, abatement of symptoms within 48 h of changing to an elemental formula
NEC associated with a known bacterial pathogen (BPNEC)	Single bacterial pathogen isolated from blood or peritoneal fluid
NEC associated with a known viral pathogen (VPNEC)	Single virus identified by culture or polymerase chain reaction from blood or other sterile bodily fluid
NEC associated with a known severe hypoxic and/or ischemic event (HIENEC)	Within 72 h after a severe hypoxic and/or ischemic event
NEC associated with recent culture negative status (ROSNEC)	Within 72 h of blood cultures that were negative (not currently on antibiotics)
NEC associated with cold stress (CLDNEC)	BW <2000 g, infant failed weaning from incubator within 72 h
NEC occurring in siblings (2XNEC)	2 or more siblings in the same genetic family acquire NEC
NEC after spontaneous intestinal perforation (SIPNEC)	Onset after surgical recovery from spontaneous intestinal perforation
NEC associated with gastroschisis (GASNEC)	Gastroschisis (preoperatively or postoperatively)
NEC associated with critical congenital heart disease (HRTNEC)	Critical congenital heart lesion (preoperatively or postoperatively)
NEC associated with a known genetic condition (GENNEC)	Either a known polymorphism or genetic condition that predisposes an infant to NEC (excluding complex congenital anomalies)
NEC associated with congenital anomaly (CANNEC)	A complex anomaly other than congenital heart disease or gastroschisis
NEC associated with a commercial product ($NEC)	A formula or other ingested commercial agent is associated with either a unique presentation or higher than normal incidence

Adapted from Gordon PV, Swanson JR, MacQueen BC, et al. A critical question for NEC researchers: can we create a consensus definition of NEC that facilitates research progress? Semin Perinatol 2017;41(1):7–14.

NEC.[7] QI strategies for NEC prevention thus far have primarily targeted the various predisposing conditions depicted in **Fig. 1**. This article reviews the evidence on which the published interventions have been based, organized by theme, as well as providing examples of successful QI interventions used in different neonatal ICU (NICUs).

SCIENTIFIC BASIS OF QUALITY IMPROVEMENT INTERVENTIONS

Intrapartum/postnatal

Delayed cord clamping

Delayed cord clamping should be part of an obstetric team's investment in any QI program targeting NEC reduction (**Box 1**). The American Academy of Pediatrics and

Box 1
Quality improvement practices

Best practices

Standardizing enteral feeding guidelines

Exclusive feedings of OMM

DM used as an alternative to formula if OMM is unavailable until an infant is past the peak time for NEC

Minimizing duration of empiric antibiotics after birth, if initiated

Avoiding antacid use in preterm infants

Implementing delayed cord clamping after birth for all infants

Practices awaiting further supportive data

Avoiding severe anemia

Feeding guidelines during PRBC transfusions

NG tube management

Probiotics

American Heart Association seventh edition of the *Textbook of Neonatal Resuscitation*[8] as well as the American College of Obstetricians and Gynecologists Committee on Obstetric Practice now recommend delayed cord clamping for 30 seconds to 60 seconds after birth in vigorous term and preterm infants.[9] This recommendation is based on the significant benefits found in preterm infants, which include reduced incidence of NEC. A 2012 Cochrane review examined 15 studies of 738 infants from 24 weeks' to 36 weeks' gestation, with delayed cord clamping from 30 seconds to 120 seconds.[10] Studies demonstrated not only less need for transfusion (7 trials; 392 infants; risk ratio [RR] 0.61 [CI, 0.46–0.81]) and less intraventricular hemorrhage (10 trials; 539 infants; RR 0.59 [CI, 0.41–0.85]) but also lower risk of NEC (5 trials; 241 infants; RR 0.62 [CI, 0.43–0.90]) with a lower risk associated with a greater placental transfusion. In addition, a single-center study comparing outcomes of deliveries compliant with delayed cord clamping (236 infants; mean GA 29.6 weeks $\pm$ 2 weeks; mean birth weight [BW] 1454 g $\pm$ 402 g) with those who were noncompliant (113 infants; mean GA 29.9 weeks $\pm$ 2.1 weeks; mean BW 1479 g $\pm$ 482 g) also demonstrated significantly lower rates of NEC (1.3% vs 5.4%; $P = .026$).[11]

Milking of the umbilical cord as an alternative to delayed cord clamping (designed to increase placental transfusion and not delay resuscitation) has also been suggested as a strategy to reduce the incidence of NEC. Reports of a QI effort describing cord milking among 158 infants (median GA 27.4 [23.1, 29.9], median BW 960 g [410, 1010]) compared with 160 historical controls (median GA 27.1 [23, 29.9], median BW 880 g [375, 2050]) revealed a significant decrease in NEC from 20% to 11% ($P<.05$).[12] There seemed to be greater benefit in those infants born less than 27 weeks' gestation although the QI study was not powered to more closely examine this subgroup of infants. Although there is a suggestion of similar improved neonatal outcomes (such as reduction in NEC) with delayed cord clamping and cord milking, further study is needed to determine benefits and risks.

In summary, delayed cord clamping is a useful component of any QI initiative to reduce NEC, although several QI initiatives have resulted in significant reductions in NEC without this intervention.[13,14] The reduction in NEC seen with delayed cord clamping may be related to the higher hemoglobin concentration, hemodynamic stability, reduction of blood transfusions at a vulnerable time, and/or transfusion of pluripotent stem cells. Delayed cord clamping is a feasible, safe, and no cost intervention at the time of delivery.[11]

Enteral Feeding

Feeding guidelines

Several investigators have demonstrated a reduction in NEC incidence with implementation of standardized feeding guidelines in their NICUs despite variability in the specifics of the guidelines (**Fig. 2**).[14–18] These guidelines have generally incorporated an early minimal enteral nutrition phase during which 10 mL/kg/d to 20 mL/kg/d of enteral nutrition have been given without increase, followed by daily advancement based on continued tolerance. As opposed to older practices in which feedings were held and infants maintained as nothing by mouth for days to weeks after birth, current regimens encourage earlier introduction with small volume feedings and are supported by basic science and clinical research.[19–21] For example, a case-control study from the Canadian Neonatal Network demonstrated an 8% increase in the odds of developing NEC for each additional day that an infant was maintained nothing by mouth, after adjusting for other confounders.[21]

The best approaches for rates of feeding advancement, fortification, and feeding during pharmacotherapy for patent ductus arteriosus (PDA) and packed red blood cell (PRBC) transfusions are still debated. This results in variation in how units have chosen to incorporate these parameters in unit feeding protocols.[13,22]

Rates of feeding advancement Due to concerns regarding excessively slow advancement and potential adverse effect on postnatal growth[23] in addition to conflicting results from published studies, centers tend to vary in their approach to feeding advances. A small randomized trial demonstrated no adverse effect of faster advancement (30 mL/kg/d vs 20 mL/kg/d).[24] Observational data exist, however, that support a negative association of rapid feeding advancement with rates of overall and fulminant NEC.[17,25]

Timing of fortification The timing of fortification of human milk (HM) also varies significantly between institutions, likely because there have been few trials evaluating this practice. A recent small randomized trial demonstrated no detrimental impact of early fortification (at 20 mL/kg/d vs 100 mL/kg/d) of enteral feedings with a liquid bovine HM fortifier on NEC, with greater protein provision over the first 4 weeks, although no effect on in-NICU growth was noted.[26] Due to the small sample size, the study was not powered to detect a difference in NEC, and further studies are needed before optimal timing of fortification can be determined.

Limiting feeding during patent ductus arteriosus treatment Some standard feeding protocols limit feeding during PDA treatment or PRBC transfusion based on a limited body of evidence, including a study of 177 very preterm infants by Clyman and colleagues[27] that demonstrated the safety of continuing trophic enteral feedings (15 mL/kg/d) during pharmacotherapy for a PDA (77% received indomethacin and 23% received ibuprofen). Infants who were randomized to continued trophic feedings reached goal enteral nutrition 3 days to 4 days faster than infants who were maintained nothing by mouth, with no difference in rates of NEC or intestinal perforation.

Limiting feeding during packed red blood cell transfusion The discussion of feeding practices before, during, and after transfusion remains unresolved. In a prospective

A

Fluid Initiation and Advancement

Initial fluids, TPN adjustments and required labs(d=days)

Birth Weight (grams)	<1000g	1000-1500g	1500-2000g	2000-2500g	>2500g
Initial TF Volume (mL/kg/d)	90-100	80-90	70-80	60	
Dextrose	Minimum GIR 4mg/kg/hr; Maximum GIR 14mg/kg/hr; Goal blood glucose 70-149mg/dL				
First Day TPN	On admission for patients <1800g				
TPN Protein Initiation	Begin protein at 2.5-3g/kg/d and advance to 4g/kg/d by DOL 2-3 unless contraindications				
TPN Protein Goal (g/kg/day)	4g	3.5-4g	3.5	3.2-3	
TPN Calorie Goal (Kcal/kg/day)	100-110				
Intralipids	Start at 0.5-3g/kg/d. Advance by 0.5-1g/kg/d.	Start at 1-2g/kg/d. Advance by 1g/kg/d.Be at goal by DOL 5			
Maximum Intralipids	3g/kg/d				
Peripheral IVFs	Dextrose concentration limit of 10% with added calcium or 12.5% with no calcium				
NPO or Feeding Delays	If infant must remain NPO or has issues with advancing feedings, make sure TPN/IL are advanced as tolerated to meet Protein, Calorie, and Intralipid goals.				

Nutrition as Feedings Advance

*Weaning of TPN/IL, fortification of feeds, oral medications **All weights are birth weight*

Feeds (mL/kg/d)		0-20	20-40	40-60	60-80	80-100	100-120	120-140	140+
Max TPN Protein (g/kg/d)	<1000g	4	4	4	3.5	3	2	1	0-0.5
	1000-1500g	4	4	3.5	3	2.5	2	1	0-0.5
	1500-2000g	3 to 3.5	3	2.5	2	1	0.5-1	0-0.5	
Max Intralipids (g/kg/d)		3	3	2.5	2	1.5	1 to off	off	
Glucose infusion rate GIR		max 13	max 11	max 9	max 7.5	max 6	max 4	trend to off	
Fortification	<1500g					At 80-100mL/kg/d ↑to 22kcal/oz, ↑to 24kcal/oz next day			Use liquid protein if <1500g
	1500-2500g				At 50-80mL/kg/d ↑to 22kcal/oz, ↑to 24kcal/oz next day				
Access							At 100-120mL/kg/d Discontinue UVC/PICC		
Vitamin A	<1000g						100mL/kg/d & on respiratory support, start 4000IU/kg/d		
	1000-1250g & on mechanical ventilation at 12hrs								
Vitamin D						Start 400IU/day			
Elemental Iron	<1500g						If DOL 14+, fortify with 3.5mg/kg/d for human milk feeds or 1.5mg/kg/d for formula feeds		
	>1500g						If DOL 14+, fortify with 2mg/kg/d for human milk feeds or 1mg/kg/d for formula feeds		
Medications							Make PO if possible		

Advancement of Enteral Feedings

GA (weeks)	Initial Rate & Advancement	150mL/kg/d over:
23-25	Increase by 10mL/kg/day	15 days
26-28	Increase by 10mL/kg/day x2 days, then increase by 15mL/kg/day	12 days
29-31	Increase by 15mL/kg/day x2 days, then increase by 20mL/kg/day	6-8 days
32-34	Increase by 20 mL/kg/day x2 days, then increase by 25-35mL/kg/day (slower advancement for lower GA)	4-6 days

B

RUMC NICU FEEDING PROTOCOL

1. Administer COLOSTRUM swabs while NPO

2. **Start feedings by 48 hours of life** with COLOSTRUM/human milk. Animal studies show that colostrum has specific impact on gut epithelium that is disrupted/ablated by feeding mature human milk or formula first.
- If NO colostrum/ human milk DOL 2 – contact peer counselor and mother
- If mother is not going to provide milk or has inadequate supply, start feedings with donor milk (check consent).
- If mother refuses donor milk, then use preterm 20 calorie formula

3. TROPHIC FEEDINGS: start as soon as possible (within first 48hrs).
- Give COLOSTRUM first – may dilute with sterile water to make 1ml total per feeding.
- Ok to give TROPHIC feedings with UAC in place.
- Do not check residuals during TROPHIC feedings unless clinical concern (abdominal distension, feeding coming up OG tube, emesis, increased apnea/bradycardia…)

4. Once feedings have been initiated, if human milk not available for brief intervals – Check with peer counselors for milk off unit, contact family and give donor milk until human milk available.

5. All VLBW (less than 1500g) infants will require UVC and/or PICC line

6. When to feed vs. not feed:
- UAC: trophic feeds
- Paralysis: continue feeds
- PDA/Indocin: trophic feeds
- Inotropes: No feeds if used to treat hypotension
- Sepsis: per clinical judgment

BIRTH WEIGHT	TROPHIC FEEDING	DAILY ADVANCEMENT	GOAL FEEDING AMOUNT at 140ml/kg/day	Days from feeds initiation to 140ml/kg/d
400-750g	1ml q4hr x 5 days	Day 6 of feedings: 1ml q2hr for 24 hr, THEN advance by 1 ml q24hr	6-9ml q2	11-14
751-1000g	1ml q2hr x 4 days	Day 5 of feedings: advance by 2ml q24hr	9-12ml q2	9-11
1001-1250g	1ml q2hr x 3 days	Day 4 of feedings: advance daily by 20ml/kg/day	12-15ml q2	10
1251-1500g (or greater if GA<33 weeks)	3ml q3hr x 3 days	Day 4 of feedings: advance daily by 20ml/kg/day	22-26ml q3	9

FORTIFICATION – human milk and donor milk
When feedings reach 100ml/kg/day then Fortify - 1packet:50ml human milk.
THEN, if stable on the next day - Fortify 1packet:25ml human milk.
FORMULA
Start with 20 calorie formula until at full feedings (140ml/kg/day).
THEN, if stable next day, change to 24 calorie/oz Formula.

Fig. 2. Examples of variation in feeding guidelines. (*A*) Monroe Carell Jr. Children's Hospital NICU at Vanderbilt University nutrition bundle protocol. (*B*) Rush University Medical Center NICU feeding protocol for infants with birthweight ≤1500 grams or gestation <33 weeks. ([*A*] *From* Stefanescu BM, Gillam-Krakauer M, Stefanescu AR, et al. Very low birth weight infant care: adherence to a new nutrition protocol improves growth outcomes and reduces infectious risk. Early Hum Dev 2016; 94:25-30; with permission.)

study with 22 infants, anemic infants less than 1250 g were unable to increase their postprandial mesenteric blood flow velocity.[28] This provided biologic plausibility for postprandial intestinal hypoperfusion that further predisposes an already immature gut to NEC. El-Dib and colleagues[29] reported a reduction from 5.3% to 1.3% in transfusion-related acute gut injury [TRAGI] after implementation of a policy to withhold feeds during transfusions. Small studies have demonstrated a reduction in transfusion associated NEC after withholding feedings during transfusion.[29,30] Christensen and colleagues[31] showed that the group of infants with TRAGI were fed larger volumes of milk in the previous 24 hours prior to NEC onset. The importance of optimizing nutrition in VLBW infants creates the need for randomized controlled trials (RCTs) to further understand the best practices with respect to feedings during PRBC transfusions.

In summary, there does not seem to be a clear best practice in terms of a specific feeding protocol but rather the introduction of uniform guidelines to minimize variability within NICUs should be considered a best practice.

Human milk—own mother's milk

OMM feedings have been associated with reductions in NEC[32–37] and are the optimal nutrition for preterm infants.[38] The protective effect is likely a result of effects from the nutritional and bioactive components in OMM. Studies in preterm infants have demonstrated reduced gut permeability with OMM compared with formula.[39] In addition, OMM provides anti-inflammatory and anti-infective components, such as commensal bacteria, oligosaccharides, anti-inflammatory cytokines, platelet-activating factor acetylhydrolase, lysozyme, lactoferrin, transforming growth factor β, and soluble CD14 as well as growth factors and stem cells, which likely counteract the risk factors for NEC.[40–46]

Clinical studies have demonstrated significant reductions in NEC when infants have received OMM of varying durations and doses. Exclusive HM feedings (OMM and/or DM) for the first 7 days[47] and exclusive OMM for the first 14 days of life[37] have been associated with significantly reduced odds of developing NEC. Other studies have identified OMM thresholds that have been associated with reduction in NEC, such as at least 50% of enteral feedings in the first 14 days,[34] greater than 50 mL/kg/d OMM over the hospitalization,[33] and a dose-dependent effect with increased survival time free of NEC with each 10% increase in OMM.[35] Given these results, QI initiatives should focus on increasing OMM feedings in NICUs.

Donor human milk

DM differs significantly from OMM due to the multiple steps required for processing, including transferring containers, freeze-thaw cycles, and pasteurization.[48] Many, but not all, of the nutritional and bioactive components of OMM are reduced in concentration and/or their activity is abolished.[49] Despite the differences between OMM and DM, a majority of studies have demonstrated reduction in NEC when DM has been used to replace formula feedings.[50–57] The strength of this literature is complicated by these studies differing significantly from one another. Some investigators have reviewed practice changes in comparison to historical cohorts, whereas others are randomized trials. In addition, a majority of studies have used DM or formula as a supplement to OMM rather than as exclusive diets.

A recent double-blind RCT in 363 VLBW infants demonstrated significantly fewer infants in the DM group developed NEC (1.7%) compared with the formula group (6.6%, $P = .02$).[55] It is unclear from the published literature if DM itself provides protection from NEC or if it is the avoidance of formula which is protective. A Cochrane review of 1070 infants found formula feeding increased the risk of NEC significantly

(RR 2.77 [95% CI, 1.40–5.46]).[53] These findings are consistent with animal studies that have demonstrated intestinal injury associated with formula exposure.[48] Given these findings, DM is increasingly used in North American NICUs when OMM is unavailable.[58] Duration of DM varies across NICUs, although a majority of institutions use a PMA criteria though 34 weeks,[58] past the peak incidence of NEC.

In summary, OMM feedings are the optimal nutrition for preterm infants and confer benefits related to reduction in risk of NEC. In addition, there seems to be a reduction in NEC when DM has been used to replace formula feedings. Those NICUs electing to use DM must remember that significant differences remain between OMM and DM with regard to non-NEC neonatal outcomes in VLBW infants.[48,55] In addition, some QI projects and research studies have begun to merge OMM and DM into a common metric, which is of concern given the significant differences in composition, associated outcomes, and costs.[14,48] Although DM may be an appropriate target for QI initiatives, it should not replace OMM as a QI priority.

Abnormal Intestinal Microbiota

Dysbiosis, or an altered gut microbiome, is thought to be a contributory factor leading to NEC. Multiple factors have an impact on bacterial colonization in a premature infant's gut. Interventions to promote healthy development of the neonatal gut microbiome have been the focus of much investigation in RCTs and cohort studies as well as QI efforts.

Antibiotic stewardship

Antibiotics have been proved to alter gut microbiome,[59,60] leading to restriction of the normal progression of microbial colonization in VLBW infants compared with healthy term infants[61] and subsequent colonization by potentially pathogenic bacteria, primarily Proteobacteria. The decisions to initiate and continue antibiotics in preterm neonates are typically based on maternal and infant clinical condition and an attending neonatologist's clinical judgment; yet, these decisions can have a great impact on the gut microbiome and risk of NEC. A large retrospective study of extremely low-BW infants from the Eunice Kennedy Shriver National Institute of Child Health and Human Development (NICHD) Neonatal Research Network demonstrated that prolonged initial empiric antibiotic treatment, defined as greater than 5 days of initial empiric antibiotic treatment with sterile culture results, was associated with the combined outcome of NEC or death as well as NEC alone. A 7% increase in the odds of developing NEC was noted for each additional day of initial empiric antibiotic treatment.[62] Similar results were found by other investigators in 2 retrospective studies,[63,64] including a case-control study, that found a significant increase in the odds of NEC with greater duration of empiric antibiotic treatment beyond 1 day to 2 days in preterm infants.[63] The current body of evidence suggests that antibiotic stewardship is an important aspect of NEC QI efforts.

Acid suppression medications

The use of medications to reduce gastric acidity has been associated with an increased risk of NEC. Histamine 2 (H_2) antagonists have been shown to alter fecal microbiota, which may predispose the immature preterm intestine to NEC.[65] In an NICHD study of 11,072 VLBW infants (787 with NEC), NEC was associated with antecedent H_2 antagonists (odds ratio [OR] 1.71; CI, 1.34–2.19; $P<.0001$).[66] A subsequent prospective multicenter study of 274 VLBW infants similarly demonstrated that among 91 infants exposed to ranitidine there was a significant risk of NEC (OR 6.6 [CI, 1.7–25]; $P = .003$). In any multifaceted QI approach to reducing the risk of NEC, data support that H_2 antagonists should be avoided in VLBW infants.[67]

Probiotics

Numerous RCTs and cohort studies have investigated the use of probiotics in preterm infants. Probiotic supplements have primarily consisted of *Bifidobacteria* species, *Lactobacillus* species, or combinations of the 2.[68–73] Meta-analyses have demonstrated reductions in NEC among infants treated with probiotics, although not all individual RCTs showed a beneficial effect.[74–78] Different results across individual trials stem from inconsistencies in design across these trials, which have been conducted in several countries and used different probiotic agents with different doses and durations of therapy. In addition, studies varied significantly in their approach to feeding with either very different or at times unspecified diets consisting of OMM, DM, and/or preterm formula.[76,79] In addition, recent cohort studies from Germany and the Netherlands demonstrate conflicting results. A significant reduction in NEC was found by Denkel and colleagues.[73] Samuels and colleagues[80] did not find a definitive effect of probiotics on NEC or death but found an interaction between diet and probiotics. Aside from the challenges related to interpreting heterogeneous studies, concerns regarding consistency and contamination of probiotic preparations, and the lack of a US Food and Drug Administration–approved product, have resulted in probiotics considered a controversial therapy in the United States.[79,81,82]

Nasogastric tube management

There have been few studies that have investigated colonization patterns of nasogastric (NG) tubes in infants. Hurrell and colleagues[83] demonstrated that gram-negative bacterial colonization increased with duration of NG tube placement in infants hospitalized in 2 NICUs. High levels of gram-negative NG tube colonization were subsequently associated with NEC, and the same organism was cultured from the peritoneum in those infants who underwent laparotomy for NEC.[84] A recent study of 94 NG tubes collected from 34 infants demonstrated 89% of NG tubes were contaminated with organisms, of which the majority were potentially pathogenic. They found that colonization occurs rapidly after insertion but found no correlation between colonization and duration that the NG tube had been in use, although the median duration was only 3.25 days.[85] These investigators are planning an RCT to investigate the impact of frequent NG tube changes on gastric contamination. Although only 1 institution has incorporated NG tube management into their NEC QI process,[13] it may be appropriate to consider based on local NEC rates and success of other implemented interventions to reduce NEC.

Other Potential Factors

Anemia and blood transfusions

PRBC transfusion in VLBW infants and its temporal relationship to developing NEC continues to be a topic of ongoing discussion. The relationship between NEC and PRBC transfusion was first described in 2006 in a retrospective study of 17 infants who developed NEC over a 17-month period.[86] Blau and colleagues[87] coined the term, TRAGI, to categorize the gut injury of anemic VLBW neonates with a temporal relationship to transfusion of PRBC, within 48 hours. Christensen and colleagues[31] similarly demonstrated TRAGI in one-third of their surgical NEC cases over a 7-year retrospective case-control study. Analysis of 23 observational, case-control studies showed an overall OR 1.95 [1.60, 2.38] between PRBC transfusion and NEC any time after transfusion and an OR 1.13 [0.99, 1.29] between PRBC transfusion and NEC within 48 hours, with an overall very low quality rating of the evidence supporting a relationship between PRBC transfusion and NEC.[88] Conversely, the following have been proposed in support of a causative relationship between NEC and PRBC transfusion within 48 hours: (1) timing of NEC after a PRBC transfusion is not random; (2) common risk factors for NEC are often absent; (3) significant anemia is present; (4) the age of the blood is slightly older in NEC cases than in controls; (5) TRAGI is not postnatal age dependent; and (6) TRAGI does not show a centering at 31 weeks' post–conception age as does non–transfusion-related NEC.[89]

Anemia of prematurity may also play a role in the potential link between NEC and PRBC transfusions.[90,91] Blau and colleagues[87] showed that the infants with TRAGI had more anemia with lower hematocrits. Similarly, a retrospective case-control study with 111 preterm infants with NEC showed that lower hematocrit levels were associated with increased odds of NEC (OR 1.10 [1.02, 1.18]).[92] In a secondary analysis of a prospective cohort study of 598 VLBW infants, the rate of NEC in a given week was significantly greater for infants with severe anemia, defined as hemoglobin less than or equal to 8 g/dL compared with infants without severe anemia.[91] Hyung and colleagues[90] found elevated levels of intestinal fatty acid binding protein, a marker of intestinal mucosal injury, both before and after PRBC transfusions. This suggests anemia may result in decreased oxygen delivery to the gastrointestinal tract allowing for an increased susceptibility to mucosal injury and necrosis. In the prospective PINT study, there was no statistically significant difference in NEC incidence between transfusion groups.[93]

Despite potential pathophysiologic rationale and findings from primarily retrospective observational studies, confounding indications for PRBC transfusions in combination with the multifactorial pathogenesis of NEC make it challenging to link transfusion to NEC.[88] The overall body of evidence is not sufficient to promote a specific practice recommendation with respect to PRBC transfusions and preventing NEC.[88] Large-scale RCTs are needed to better evaluate the plausibility of this temporal relationship and the role of PRBC transfusions in prevention of NEC.

PROVEN QUALITY IMPROVEMENT SUCCESS

Various QI efforts have demonstrated a decrease in the incidence of NEC. Most efforts have focused on standardizing feeding protocols and promotion of exclusive HM nutrition (**Table 2**).[7,11,13,14,22,94–97] Despite the limited and conflicting evidence regarding strategies for prevention, early diagnosis, and targeted treatment, QI remains a reliable and worthwhile approach to decrease the incidence of NEC in VLBW infants.

As seen in Table 2, the QI projects focused on NEC reduction range in size from 232 infants in a single center to 58,555 infants in a multicenter collaborative with 330 NICUs. Across these projects, a clear aim statement is defined and historical data are reviewed to differentiate the impact of implementation of better clinical practices from the baseline to intervention and sustain phases. These projects acknowledged the importance of continuous short interval data monitoring, which allow for rapid test of change and learning through Plan-Do-Study-Act (PDSA) cycles.[22] For example, the authors' experience at Rush University Children's Hospital demonstrated the importance of continuous data monitoring and learning through PDSA cycles when initial implementation of a standardized feeding protocol did not reduce the NICU's NEC incidence in VLBW infants, as had been anticipated from previous QI publications. This observation led the authors to investigate additional risk factors for NEC that were relevant to the NICU, revealing a change in NG tube practice at the time of implementation of the feeding protocol. This observation prompted the addition of another key driver for change that addressed the hygienic handling of NG tubes.[13] With implementation of a range of interventions, the authors reduced NEC incidence

Table 2
Necrotizing enterocolitis quality improvement projects

Authors	Time Frame	Setting	Outcome Measure	Results: Necrotizing Enterocolitis Incidence	Drivers and Interventions	Donor Milk
Aziz et al,[11] 2012	2008–2009	480 infants 1 center GA <33 wk	DCC compliance (primary) NEC incidence (secondary)	5.4% to 1.3%	Implement DCC for 45 s Provide obstetric and neonatal staff education and visuals Create algorithm for eligible and noneligible infants Documentation of compliance by NICU staff	N/A
Lee et al,[96] 2012	2009–2011	1833 infants 11 centers BW 401–1500 g or GA 22–29 wk	BF rates at discharge (primary) NEC incidence (secondary)	7% to 2.4%	Implement education and advocacy for provision of BM Establish and maintain appropriate maternal milk supply Establish consistent and comprehensive nutritional monitoring program	Available
Patel et al,[13] 2014	2009–2011	232 infants 1 center VLBW infants	NEC incidence	10% to 2.9%	Implement feeding guideline Reduce NG tube indwelling time	Available 2013
Lee et al,[97] 2014	2008–2012	6026 infants 25 Canadian NICUs GA <29 wk	NEC (multiple morbidities)	10% vs 8% 0.73 OR (95% CI, 0.52–0.98)	Establish feeding guideline Introduce early feeding Standardize use of DM Promote use of colostrum or enhanced expressed breast milk Establish early total parenteral nutrition Standardize hold enteral feeds during PRBC transfusions Establish DCC practice Decrease nosocomial infections	Available

(*continued on next page*)

Table 2
(continued)

Authors	Time Frame	Setting	Outcome Measure	Results: Necrotizing Enterocolitis Incidence	Drivers and Interventions	Donor Milk
Alshaikh et al,[94] 2015	2009–2013	454 infants 1 center GA <32 wk	NEC incidence	8.9% to 4.8%	Improve rate of maternal BF Increase use of colostrum for trophic feeds Shorten time to introduction of trophic feeds Standardize education and training for lactation consultants Standardize education materials for mothers (written and DVD) Standardize education and training for nursing staff Decrease time lapse after delivery for mother to meet lactation specialist Establish antepartum education	Available Excluded from outcome
Ellsbury et al,[95] 2016	2009–2013	58,555 infants 330 centers VLBW infants	NEC (multiple morbidities)	6.6% to 3.9%	Increase HM use Standardize feeding protocols Promote early protein in intravenous fluids Reduce H_2 antagonist usage Decrease nosocomial infections Establish antibiotics stewardship	Available
Stefanescu et al,[14] 2016	2011–2013	299 infants 1 center VLBW infants	Growth (primary) NEC (secondary) Other morbidities BF rates at discharge	6% to 2%	Standardize parenteral and enteral nutrition protocols Standardize fortification Early HM feedings (both OMM and DM) Earlier discontinuation of central lines	Available
Talavera et al,[22] 2016	2010–2013	606 infants 8 centers VLBW infants	NEC incidence	8% to <4%	Standardize early HM feedings Standardize conservative feeding guideline during blood transfusions and indomethacin Restriction of ranitidine in VLBW infants <1500 g and <28 wk PMA	Available

Abbreviations: BF, breastfeeding; BM, breast milk; DCC, delayed cord clamping.

from 10% to 2.9%. The authors' QI effort has continued with additional PDSA cycles focused on feeding guidelines during PRBC transfusions (implemented in 2012) and DM feedings (implemented in 2013). The authors' unit's low incidence of NEC was sustained through 2016.

A common component across all these QI projects is the formation of an interdisciplinary team that includes physicians, nurses, neonatal nutritionists, and lactation specialists. In some cases, interdisciplinary representation may cross beyond NICU boundaries. Aziz and colleagues[11] demonstrated collaboration with the obstetric front-line staff to promote education and implement delayed cord clamping in infants less than 33 weeks' GA after which they observed a reduction in NEC incidence from 5.4% to 1.3% as a secondary outcome. The California Perinatal Quality of Care Collaborative decreased the incidence of NEC in VLBW infants from 7% to 2.4% in less than 2 years by increasing breast milk use.[96] The investigators conducted follow-up interviews of the participating NICUs to characterize the perceived factors associated with sustained improvement and revealed that, among other things, physician involvement with interdisciplinary teams was key to the sustainable success of this multicenter collaborative effort.[98]

SUMMARY

Best practice implementation (see **Box 1**), driven by PDSA cycles and continuous data monitoring, continue to show successful and sustainable improvements in VLBW infant outcomes, including NEC. Variation in NEC incidence among centers validates the importance of continued QI and collaboration to determine best practices. Although new strategies for prevention, diagnosis, and treatment of NEC continue to be investigated, efforts should be focused on QI. Consistent findings across published accounts of QI efforts aimed at reducing NEC demonstrate that interventions aimed at improving consistency in feeding advancement, increasing HM use, and decreasing antibiotic and H_2 antagonist usage decrease the incidence of NEC.

REFERENCES

1. Caplan MS, Fanaroff A. Necrotizing: a historical perspective. Semin Perinatol 2017;41(1):2–6.
2. Patel RM, Denning PW. Intestinal microbiota and its relationship with necrotizing enterocolitis. Pediatr Res 2015;78(3):232–8.
3. Neu J, Walker WA. Necrotizing enterocolitis. N Engl J Med 2011;364(3):255–64.
4. Gordon PV, Swanson JR, MacQueen BC, et al. A critical question for NEC researchers: can we create a consensus definition of NEC that facilitates research progress? Semin Perinatol 2017;41(1):7–14.
5. Gordon PV, Clark R, Swanson JR, et al. Can a national dataset generate a nomogram for necrotizing enterocolitis onset? J Perinatol 2014;34(10):732–5.
6. Horbar JD, Edwards EM, Greenberg LT, et al. Variation in performance of neonatal intensive care units in the United States. JAMA Pediatr 2017;171(3): e164396.
7. Kim JH. Necrotizing enterocolitis: the road to zero. Semin Fetal Neonatal Med 2014;19(1):39–44.
8. Weiner GM, Zaichkin J, editors. Textbook of neonatal resuscitation (NRP). 7th edition. Elk Grove Village (IL): American Academy of Pediatrics and American Heart Association; 2016.
9. ACOG. Committee opinion no. 684. Delayed umbilical cord clamping after birth. Obstet Gynecol 2017;129(1):e5–10.

10. Rabe H, Diaz-Rossello JL, Duley L, et al. Effect of timing of umbilical cord clamping and other strategies to influence placental transfusion at preterm birth on maternal and infant outcomes. Cochrane Database Syst Rev 2012;(8):CD003248.
11. Aziz K, Chinnery H, Lacaze-Masmonteil T. A single-center experience of implementing delayed cord clamping in babies born at less than 33 weeks' gestational age. Adv Neonatal Care 2012;12(6):371–6.
12. Patel S, Clark EA, Rodriguez CE, et al. Effect of umbilical cord milking on morbidity and survival in extremely low gestational age neonates. Am J Obstet Gynecol 2014;211(5):519.e1-e7.
13. Patel AL, Trivedi S, Parikh NM, et al. Reducing necrotizing enterocolitis in very low birth weight infants using quality improvement methods. J Perinatol 2014;34: 850–7.
14. Stefanescu BM, Gillam-Krakauer M, Stefanescu AR, et al. Very low birth weight infant care: adherence to a new nutrition protocol improves growth outcomes and reduces infectious risk. Early Hum Dev 2016;94:25–30.
15. Patole S, McGlone L, Muller R. Virtual elimination of necrotising enterocolitis for 5 years - reasons? Med Hypotheses 2003;61(5–6):617–22.
16. Patole SK, de Klerk N. Impact of standardised feeding regimens on incidence of neonatal necrotising enterocolitis: a systematic review and meta-analysis of observational studies. Arch Dis Child Fetal Neonatal Ed 2005;90(2):F147–51.
17. Henderson G, Craig S, Brocklehurst P, et al. Enteral feeding regimens and necrotising enterocolitis in preterm infants: a multicentre case-control study. Arch Dis Child Fetal Neonatal Ed 2009;94(2):F120–3.
18. Viswanathan S, McNelis K, Super D, et al. Standardized slow enteral feeding protocol and the incidence of necrotizing enterocolitis in extremely low birth weight infants. JPEN J Parenter Enteral Nutr 2015;39(6):644–54.
19. Kansagra K, Stoll B, Rognerud C, et al. Total parenteral nutrition adversely affects gut barrier function in neonatal piglets. Am J Physiol Gastrointest Liver Physiol 2003;285(6):G1162–70.
20. Rouwet EV, Heineman E, Buurman WA, et al. Intestinal permeability and carrier-mediated monosaccharide absorption in preterm neonates during the early postnatal period. Pediatr Res 2002;51(1):64–70.
21. Kirtsman M, Yoon EW, Ojah C, et al. Nil-per-os days and necrotizing enterocolitis in extremely preterm infants. Am J Perinatol 2014;32(8):785–94.
22. Talavera MM, Bixler G, Cozzi C, et al. Quality improvement initiative to reduce the necrotizing enterocolitis rate in premature infants. Pediatrics 2016;137(5) [pii:e20151119].
23. Morgan J, Young L, McGuire W. Slow advancement of enteral feed volumes to prevent necrotising enterocolitis in very low birth weight infants. Cochrane Database Syst Rev 2015;(10):CD001241.
24. Karagol BS, Zenciroglu A, Okumus N, et al. Randomized controlled trial of slow vs rapid enteral feeding advancements on the clinical outcomes of preterm infants with birth weight 750-1250 g. JPEN 2013;37(2):223–8.
25. Lambert DK, Christensen RD, Baer VL, et al. Fulminant necrotizing enterocolitis in a multihospital healthcare system. J Perinatol 2012;32(3):194–8.
26. Shah SD, Dereddy N, Jones TL, et al. Early versus delayed human milk fortification in very low birth weight infants-A randomized controlled trial. J Pediatr 2016; 174:126–31.e1.
27. Clyman R, Wickremasinghe A, Jhaveri N, et al. Enteral feeding during indomethacin and ibuprofen treatment of a patent ductus arteriosus. J Pediatr 2013;163(2): 406–11.

28. Krimmel GA, Baker R, Yanowitz TD. Blood transfusion alters the superior mesenteric artery blood flow velocity response to feeding in premature infants. Am J Perinatol 2009;26(2):99–105.
29. El-Dib M, Narang S, Lee E, et al. Red blood cell transfusion, feeding and necrotizing enterocolitis in preterm infants. J Perinatol 2011;31(3):183–7.
30. Mohamed A, Shah PS. Transfusion associated necrotizing enterocolitis: a meta-analysis of observational data. Pediatrics 2012;129(3):529–40.
31. Christensen RD, Lambert DK, Henry E, et al. Is "transfusion-associated necrotizing enterocolitis" an authentic pathogenic entity? Transfusion 2010;50(5):1106–12.
32. Lucas A, Cole TJ. Breast milk and neonatal necrotising enterocolitis. Lancet 1990;336:1519–23.
33. Schanler RJ, Shulman RJ, Lau C. Feeding strategies for premature infants: beneficial outcomes of feeding fortified human milk versus preterm formula. Pediatrics 1999;103:1150–7.
34. Sisk PM, Lovelady CA, Dillard RG, et al. Early human milk feeding is associated with a lower risk of necrotizing enterocolitis in very low birth weight infants. J Perinatol 2007;27:428–33.
35. Meinzen-Derr J, Poindexter B, Wrage L, et al. Role of human milk in extremely low birth weight infants' risk of necrotizing enterocolitis or death. J Perinatol 2009;29(1):57–62.
36. Corpeleijn WE, Kouwenhoven SM, Pappa MC, et al. Intake of own mother's milk during the first days of life is associated with decreased morbidity and mortality in very low birth weight infants during the first 60 days of life. Neonatology 2012;102(4):276–81.
37. Johnson TJ, Patel AL, Bigger HR, et al. Cost savings of human milk as a strategy to reduce the incidence of necrotizing enterocolitis in very low birth weight infants. Neonatology 2015;107(4):271–6.
38. Eidelman AI, Schanler RJ. Breastfeeding and the use of human milk. Pediatrics 2012;129(3):e827–41.
39. Taylor SN, Basile LA, Ebeling M, et al. Intestinal permeability in preterm infants by feeding type: mother's milk versus formula. Breastfeed Med 2009;4(1):11–5.
40. Jeurink PV, van Bergenhenegouwen J, Jimenez E, et al. Human milk: a source of more life than we imagine. Benef Microbes 2013;4(1):17–30.
41. Collado MC, Santaella M, Mira-Pascual L, et al. Longitudinal study of cytokine expression, lipid profile and neuronal growth factors in human breast milk from term and preterm deliveries. Nutrients 2015;7(10):8577–91.
42. Underwood MA, Gaerlan S, De Leoz ML, et al. Human milk oligosaccharides in premature infants: absorption, excretion, and influence on the intestinal microbiota. Pediatr Res 2015;78(6):670–7.
43. Labeta MO, Vidal K, Nores JE, et al. Innate recognition of bacteria in human milk is mediated by a milk-derived highly expressed pattern recognition receptor, soluble CD14. J Exp Med 2000;191(10):1807–12.
44. Dvorak B, Fituch CC, Williams CS, et al. Concentrations of epidermal growth factor and transforming growth factor-alpha in preterm milk. Adv Exp Med Biol 2004;554:407–9.
45. Hassiotou F, Hartmann PE. At the dawn of a new discovery: the potential of breast milk stem cells. Adv Nutr 2014;5(6):770–8.
46. Lonnerdal B. Bioactive proteins in human milk: mechanisms of action. J Pediatr 2010;156:S26–30.

47. Kimak KS, de Castro Antunes MM, Braga TD, et al. Influence of enteral nutrition on occurrences of necrotizing enterocolitis in very-low-birth-weight infants. J Pediatr Gastroenterol Nutr 2015;61(4):445–50.
48. Meier PP, Patel A, Esquerra-Zwiers A. Donor human milk update: evidence, mechanisms and priorities for research and practice. J Pediatr 2017;180:15–21.
49. Underwood M, Scoble J. Human milk and the premature infant: focus on the use of pasteurized donor human milk in the NICU. In: Rajendra R, Preedy V, Patel V, editors. Diet and nutrition in critical care. New York: Springer-Verlag; 2015.
50. Schanler RJ, Lau C, Hurst NM, et al. Randomized trial of donor human milk versus preterm formula as substitutes for mothers' own milk in the feeding of extremely premature infants. Pediatrics 2005;116(2):400–6.
51. Sullivan S, Schanler RJ, Kim JH, et al. An exclusively human milk-based diet is associated with a lower rate of necrotizing enterocolitis than a diet of human milk and bovine milk-based products. J Pediatr 2010;156(4):562–7.e1.
52. Cristofalo EA, Schanler RJ, Blanco CL, et al. Randomized trial of exclusive human milk versus preterm formula diets in extremely premature infants. J Pediatr 2013; 163:1592–5.
53. Quigley M, McGuire W. Formula versus donor breast milk for feeding preterm or low birth weight infants. Cochrane Database Syst Rev 2014;(4):CD002971.
54. Kantorowska A, Wei JC, Cohen RS, et al. Impact of donor milk availability on breast milk use and necrotizing enterocolitis rates. Pediatrics 2016;137(3):1–8.
55. O'Connor DL, Gibbins S, Kiss A, et al. Effect of supplemental donor human milk compared with preterm formula on neurodevelopment of very low-birth-weight infants at 18 months: a randomized clinical trial. JAMA 2016;316(18):1897–905.
56. Corpeleijn WE, de Waard M, Christmann V, et al. Effect of donor milk on severe infections and mortality in very low-birth-weight infants: the early nutrition study randomized clinical trial. JAMA Pediatr 2016;170(7):654–61.
57. Sisk PM, Lambeth TM, Rojas MA, et al. Necrotizing enterocolitis and growth in preterm infants fed predominantly maternal milk, pasteurized donor milk, or preterm formula: a retrospective study. Am J Perinatol 2016. http://dx.doi.org/10.1055/s-0036-1597326.
58. Hagadorn JI, Brownell EA, Lussier MM, et al. Variability of criteria for pasteurized donor human milk use: a survey of U.S. neonatal ICU medical directors. JPEN 2014;40(3):326–33.
59. Gewolb IH, Schwalbe RS, Taciak VL, et al. Stool microflora in extremely low birthweight infants. Arch Dis Child Fetal Neonatal Ed 1999;80(3):167–73.
60. Greenwood C, Morrow AL, Lagomarcino AJ, et al. Early empiric antibiotic use in preterm infants is associated with lower bacterial diversity and higher relative abundance of enterobacter. J Pediatr 2014;165(1):23–9.
61. Schwiertz A, Gruhl B, Lobnitz M. Development of the intestinal bacterial composition in hospitalized preterm infants in comparison with breast-fed, full-term infants. Pediatr Res 2003;54(3):393–9.
62. Cotten CM, Taylor S, Stoll B, et al. Prolonged duration of initial empirical antibiotic treatment is associated with increased rates of necrotizing enterocolitis and death for extremely low birth weight infants. Pediatrics 2009;123(1):58–66.
63. Alexander VN, Northrup V, Bizzarro MJ. Antibiotic exposure in the newborn intensive care unit and the risk of necrotizing enterocolitis. J Pediatr 2011;159:392–7.
64. Kuppala VS, Meinzen-Derr J, Morrow AL, et al. Prolonged initial empirical antibiotic treatment is associated with adverse outcomes in premature infants. J Pediatr 2011;159(5):720–5.

65. Gupta RW, Tran L, Norori J, et al. Histamine-2 receptor blockers alter the fecal microbiota in premature infants. J Pediatr Gastroenterol Nutr 2013;56(4):397–400.
66. Guillet R, Stoll BJ, Cotten CM, et al. Association of H2-blocker therapy and higher incidence of necrotizing enterocolitis in very low birth weight infants. Pediatrics 2006;117(2):e137–42.
67. Terrin G, Passariello A, De Curtis M, et al. Ranitidine is associated with infections, necrotizing enterocolitis, and fatal outcome in newborns. Pediatrics 2012;129(1): e40–5.
68. Repa A, Thanhaeuser M, Endress D, et al. Probiotics (lactobacillus acidophilus and bifidobacterium bifidum) prevent NEC in VLBW infants fed breast milk but not formula. Pediatr Res 2015;77(2):381–8.
69. Dilli D, Aydin B, Fettah ND, et al. The ProPre-save study: effects of probiotics and prebiotics alone or combined on necrotizing enterocolitis in very low birth weight infants. J Pediatr 2015;166(3):545–51.e1.
70. Janvier A, Malo J, Barrington KJ. Cohort study of probiotics in a North American neonatal intensive care unit. J Pediatr 2014;164(5):980–5.
71. Bin-Nun A, Bromiker R, Wilschanski M, et al. Oral probiotics prevent necrotizing enterocolitis in very low birth weight neonates. J Pediatr 2005;147(2):192–6.
72. Lin HC, Su BH, Chen AC, et al. Oral probiotics reduce the incidence and severity of necrotizing enterocolitis in very low birth weight infants. Pediatrics 2005;115(1):1–4.
73. Denkel LA, Schwab F, Garten L, et al. Protective effect of dual-strain probiotics in preterm infants: a multi-center time series analysis. PLoS One 2016;11(6): e0158136.
74. Deshpande G, Rao S, Patole S, et al. Updated meta-analysis of probiotics for preventing necrotizing enterocolitis in preterm neonates. Pediatrics 2010;125(5): 921–30.
75. Costeloe K, Hardy P, Juszczak E, et al, Probiotics in Preterm Infants Study Collaborative Group. Bifidobacterium breve BBG-001 in very preterm infants: a randomised controlled phase 3 trial. Lancet 2016;387:649–60.
76. Embleton ND, Zalewski S, Berrington JE. Probiotics for prevention of necrotizing enterocolitis and sepsis in preterm infants. Curr Opin Infect Dis 2016;29(3): 256–61.
77. Aceti A, Gori D, Barone G, et al. Probiotics for prevention of necrotizing enterocolitis in preterm infants: systematic review and meta-analysis. Ital J Pediatr 2015; 41:89.
78. AlFaleh K, Anabrees J. Probiotics for prevention of necrotizing enterocolitis in preterm infants. Cochrane Database Syst Rev 2014;(4):CD005496.
79. Underwood MA. Impact of probiotics on necrotizing enterocolitis. Semin Perinatol 2017;41(1):41–51.
80. Samuels N, van de Graaf R, Been JV, et al. Necrotising enterocolitis and mortality in preterm infants after introduction of probiotics: a quasi-experimental study. Sci Rep 2016;6:31643.
81. Neu J. Probiotics and necrotizing enterocolitis. Clin Perinatol 2014;41(4):967–78.
82. Tarnow-Mordi W, Soll RF. Probiotic supplementation in preterm infants: it is time to change practice. J Pediatr 2014;164(5):959–60.
83. Hurrell E, Kucerova E, Loughlin M, et al. Neonatal enteral feeding tubes as loci for colonisation by members of the enterobacteriaceae. BMC Infect Dis 2009;9:146.
84. Mehall JR, Kite CA, Saltzman DA, et al. Prospective study of the incidence and complications of bacterial contamination of enteral feeding in neonates. J Pediatr Surg 2002;37(8):1177–82.

85. Petersen SM, Greisen G, Krogfelt KA. Nasogastric feeding tubes from a neonatal department yield high concentrations of potentially pathogenic bacteria- even 1 d after insertion. Pediatr Res 2016;80(3):395–400.
86. Mally P, Golombek SG, Mishra R, et al. Association of necrotizing enterocolitis with elective packed red blood cell transfusions in stable, growing, premature neonates. Am J Perinatol 2006;23(8):451–8.
87. Blau J, Calo JM, Dozor D, et al. Transfusion-related acute gut injury: necrotizing enterocolitis in very low birth weight neonates after packed red blood cell transfusion. J Pediatr 2011;158(3):403–9.
88. Hay S, Zupancic JA, Flannery DD, et al. Should we believe in transfusion-associated enterocolitis? applying a GRADE to the literature. Semin Perinatol 2017;41(1):80–91.
89. La Gamma EF, Blau J. Transfusion-related acute gut injury: feeding, flora, flow, and barrier defense. Semin Perinatol 2012;36(4):294–305.
90. Hyung N, Campwala I, Boskovic DS, et al. The relationship of red blood cell transfusion to intestinal mucosal injury in premature infants. J Pediatr Surg 2016. http://dx.doi.org/10.1016/j.jpedsurg.2016.10.049 [pii:S0022–3468(16)30531-0].
91. Patel RM, Knezevic A, Shenvi N, et al. Association of red blood cell transfusion, anemia, and necrotizing enterocolitis in very low-birth-weight infants. JAMA 2016; 315(9):889–97.
92. Singh R, Visintainer PF, Frantz ID 3rd, et al. Association of necrotizing enterocolitis with anemia and packed red blood cell transfusions in preterm infants. J Perinatol 2011;31(3):176–82.
93. Kirpalani H, Whyte RK, Andersen C, et al. The premature infants in need of transfusion (PINT) study: a randomized, controlled trial of a restrictive (low) versus liberal (high) transfusion threshold for extremely low birth weight infants. J Pediatr 2006;149(3):301–7.
94. Alshaikh B, Kostecky L, Blachly N, et al. Effect of a quality improvement project to use exclusive mother's own milk on rate of necrotizing enterocolitis in preterm infants. Breastfeed Med 2015;10(7):355–61.
95. Ellsbury DL, Clark RH, Ursprung R, et al. A multifaceted approach to improving outcomes in the NICU: the Pediatrix 100 000 babies campaign. Pediatrics 2016;137(4) [pii:e20150389].
96. Lee HC, Kurtin PS, Wight NE, et al. A quality improvement project to increase breast milk use in very low birth weight infants. Pediatrics 2012;130(6):e1679–87.
97. Lee SK, Shah PS, Singhal N, et al. Association of a quality improvement program with neonatal outcomes in extremely preterm infants: a prospective cohort study. CMAJ 2014;186(13):E485–94.
98. Stone S, Lee HC, Sharek PJ. Perceived factors associated with sustained improvement following participation in a multicenter quality improvement collaborative. Jt Comm J Qual Patient Saf 2016;42(7):309–15.

Using Quality Improvement Tools to Reduce Chronic Lung Disease

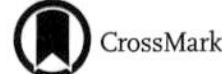

Alan Peter Picarillo, MD[a,*], Waldemar Carlo, MD[b]

KEYWORDS

- Chronic lung disease • Respiratory care • Potentially better practices
- Key driver diagram • Quality improvement

KEY POINTS

- Overall chronic lung disease (CLD) rates have not decreased appreciably in the past 20 years when compared to other neonatal morbidities and new approaches may need to be taken.
- Studies have demonstrated reduction in CLD by use of following strategies: avoidance of intubation by application of early CPAP/non-invasive ventilation, selective use of surfactant, initiation of caffeine, gentle ventilation and extubation strategies for intubated infants.
- Development of a local quality improvement initiative using the best available evidence, along with multidisciplinary involvement of team members can lead to success in educing CLD rates.

INTRODUCTION

Despite the increased use of exogenous surfactant administration, increased access to antenatal steroids for mothers threatening preterm delivery, and substantial advancements in respiratory care, the overall incidence of chronic lung disease (CLD) has remained stubbornly elevated in the very low birthweight (VLBW) population over the past two decades.[1] During this time period, other improvements in medical care have led to substantial decreases in the incidence of other morbidities of VLBW infants, such as hospital-acquired bloodstream infections, necrotizing enterocolitis (NEC), severe interventricular hemorrhage, and severe retinopathy of prematurity.

CLD was first described by Northway and colleagues[2] in 1967, and these early cases were usually seen in premature infants with severe respiratory distress syndrome (RDS) who received positive pressure ventilation and oxygen administration. This chronic

[a] Maine Neonatology Associates, Barbara Bush Children's Hospital, Maine Medical Center, 22 Bramhall Street, Portland, ME 04102, USA; [b] Division of Neonatology, University of Alabama-Birmingham, 1700 6th Avenue South, 9380 176F WIC, Birmingham, AL 35249, USA
* Corresponding author.
E-mail address: Alan.Picarillo@shcr.com

Clin Perinatol 44 (2017) 701–712
http://dx.doi.org/10.1016/j.clp.2017.05.010 perinatology.theclinics.com

pulmonary disease was descriptively named bronchopulmonary dysplasia (BPD) because of the pathologic changes of injury and cellular repair of the parenchyma of the lung tissue, coupled with alterations in growth of the developing lung. Before the advent of mechanical ventilation, infants with RDS had high mortality rates because it was the leading cause of death in live-born premature infants; after the introduction of mechanical ventilation in neonatal care, BPD was seen primarily as a disease of mechanically ventilated late preterm infants. In modern times, because of advancements in neonatal care, infants at this gestation now rarely have severe pulmonary-related morbidity, and CLD is primarily seen in smaller preterm infants.

CLD is currently defined as need for supplemental oxygen for infants at 36 weeks corrected postmenstrual age,[3] although there remains a spectrum of severity of illness for infants with this diagnosis. Newer definitions have been proposed to reflect this reality with the following classification: mild CLD is need for supplemental oxygen at 28 days, but not at 36 weeks post-menstrual age (PMA); moderate BPD is need for supplemental oxygen at 28 days and less than 30% oxygen at 36 weeks PMA; and severe BPD is need for supplemental oxygen at 28 days and greater than 30% oxygen at 36 weeks PMA and/or positive pressure ventilation at 36 weeks PMA.[4]

Quality improvement (QI) projects have become a mainstay of neonatal care over the past decade, with an increasing number of publications devoted to this topic. Neonatal intensive care units (NICUs) are well positioned for QI projects because of a long-standing history of participation in data collection, data benchmarking, and collaborative learning opportunities that exist throughout neonatology.[5]

Borrowing liberally from manufacturing and other industries, medicine has started to embrace the theory and methodology of QI science and how to apply that science to their daily work in improving the care of infants and families in their respective NICUs.

There have been several single-center and multicenter publications that have demonstrated QI projects leading to a reduction in CLD,[6–8] but there has been no sustained overall decrease in CLD rates in VLBW infants in large national data sets.[1,9,10] Many interventions that are described at the unit-level have either not been translatable or have not been successful in a broad application across a multitude of NICUs. This disparity between successful local initiatives and lack of widespread improvement likely highlights the importance of local context. Although any QI effort needs to structure its measures and interventions to the local environment, this may be particularly true for neonatal respiratory care, where the complex nature of CLD requires specific interventions and culture change that may not be easily translated from one NICU to another.[11]

This article examines several strategies to reduce CLD in premature infants. It is hoped that the information provided is useful to neonatal providers seeking to evaluate or improve respiratory care practices in their NICU with a goal of reducing the burden of CLD in their patients and their families.

QUALITY IMPROVEMENT FOR CHRONIC LUNG DISEASE: GENERAL CONSIDERATIONS

A broad and expansive description of QI science and methods has been discussed extensively in other articles and is not included here. However, several common principles are important to apply when focusing on QI for CLD reduction. A specific QI project for CLD, similar to other projects, must be based on best available evidence in the medical literature, expert recommendations, or based on work by previous QI initiatives. Clinical practices that have the potential to improve the outcomes of neonatal care are known as potentially better practices (PBPs).[12]

These PBPs are existing recommendations or protocols that have the potential to improve the care and change the outcome of the specific clinical project. They are tested, modified, and changed to fit each individual NICU microsystem in which they are introduced; not all PBPs work for each and every unit. Examples of specific PBPs vary for reducing the incidence of CLD or lung injury, but most include the use of early continuous positive airway pressure (CPAP), caffeine use in specific populations, selective surfactant use, minimization of the duration of mechanical ventilation, and gentle ventilation strategies.

Once a unit-based multidisciplinary team (including parent or family members) has been established and executive leadership buy-in obtained by the team, progression to the QI project involves the choosing of a specific aim or aims from a list of accepted PBPs or toolkits, many of which are available in previously published QI initiatives or retrieved online. Construction of tools, such as key driver diagrams, can help structure the team and allow for all members to contribute and understand the rationale for new changes to practice that are being introduced.

QUALITY IMPROVEMENT FOR CHRONIC LUNG DISEASE: SPECIFIC STRATEGIES

Several specific strategies have evidence supporting their use in improvement initiatives to reduce CLD. Some of these are summarized next, and **Table 1** provides an overview of how these strategies can be used in the context of a local QI effort.

Early Continuous Positive Airway Pressure

Multiple trials have proven the benefit of early nasal CPAP in the delivery room for initial respiratory stabilization of the preterm and even the extremely preterm infant,[13–15] with a combined reduction in death or CLD. Even the most preterm infant at 24 to 25 weeks gestation has shown benefit from this approach with a lower mortality rate in the COIN (Continuous Positive Airway Pressure or Intubation at Birth) trial when compared with initial planned intubation/mechanical ventilation group. CPAP started soon after birth is a strategy that seems to reduce CLD/death and is an accepted alternative to prophylactic surfactant approach.

After the aim statement has been created by the team, measurement for this specific intervention needs to be chosen, with common measurement point consisting of percent of infants who receive nasal CPAP before positive pressure ventilation via an endotracheal tube. A potential complication of earlier CPAP use is higher risk of pneumothorax. In the COIN trial, a higher pneumothorax rate was seen in the CPAP group compared with the immediate intubation group, but this was not seen in other trials, and was not significantly different between the two groups in meta-analysis. Nevertheless, tracking pneumothorax rates as a balancing measure should be considered.

Certain barriers exist for starting CPAP soon after birth. The most common barrier identified is the belief that VLBW infants, especially extremely low birth weight infants, require immediate intubation and surfactant therapy. However, there have been several trials that do not lend support to this approach as being superior to a nasal CPAP-first approach.[13,16–18]

One strategy that can help address staff concerns includes the development of a consensus guideline with specific criteria for delivery room management of premature infants with noninvasive ventilation. Participation of all team members including physicians, neonatal nurse practitioners, neonatal nurses, respiratory therapists, family members, and other allied health professionals would allow for locally constructed guidelines based on a shared approach and would be extremely effective in

Table 1
Specific strategies for a quality improvement initiative to reduce chronic lung disease

	Intervention	Process Measure	Balancing Measure	PDSA/Test of Change	Barriers to Change
Early CPAP	Early CPAP in delivery room for infants that meet criteria	Number of infants CPAP attempted in the delivery room	Pneumothorax	Apply early CPAP to spontaneously breathing infant in delivery room	Preconceived notion that infants <28 wk need to be ventilated at birth
Selective surfactant	Develop criteria for INSURE method	Number of infants who meet criteria but were not extubated	Pneumothorax	Develop criteria for intubation and surfactant administration	Practice patterns to leave infants intubated for a period of time following surfactant
Caffeine	Start caffeine on infants when weaning from ventilator	Number of infants who were started on caffeine	Number of intubated infants still on caffeine >7 d	Develop protocol with standard caffeine dosing for initiation and maintenance	Fear of increased rates of NEC
Gentle ventilation	Reduction of tidal volume to specified daily target	Daily audits on ventilator setting with recorded tidal volumes	Number of ventilator changes	Develop a specific tidal volume target	Inability to accurately measure tidal volumes
Extubation guidelines	Develop criteria for extubation of ventilated infants	Attempt SBT on all infants before extubation	Number of reintubations	Develop passing criteria for SBT for infants ready for extubation	Previous practice of allowing infant to remain ventilated "vent to grow"

Abbreviations: INSURE, intubate, surfactant, extubate; PDSA, Plan, Do, Study, Act; SBT, spontaneous breathing test.

overcoming staff resistance or staff perceptions regarding the need for immediate intubation.[19] Based on best available evidence and this local consensus-driven process, each NICU team should detail specific criteria for infants that may be appropriate candidates for early CPAP in their NICU, based on gestational age, presence of antenatal steroid administration, and other factors, and should then prospectively collect process and outcomes data closely, along with prompt feedback to team members.

Selective Surfactant Use

Surfactant-replacement therapy has been an effective mainstay therapy for RDS in neonates and has been shown to decrease mortality, combined outcome of death/CLD, and pneumothoraces.[20,21] Given the evidence described supporting early CPAP as an improvement strategy for very preterm infants, the role of surfactant must be considered differently. Earlier studies advocated for prophylactic surfactant, but more recent data demonstrated that early CPAP in the delivery room versus prophylactic surfactant has improved outcomes (lower death/CLD combined outcome) when compared with CPAP alone.[18] In the SUPPORT (Surfactant, Positive Pressure and Oxygenation Randomized Trial) trial,[13] infants 24 to 25 weeks who were randomized to CPAP had a lower mortality rate than infants who were intubated and received prophylactic surfactant.

Based on these data, current guidelines advise noninvasive ventilation as a PBP in the delivery room, but if the neonate requires intubation and mechanical ventilation, then administration of surfactant within the first 3 hours of life reduces mortality and morbidity associated with RDS.[20]

In addition, techniques to avoid prolonged positive ventilation and the concomitant damage to lung tissue, such as intubate-surfactant-extubate and less invasive surfactant administration, may reduce CLD and the need for ventilation[22–24]

Development of guidelines and workflow to introduce early CPAP/noninvasive ventilation in the delivery room with previously agreed on indication for administration of rescue surfactant is an important component to selective surfactant use in a NICU. Measurement of how many infants at a specified gestational age have an attempt at noninvasive ventilation allows for the unit-based QI team to further refine their protocols to stratify which infants are successful with this approach. Having a unit-based approach[19] to the use of intubation and surfactant-replacement therapy based on agreed on parameters (eg, pH <7.2; F_{IO_2} >40%; increased work of breathing) and prospectively collecting data on compliance with the parameters to give feedback to providers is valuable. An example of such an approach is given in **Fig. 1**. Also, it is important to collect data on balancing measures, such as pneumothoraces, to confirm that the local change in practice is not leading to worse outcomes.

Caffeine

Apnea is a common occurrence in NICUs, especially prevalent in VLBW infants less than 32 weeks gestation.[12] The CAP (Caffeine for Apnea of Prematurity) trial demonstrated that infants less than 1250 g who did not receive caffeine treatment had increased CLD and additional short-term and long-term morbidities.[25] In addition, infants who received caffeine in this trial had decreased time on ventilator support, decreased postnatal corticosteroid use, and decreased oxygen use when compared with the placebo group. Long-term developmental outcomes did not differ between in the two groups,[26] but the short-term pulmonary benefits of caffeine treatment were important.

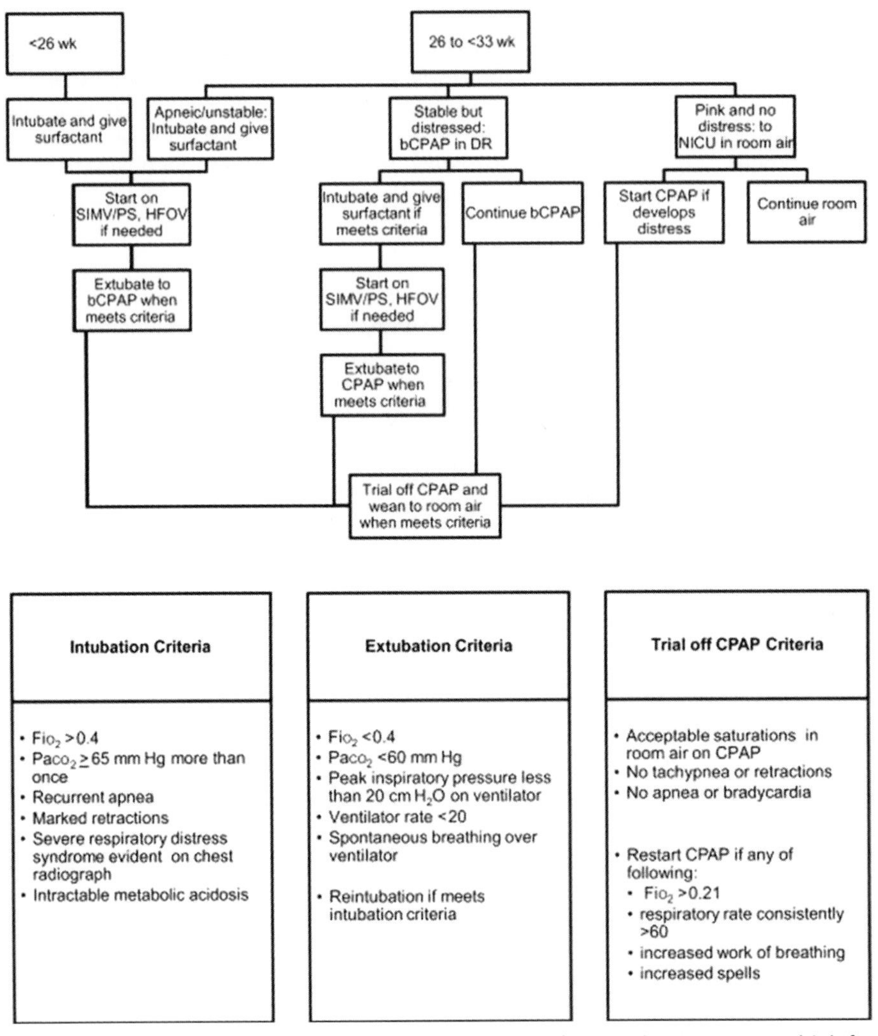

Fig. 1. Respiratory management of infants. FIO_2, fraction of inspired oxygen; HFOV, high frequency oscillatory ventilation; SIMV/PS, synchronized intermittent mandatory ventilation/pressure support. (*From* Levesque BM, Kalish LA, LaPierre J, et al. Impact of implementing 5 potentially better respiratory practices on neonatal outcomes and costs. Pediatrics 2011;128(1):e221; with permission.)

NICUs should consider establishment of a local guideline for caffeine administration, in consultation with hospital pharmacists. Specific components of this guideline should include initiation of caffeine when weaning from the ventilator, dosing caffeine with a standard loading dose and maintenance dose, and conversion of intravenous caffeine to enteral when a certain volume of feeds are reached. Such measurements as number of eligible infants who received caffeine or the time from birth when caffeine was first received by the infant are metrics that can be tracked by teams that use this as a process measure. Barriers, such as the fear of increased rates of NEC with administration of methylxanthines, have not been noted in larger studies.[25]

Gentle Ventilation (Low Tidal Volume/Permissive Hypercapnea)

During mechanical ventilation of an infant, a balance must be achieved where the infant is provided with the lowest possible inspiratory pressure to minimize volutrauma, but enough pressure to ensure adequate gas exchange. Expiratory tidal volume may be measured by the ventilator and a goal of no more than 4 to 6 mL/kg. The respiratory system of premature infants with RDS has low lung compliance, coupled with low resistance, which leads to a short time constant. To take advantage of these characteristics in a recently delivered infant, optimal ventilation with short inspiratory times and fast rates results in less air leak syndromes and nonsignificant mortality when compared with infants ventilated with slow rates and long inspiratory times.[27]

Permissive hypercapnia is a ventilatory strategy that may reduce injury to the developing lung through a variety of mechanisms. Data based on the current literature, pertinent physiologic rationale, and experimental research demonstrate that permissive hypercapnia may be beneficial. Several trials suggest that a strategy of permissive hypercapnia (usually limited by a pH of at least 7.2) started early, before initiation of mechanical ventilation, combined with prolonged permissive hypercapnia during mechanical ventilation optimizes pulmonary/survival benefits and seems to be safe in neonates.[13,28] These data support the use of permissive hypercapnia as an alternative to traditional ventilator support strategies that aim to maintain normocapnia. Further research is necessary to elucidate better strategies of permissive hypercapnia, such as target CO_2 levels, duration of the intervention, and minimal tidal volume ventilation.

QI projects centered on gentle ventilation and permissive hypercapnia can have an aim to reduce tidal volume of the infant to a specific target (eg, <4–6 mL/kg) and mildly elevated P_{CO_2} (≤65 mm Hg) to mechanically ventilated infants. Daily audits of ventilated infants (tidal volumes with accompanying ventilator settings and P_{CO_2} levels) with feedback given to provider and team allows for needed adjustments to be made in the PDSA (Plan, Do, Study, Act) cycles of this specific initiative. Barriers to this test of change include a tradition of long-standing ventilator settings with resistance of low inspiratory pressures and high ventilator rates, along with providing normocapnia to ventilated infants; education to all team members (physicians, nursing, respiratory therapists, and families) on this approach may ease its adoption and acceptance.

Extubation Strategies and Protocols

One of the most difficult decisions in a NICU involved the timing of weaning and extubation for a mechanically ventilated infant. The potential success of rapid weaning and extubation needs to be weighed against the potential negative outcome of an infant who may develop clinical deterioration and then require subsequent reintubation shortly after being extubated.

High level of evidence and standard criteria for extubation guidelines in neonatal medicine do not exist. The decision to extubate an infant is usually left to the clinical team who may not have defined criteria for extubation readiness. In the absence of defined extubation criteria, infants may remain ventilated longer than needed, along with a potential for ventilator-induced volutrauma. Some researchers have evaluated the utility of a spontaneous breathing test (SBT) to select and predict VLBW infants who may have greater success with extubation. The SBT is a 3-minute period of endotracheal intubation and infants who are successful are then extubated. Most infants who were successful with the SBT remained extubated, with 22% of this cohort needing reintubation,[29] but further studies are needed to evaluate the diagnostic accuracy of this test.

Another bedside test that has been evaluated for extubation readiness is the minute ventilation test (MVT), where the minute ventilation on endotracheal CPAP alone must be greater than 50% of the minute volume of mechanical ventilation. In one small study,[30] infants who were extubated according to success of an MVT were extubated several hours earlier (8 vs 36 hours) when compared with those infants who were evaluated clinically; the extubation rates in both groups were similar.

Creation a local protocol for extubation readiness can incorporate existing bedside tests, such as SBT or MVT, with defined criteria (eg, pH >7.2; P_{CO_2} <60 mm Hg; F_{IO_2} <40%; MAP (mean airway pressure) <7; caffeine administration to infant) to successfully extubate a mechanically ventilated infant (see **Fig. 1**). Success or failures of each eligible infant, along with an assessment of process measures and potential refinement of protocol based on rapid PDSA cycles, allows for the team to accept the protocol or amend it as needed to fit the clinical microsystem of the NICU. Barriers to extubation success include prior practice of prolonged intubation to let a VLBW infant rest and "vent to grow," along with fear of potential reintubation.

Other Strategies

Multiple other care practices may impact the development of BPD, and may be amenable to improvement initiatives. These include systemic corticosteroids, fluid restriction, diuretics, use of vitamin A, noninvasive positive pressure ventilation, and oxygen saturation targeting. Although these are not reviewed in detail here, in general, a lack of compelling data on efficacy, a lack of long-term data on outcomes, or other concerns limit the potential widespread use of these interventions as improvement strategies. For example, although controversial, systemic corticosteroids have shown a reduction in CLD, but with an unacceptable increased risk in cerebral palsy. Although there may be data that delayed use of systemic corticosteroids (>7 days of age) has less short-term morbidities than early (<7 days of age) systemic corticosteroids, the limited follow-up data give pause to routine administration of steroids, and in cases where it is given the dose and duration should be minimized during the treatment course.[31] Inhaled corticosteroids have shown reduced CLD in a recent meta-analysis, but long-term follow-up data are not yet available.[32]

DEVELOPING A QUALITY IMPROVEMENT INITIATIVE FOR CHRONIC LUNG DISEASE

There have been many collaborative efforts to reduce CLD over the past decade leading to site-specific reductions in CLD. With any type of QI project, there is always concern that improvement is related to the Hawthorne effect, but the powerful effect of culture change and increased teamwork with all involved disciplines to implement process change cannot be understated. Local development of a collaborative QI project should include interventions, process measures, balancing measures, tests of change, and barriers to change (see **Table 1**). This process should be multidisciplinary and also include the parent voice to make sure that the changes proposed by the group for the initiative not only is evidence-based, but is patient focused.

Development of a key driver diagram allows for the project to have a visual representation of a structured improvement roadmap. The construction of these diagrams details the project planning with keeping a focus on factors that allow the team to realize the project aim. This diagram organizes the improvement aim, the key drivers (the "what" needed to accomplish that aim), and the interventions (the "how" [change concepts], also known as secondary drivers) into a learning and communication framework. An example of a key driver diagram for surfactant administration is shown in **Fig. 2**.

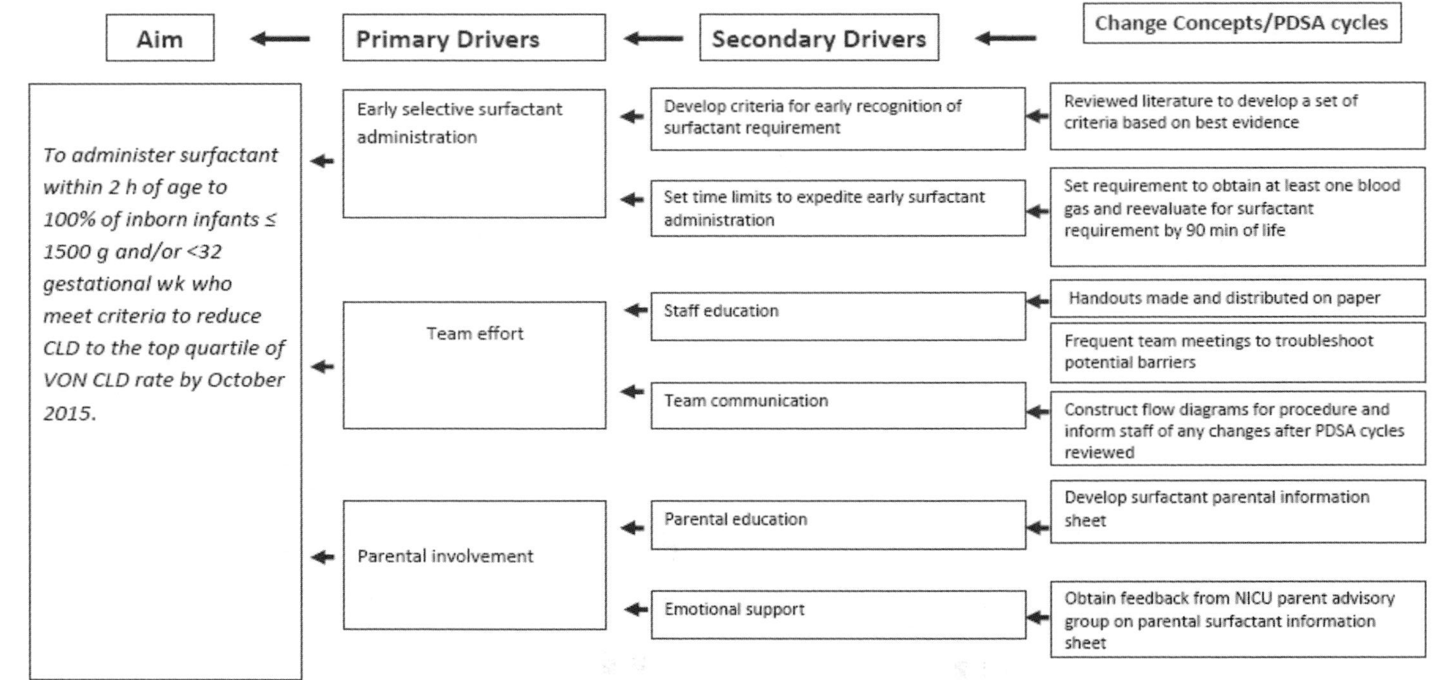

Fig. 2. Example of a key driver diagram for surfactant administration. PDSA, Plan, Do, Study, Act; VON, Vermont-Oxford Network.

Examples of Quality Improvement Initiatives

A large cluster-randomized trial performed by the National Institute of Child Health and Human Development Neonatal Research Network for prevention of CLD in infants less than 1250 g saw no improvement in survival free of CLD in a cohort of greater than 4000 patients. The centers that were randomized to the intervention group included adoption of PBPs from the benchmark centers that were recognized for having high rates of CLD-free survival in this population. The authors believed that although the intervention centers adopted care practice from benchmark institutions, the possibility of no significant decrease in the outcome may have been because there was only weak evidence supporting some of the new practices that were introduced.[6]

Conversely, in the Vermont-Oxford Breathsavers group, 19 hospitals participated in the adoption of PBPs during a 2-year collaborative QI project, consisting of close to 3600 VLBW infants during the collaborative time periods. Most (15 of 19) hospitals saw a decrease in the CLD rates during this project, and the pooled data across the collaborative demonstrated a statistically significant reduction in CLD rates and a statistically significant increase in VLBW infants who survived free of CLD.[8]

In addition, there have been publications of single-center experiences that have demonstrated reduction in CLD rates by implementation of pre-existing PBPs in addition to site-specific improvement bundles. One center instituted a bundle of practices to reduce CLD, including a site visit to a nearby NICU with a low CLD rate. By the addition of a series of new practices around respiratory care, this NICU was able to achieve a 50% reduction (46.5% to 20.5%) in rates of CLD over a 2-year time period that was sustained.[7] Another center implemented five PBPs centered around noninvasive ventilation (bubble CPAP) and strict intubation and extubation criteria and demonstrated a reduction in CLD rates from 17% preintervention to 8% postintervention.[19]

SUMMARY

Rates of CLD in VLBW infants have not decreased at the same pace as other neonatal morbidities during the past 20 years. Multifactorial causes of CLD make this common morbidity difficult to reduce, although there have been several individual QI projects in individual NICUs that have had success, but the lessons learned in these single centers have not been adopted by most NICUs. Building on the PBPs incorporated by these NICUs that were successful in lowering their rates of CLD, a road map for lower rates of CLD exists for NICUs that are struggling with rates of CLD that are higher than they would expect.

A comprehensive QI project incorporating all or a portion of PBPs, such as the use of early CPAP, caffeine use in specific populations, selective surfactant use, minimization of the duration of mechanical ventilation, and gentle ventilation strategies, can lead to a successful reduction in CLD rates. As more and more NICUs incorporate these new strategies into their daily work, establishing protocols to ensure safe and effective ventilatory care, we believe that CLD can join the reductions seen in nosocomial infections, interventricular hemorrhage, and NEC that have been realized in VLBW infants over the past 20 years.

REFERENCES

1. Horbar JD, Edwards EM, Greenberg LT, et al. Variation in performance of neonatal intensive care units in the United States. JAMA Pediatr 2017;171(3): e164396.

2. Northway WH Jr, Rosan RC, Porter DY. Pulmonary disease following respirator therapy of hyaline-membrane disease. Bronchopulmonary dysplasia. N Engl J Med 1967;276:357–68.
3. Shennan AT, Dunn MS, Ohlsson A, et al. Abnormal pulmonary outcomes in premature infants: prediction from oxygen requirement in the neonatal period. Pediatrics 1988;82:527–32.
4. Jobe AH, Bancalari E. Bronchopulmonary dysplasia. Am J Respir Crit Care Med 2001;163(7):1723–9.
5. Swanson J, Perlman S. Roadmap to a successful quality improvement project. J Perinatol 2017;37(2):112–5.
6. Walsh M, Laptook A, Kazzi SN, et al. A cluster-randomized trial of benchmarking and multimodal quality improvement to improve rates of survival free of bronchopulmonary dysplasia for infants with birth weights of less than 1250 grams. Pediatrics 2007;119(5):876–90.
7. Birenbaum H, Dentry A, Cirelli J, et al. Reduction in the incidence of chronic lung disease in very low birth weight infants: results of a quality improvement process in a tertiary level NICU. Pediatrics 2009;123:44–50.
8. Payne NR, LaCorte M, Sun S, et al, Breathsavers Group. Evaluation and development of potentially better practices to reduce bronchopulmonary dysplasia in very low birth weight infants. Pediatrics 2006;118(Suppl 2):S65–72.
9. Stoll BJ, Hansen NI, Bell EF, et al. Neonatal outcomes of extremely preterm infants from the NICHD neonatal research network. Pediatrics 2010;126(3):443–56.
10. Isayama T, Lee SK, Mori R, et al, Canadian Neonatal Network, Neonatal Research Network of Japan. Comparison of mortality and morbidity of very low birth weight infants between Canada and Japan. Pediatrics 2012;130(4):e957–65.
11. Institute of Medicine (IOM). Crossing the quality chasm: a new health system for the 21st century. Washington, DC: National Academy Press; 2001.
12. Horbar JD, Plsek PE, Leahy K, NIC/Q 2000. NIC/Q 2000: establishing habits for improvement in neonatal intensive care units. Pediatrics 2003;111(4 Pt 2):e397–410.
13. SUPPORT Study Group of the Eunice Kennedy Shriver NICHD Neonatal Research Network, Finer NN, Carlo WA, et al. Early CPAP versus surfactant in extremely preterm infants. N Engl J Med 2010;362(21):1970–9.
14. Verder H, Albertsen P, Ebbesen F, et al. Nasal continuous positive airway pressure and early surfactant therapy for respiratory distress syndrome in newborns of less than 30 weeks' gestation. Pediatrics 1999;103:E24.
15. Schmölzer GM, Kumar M, Pichler G, et al. Non-invasive versus invasive respiratory support in preterm infants at birth: systematic review and meta-analysis [review]. BMJ 2013;347:f5980 [Erratum appears in BMJ 2014;348:g58].
16. Morley CJ, Davis PG, Doyle LW, et al, COIN Trial Investigators. Nasal CPAP or intubation at birth for very preterm infants. N Engl J Med 2008;358:700–8.
17. Dunn MS, Kaempf J, de Klerk A, et al, Vermont Oxford Network DRM Study Group. Randomized trial comparing 3 approaches to the initial respiratory management of preterm neonates. Pediatrics 2011;128(5):e1069–76.
18. Rojas-Reyes MX, Morley CJ, Soll R. Prophylactic versus selective use of surfactant in preventing morbidity and mortality in preterm infants. Cochrane Database Syst Rev 2012:CD000510.
19. Levesque BM, Kalish LA, LaPierre J, et al. Impact of implementing 5 potentially better respiratory practices on neonatal outcomes and costs. Pediatrics 2011;128(1):e218–26.

20. Soll R, Ozek E. Prophylactic protein free synthetic surfactant for preventing morbidity and mortality in preterm infants. Cochrane Database Syst Rev 2010;(1):CD001079.
21. Cummings JJ, Polin RA, Committee on Fetus and Newborn, American Academy of Pediatrics. Noninvasive respiratory support. Pediatrics 2016;137(1). http://dx.doi.org/10.1542/peds.2015-3758.
22. Stevens TP, Harrington EW, Blennow M, et al. Early surfactant administration with brief ventilation vs. selective surfactant and continued mechanical ventilation for preterm infants with or at risk for respiratory distress syndrome. Cochrane Database Syst Rev 2007;(4):CD003063.
23. Göpel W, Kribs A, Ziegler A, et al. Avoidance of mechanical ventilation by surfactant treatment of spontaneously breathing preterm infants (AMV): an open-label, randomised, controlled trial. Lancet 2011;378:1627–34.
24. Barrington K, Finer N. The natural history of the appearance of apnea of prematurity. Pediatr Res 1991;29(4 Pt 1):372–5.
25. Schmidt B, Roberts RS, Davis P, et al, Caffeine for Apnea of Prematurity Trial Group. Caffeine therapy for apnea of prematurity. N Engl J Med 2006;354(20): 2112–21.
26. Schmidt B, Anderson PJ, Doyle LW, et al, Caffeine for Apnea of Prematurity (CAP) Trial Investigators. Survival without disability to age 5 years after neonatal caffeine therapy for apnea of prematurity. JAMA 2012;307(3):275–82.
27. Kamlin C, Davis PG. Long versus short inspiratory times in neonates receiving mechanical ventilation. Cochrane Database Syst Rev 2004;(4):CD004503.
28. Carlo WA, Stark AR, Bauer C, et al. Effects of minimal ventilation in a multicenter randomized controlled trial of ventilator support and early corticosteroid therapy in extremely low birthweight infants. Pediatrics 1999;104(3 Suppl):738–9.
29. Kamlin CO, Davis PG, Argus B, et al. A trial of spontaneous breathing to determine the readiness for extubation in very low birth weight infants: a prospective evaluation. Arch Dis Child Fetal Neonatal Ed 2008;93(4):F305–6.
30. Gillespie LM, White SD, Sinha SK, et al. Usefulness of the minute ventilation test in predicting successful extubation in newborn infants: a randomized controlled trial. J Perinatol 2003;23(3):205–7.
31. Doyle LW, Ehrenkranz RA, Halliday HL. Late (>7 days) postnatal corticosteroids for chronic lung disease in preterm infants. Cochrane Database Syst Rev 2014;(5):CD001145.
32. Shinwell ES, Portnov I, Meerpohl JJ, et al. Inhaled corticosteroids for bronchopulmonary dysplasia: a meta-analysis. Pediatrics 2016;138(6) [pii:e20162511].

Alarm Safety and Alarm Fatigue

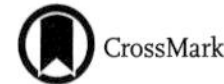

Kendall R. Johnson, MD[a,b], James I. Hagadorn, MD, MS[a,b], David W. Sink, MD[a,b,*]

KEYWORDS

- Clinical alarms • Alarm fatigue • Alarm safety • Quality improvement
- Neonatal intensive care

KEY POINTS

- The proliferation of alarming devices in neonatal intensive care (NICU) has created significant risk of patient harm due to alarm desensitization and missed alarms.
- A large proportion of clinical alarms in NICUs are nonactionable, creating a cry wolf phenomenon that promotes alarm fatigue.
- Safe alarm practices require attention to device functionality, alarm settings, staff operating the devices, patient condition, and environment of care.
- Sound quality improvement methods can significantly reduce clinical alarm burden and enhance alarm safety.

THE ALARM SAFETY PROBLEM

Medical device alarms present care providers with a dilemma: they contribute crucially to effective patient care; however, they may also cause unintended adverse consequences. Safe and effective use of device alarms requires an understanding of the technology sufficiently clear to balance inherent benefits and risks. For some patients in intensive care settings, the number of alarm signals may reach several hundred per day, creating such a high alarm burden that desensitized staff may miss, devalue, ignore, or disable alarm signals.[1] Alarm desensitization, or alarm fatigue, is a multifactorial problem related to the rapid proliferation of alarming devices, use of alarm limits that are unnecessarily narrow or not standardized, and exacerbated by high rates of false or nonactionable alarms.[2] Many organizations have called attention to alarm safety as an important issue, including the Joint Commission, the Emergency Care Research Institute, and the Association for the Advancement of Medical

---

Disclosure Statement: The authors have no financial conflicts of interest to disclose.

[a] Department of Pediatrics, University of Connecticut School of Medicine, 263 Farmington Avenue, Farmington, CT 06030, USA; [b] Division of Neonatology, Connecticut Children's Medical Center, 282 Washington Street, Hartford, CT 06106, USA

* Corresponding author. Connecticut Children's Medical Center, 282 Washington Street, Hartford, CT 06106.

E-mail address: dsink@connecticutchildrens.org

Clin Perinatol 44 (2017) 713–728

http://dx.doi.org/10.1016/j.clp.2017.05.005

Instrumentation.[1,3,4] In June 2013, The Joint Commission approved a new National Patient Safety Goal on clinical alarm safety for hospitals (**Box 1**). This safety goal was prompted by a series of 98 alarm-related sentinel events reported to The Joint Commission from 2009 to 2012. Eighty of these events resulted in death, 13 in permanent loss of function, and 5 in unexpected additional care or extended hospitalizations.

Medical Device Alarms in the Neonatal Intensive Care Unit

In neonatal intensive care units (NICUs), cardiorespiratory events with vital sign fluctuation, especially in preterm infants, contribute significantly to alarm burden. Alarm fatigue or desensitization may develop when frequent oxygen saturation (SpO_2) or heart rate alarms sound, yet the events self-resolve before clinical action is needed. In a 2002 study of nurse responses to NICU cardiorespiratory alarms, each monitor alerted 16.7 times per hour and most were SpO_2 alarms.[5] In baseline measures in Connecticut Children's NICUs, staff experienced 11.9 SpO_2 alarms per very low birth weight (VLBW; <1500g) infant per hour. Based on typical nurse assignments in the open bay NICU rooms, the authors estimate each of our nurses was exposed to an SpO_2 alarm nearly every minute of their shift. This estimate did not include other cardiorespiratory alarms or alarms from other devices, such as pumps or ventilators.

MONITORED SYSTEMS AND ALARM RESPONSE

Human Factors and Alarms

Human response to clinical alarms has correlates in other fields, including aviation, nuclear power, and many others. A significant body of human factors research exists related to alarms. Binary alarm systems are automated decision aids that classify current condition into either normal or critical. The positive predictive value (PPV) of an

Box 1
Elements of performance for the Joint Commission's 2014 National Patient Safety Goal 06.01.01

1. As of July 1, 2014, leaders establish alarm system safety as a hospital priority.
2. During 2014, identify the most important alarm signals to manage based on the following:
   - Input from the medical staff and clinical departments
   - Risk to patients if the alarm signal is not attended to or if it malfunctions
   - Whether specific alarm signals are needed or unnecessarily contribute to alarm noise and alarm fatigue
   - Potential for patient harm based on internal incident history
   - Published best practices and guidelines.
3. As of January 1, 2016, establish policies and procedures for managing the alarms identified in 2 (above) that, at a minimum, address the following:
   - Clinically appropriate settings for alarm signals
   - When alarm signals can be disabled
   - When alarm parameters can be changed
   - Who in the organization has the authority to set alarm parameters
   - Who in the organization has the authority to change alarm parameters
   - Who in the organization has the authority to set alarm parameters to the off setting
   - Monitoring and responding to alarm signals
   - Checking individual alarm signals for accurate settings, proper operation, and detectability.
4. As of January 1, 2016, educate staff and licensed independent practitioners about the purpose and proper operation of alarm systems for which they are responsible.

alarm system represents the probability that there is a true critical event in case of an alarm: PPV = true alarms/(true alarms + false alarms).[6] When PPV is low, operator responses are more delayed and alarms are more often ignored.[6,7] Monitors designed to warn an operator of a dangerous condition typically have alarms set to a high sensitivity; however, if prevalence of the dangerous condition is low, this leads to low PPV with more false positive alarms relative to true positive alarms. When operators know that an alarm is likely to reflect a critical event (high PPV), they tend to respond to all alarms. However, when the PPV is low, operators may become desensitized and ignore or overlook the warnings. Alarm response rates seem to match closely what operators expect to be the probability of true alarms (probability matching).[8]

Decision-making becomes more complex if operators are able to reduce uncertainty related to an alarm by cross-checking its validity with other available information. Operators then have 3 alternatives to respond to an alarm: directly respond, ignore, or cross-check before deciding how to respond. Operators with real-time alarm validity information may respond less frequently but more appropriately to alarms.[9] A common form of cross-checking in the NICU occurs when nurses visually check the pulse waveform on oximeter displays to help determine whether a saturation alarm is real or an artifact of poor probe signal.

Complex work such as nursing care in the NICU involves ongoing attention to primary tasks (eg, patient assessments, medication administration) and to intermittent secondary tasks such as responding to alarms. In such dual-task systems, time and effort spent responding to alarms detracts from the primary tasks. As primary task workload increases, alarm task performance typically worsens, particularly when alarm reliability is low.[9,10] Alarm response rates in such cases may be low because the operator must choose an action based on relative urgency of the primary and secondary tasks. Alarm signal sounds that are reliably different in their urgency may help operators quickly assess need for immediate transition to the alarm task versus completion of a primary task followed by attention to the alarm.[11]

Medical Device Alarm Standardization

The International Electrotechnical Commission (IEC) is a worldwide organization that promotes international standardization in electronic fields. In 2006, in response to clinicians' discontent with alarm signals, particularly with the frequency of false positive or false negative alarms, the IEC developed standards for alarm systems in medical electrical equipment and medical electrical systems.[12] The standards intended to reduce the proliferation of alarm signals in clinical settings, minimize distraction, and increase usability of clinical alarm systems. Standardized alarm nomenclature and definitions were applied (**Table 1**). Audible alarm signal specifications, including priority indicators, were suggested to improve consistency across manufacturers and health care systems such that clinicians would recognize similar alarm sounds regardless of setting. Manufacturer compliance with the standard is voluntary; however, legal and economic pressures should increasingly bring compliant devices to hospitals.

Neonatal Intensive Care Unit Alarm Environment

Physiologic monitor alarm configuration

Cardiorespiratory monitors, applied almost universally to NICU patients, continuously assess multiple physiologic variables and display values at the bedside and/or remotely via centralized displays. Various alarm conditions may arise in these devices, such as low or high heart rate, respiratory rate, SpO_2, blood pressure, electrocardiogram (EKG) rhythm abnormalities, and even poor signal quality or other technical

Table 1
Alarm nomenclature: selected International Electrotechnical Commission standard terms

Term	Definition
Alarm system	Parts of medical electrical equipment or a medical electrical system that detect alarm conditions and, as appropriate, generate alarm signals
Alarm signal	Type of signal generated by the alarm system to indicate the presence (or occurrence) of an alarm condition
Alarm condition	State of the alarm system when it has determined that a potential or actual hazardous situation exists for which operator notification is required
Alarm signal generation delay	Time from the onset of an alarm condition to the generation of its alarm signals
Alarm limit	Threshold used by an alarm system to determine an alarm condition
Alarm settings	Alarm system configuration, including but not limited to alarm limits, characteristics of any alarm signal inactivation states, and the values of variables or parameters that determine the function of the alarm system
Default alarm preset	Alarm preset that can be activated by the alarm system without operator action Note: alarm presets configured by the manufacturer or responsible organization are possible types of default alarm presets
High-priority	Indicating that immediate operator response is required
Medium priority	Indicating that prompt operator response is required
Low-priority	Indicating that operator awareness is required
Escalation	Process by which an alarm system increases the priority of an alarm condition or increases the sense of urgency of an alarm signal
Intelligent alarm system	Alarm system that makes logical decisions based on monitored information without operator intervention
Nonlatching alarm signal	Alarm signal that automatically stops being generated when its associated triggering event no longer exists

From Commission IE. IEC 60601-1-8:2006. Medical electrical equipment — Part 1-8: General requirements for basic safety and essential performance — Collateral standard: General requirements, tests and guidance for alarm systems in medical electrical equipment and medical electrical systems 2006. The author thanks the International Electrotechnical Commission (IEC) for permission to reproduce Information from its International Standards.

alarms. Alarm limits are set to alert clinicians of potentially or actually dangerous conditions that require assessment and possibly intervention. Audible alarm signals may be set to stop when the alarm condition ends without requiring a clinician to manually acknowledge the alarm. Such nonlatching alarms are appropriate when alerting nurses to conditions that often self-resolve in NICU patients, such as low or high SpO_2 or heart rate.

The alarm configuration on NICU monitors typically includes alarm settings that may be manufacturer-configured presets, hospital-configured presets, operator-configured presets, or adjustable settings. Presets may include settings for alarm limits, alarm signal generation delays, latching, and alarm escalation (see **Table 1**). It may be preferable to allow nurse adjustments to settings such as SpO_2 or respiratory rate alarm limits to individualize care to certain patient populations (eg, VLBW, cyanotic heart disease). However, organization-configured presets may be desirable to standardize most other alarm settings and prevent individual operator changes to settings (ie, alarm delays or escalation algorithms).

Other neonatal intensive care unit alarming devices

Modern NICUs use a broad array of electronic devices that use 1 or more audible alarms. Mechanical ventilators produce a variety of alarm signals, such as low or high delivered pressure, volume, minute ventilation, abnormal gas humidity, or mechanical malfunction. Redundant alarm signals may occasionally arise, such as high respiratory rate alarm signals from both the ventilator and cardiorespiratory monitor. Each device could also have different limits set for the same physiologic variable, whether through presets or manual settings entered by different clinicians. Other NICU alarms and alarming devices include those listed in **Box 2**.

Alarm Response in Intensive Care Units

NICUs and other ICUs often experience a high number of alarms with low validity. Reported proportion of clinical alarms requiring intervention or action varies from less than 1% to 36%.[13] Two studies in pediatric ICUs found less than 10% of clinical alarms resulted in a change in care, with the PPV for individual devices as low as 1% for pulse oximeters and 3% in ventilators.[14,15] The high burden of NICU alarms affects the ability of nurses to both respond to alarms and perform their primary tasks in patient care, assessments, medication administration, infant feeding, documentation, and so forth. Probabilities for nurse response to an alarm depend on the causes of the alarm, its duration, and the characteristics of the patient.[5] Short-lived alarms may be filtered out, presumably through a learned behavior regarding self-limited alarm conditions in their population (ie, brief bradycardia or desaturation events).

QUALITY IMPROVEMENT EFFORTS PROMOTING ALARM SAFETY

Key Drivers of Alarm Fatigue

Many factors contribute to clinical alarm burden and alarm fatigue. Quality improvement (QI) efforts to address alarm fatigue may benefit from classification of such factors into a key driver diagram (**Fig. 1**).

Primary Driver: Devices

There may be situations in which alarming devices are used unnecessarily. A stable term infant treated for hypoglycemia may not require pulse oximetry monitoring. Unnecessary oximetry monitoring in a vigorous infant likely begets motion artifact and false alarms. Similarly, the device may be necessary, although a specific alarm within the device is not, such a high-SpO_2 alarm for a patient in room air. Devices not meeting standards or lacking sensor reliability may increase false alarms due to artifact signals. Devices emitting unprioritized alarm signals for low-priority events prevent nurses from appropriately triaging their actions. Alarm fatigue due to lower priority alarms may be reduced by extending the alarm delay, changing to visual alerts, or even considering eliminating the alarm altogether. False alarms due to defective EKG leads or oximetry probes, motion, or light interfering with probes, also contribute heavily to alarm fatigue.[16,17]

Primary Driver: Alarm Settings

Device alarm settings, including alarm limits, alarm delays, and alarm latching, each have significant impact on alarm burden. Evidence for optimal alarm settings for neonates is limited, generally arising from retrospective studies correlating frequency and

Box 2
List of common neonatal intensive care unit alarms and alarm devices

Pulse oximeters

EKG or arrhythmia

Apnea monitors

Invasive blood pressure

Central monitoring station

Secondary alarm escalation system

Infusion pumps

Enteral feeding pumps

Radiant warmers

Incubators

Continuous or bilevel positive airway pressure or delivery devices

Ventilator pressure

Ventilator tidal volume

Ventilator respiratory rate

Ventilator apnea

Ventilator minute ventilation

Transcutaneous carbon dioxide (CO_2) monitors

End-tidal CO_2 monitors

Near-infrared spectroscopy monitors

Cooling blanket or devices

Oxygen humidification devices

Amplitude-integrated electroencephalography monitors

Extracorporeal membrane oxygenators

Ventricular-assist devices

Breastmilk warmers

Nurse call system

Personal pagers

Mobile notification systems

Code blue alert

Delivery room emergency alert

Infant security bands

Panic button or security alert

duration of cardiorespiratory event with outcomes, creating questions of associative rather than causal relationships. However, some guidance may come from recent studies leveraging technical advances in device data collection and analysis. Di Fiore and colleagues[18] noted a higher incidence of hypoxemic events with SpO_2 equal to or less than 80 for equal to or greater than 10 seconds was associated with increased adjusted risk for severe retinopathy of prematurity (ROP) requiring laser therapy. Study

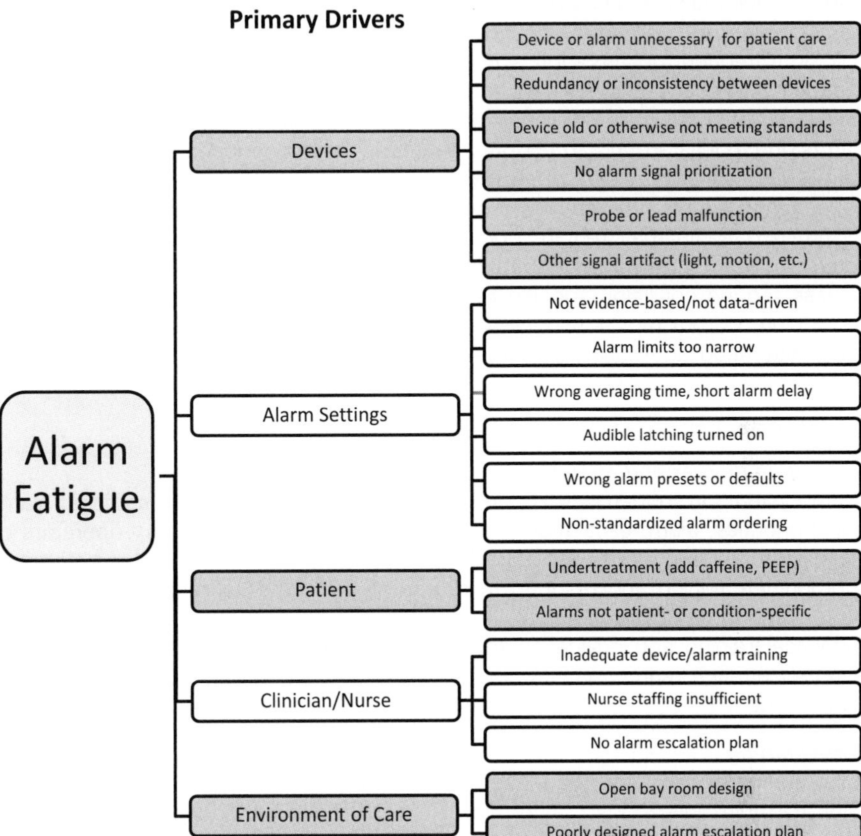

Fig. 1. Key driver diagram of primary and secondary drivers which may serve as leverage points to address alarm fatigue.

guidelines suggested a delay of 30 seconds before the clinician adjusts the fraction of inspired oxygen (FiO_2). Using data from the Canadian Oxygen Trial,[19] investigators found that prolonged hypoxemic episodes, with SpO_2 less than 80% lasting at least 1 minute during the first 2 to 3 months after birth were associated with adverse 18-month outcomes.[20] Such data may help guide practical decisions such as which low-SpO_2 alarm limit and alarm delay settings are likely to optimize patient outcomes and minimize alarm fatigue.

An analysis of adult intensive care unit (ICU) SpO_2 data suggested that reducing the low-alarm limit and increasing the alarm delay both reduced alarm frequency.[21] In this study, the alarm rate varied among patients and within individual patients over time, suggesting potential importance of individualizing alarm settings based on patient condition. In the NICU, alarm limits individualized for age or condition (eg, cyanotic heart disease) may be accomplished through monitor default profiles or by using standardized alarm order sets. Other alarm settings, such as alarm delays, averaging time (for SpO_2), or alarm latching, may not be modifiable by end users. In such cases, unit-based or institution-based settings may require clinical engineering or even assistance from the device vendor to change.

Primary Driver: Patients

Alarm burden may also increase in situations in which patients become more unstable or are undertreated for their condition. An infant with worsening lung compliance and more frequent desaturation alarms may be in need of additional positive end-expiratory pressure. Such treatment improves the patient's condition and also may reduce oximeter alarms by stabilizing pulmonary status. Low-minute ventilation alarms due to leak around an endotracheal tube may be reduced by a more appropriately sized endotracheal tube or by considering noninvasive respiratory support. Apnea alarms may be reduced with more appropriate caffeine dosing.

Certain patients may require condition-specific alarm settings so alarms that occur will be meaningful and actionable.[2] Patients with cyanotic congenital heart disease require condition-specific SpO_2 lower and upper alarm limits, which are very different from most other NICU patients. Older infants still remaining in the NICU may need age-based adjustments for heart rate and respiratory rate alarm limits.

Primary Driver: Clinicians or Nurses

Training on devices and alarms

Alarm systems in modern NICUs are complex, with multiple alarm settings, alarm signal priorities, alarm escalation algorithms, and so forth. As primary operators of these systems, NICU nurses need adequate training and ongoing user support to appropriately set up and respond to device alarms. When surveyed, 60% of ICU nurses reported needing more monitor training to properly manage alarms.[22] Alarm in-service training and device alarm system job aides, developed in coordination with clinical engineering, may improve alarm setting compliance[23] and even reduce alarm burden.[24]

Nurse staffing

Nurse staffing and oximeter alarm management may have related effects on SpO_2 stability. In a multicenter study, changes in an infant's alarm limits had a greater impact on SpO_2 target achievement when the nurse cared for only 1 infant compared with when the nurse cared for multiple infants.[25]

Primary Driver: Environment of Care

When a nurse encounters an alarm in a patient while engaged in a separate high-priority task, alarm escalation systems direct the alarm to a secondary responder if the primary nurse is unable to respond promptly. Alarm escalation algorithms with pagers to acknowledge or escalate to another nurse have decreased alarm frequency and duration in ICUs.[26] Such systems can help maintain prompt response times in single-patient room NICUs.[27]

Alarm Safety Team Composition

The success of an alarm safety improvement effort depends heavily on assembling the right people into the project team. **Table 2** shows an example of such a team and their roles.

Potentially Better Alarm Practices

In health care QI, a potentially better practice (PBP) is a practice that has been shown to improve outcomes in 1 or more settings, and that can be locally adapted and implemented with a reasonable expectation for improvement in a new setting.[28] There are many examples in the literature of development and implementation of PBPs in the

Table 2
Alarm safety team

Team Members	Roles
Project sponsorship	Link QI team to senior management, financial support
Clinical leadership	Has authority to test and implement change
Day-to-day leadership	Lead QI team and ensure task completion
Technical expertise:	Deep knowledge of process or area in question
Nurses	Clarify alarm impact on daily workflow Prioritize alarms to balance patient safety and alarm fatigue Identify which alarms contribute most to alarm burden and alarm fatigue Identify which alarms are nonactionable
Physician	Expert on physiology of alarm conditions Guide development of evidence-based, data-driven alarm settings
Respiratory therapist	Expert in ventilator alarms and settings Identify nuisance or duplicated alarms Set prioritization of respiratory alarms
Clinical engineering	Expert in device features, limitations Access to institutional default settings not available to end users
Clinical educator	Train staff on alarm systems and alarm policies or procedures
Consultants:	Expertise likely to be tapped periodically
Patients and families	Unique perspective on alarms: often emotionally affected by frequent false or nuisance alarms that staff may disregard Help develop parent education on alarms: self-resolving alarm conditions, alarm priorities, and balance between alarm sensitivity and alarm fatigue.
Information technology	Networking alarms as in alarm escalation systems Resource for alarm and clinical data reporting, QI metrics
Risk management	Risk implications of alarm systems
Device manufacturers	Device alarm functionality, untapped features or upgrades Share success stories from other institutions using the devices Customer-driven improvements in devices

NICU setting.[28–32] The process for PBP development may include literature review, stakeholder surveys, key driver process analysis, and benchmarking through comparison with high-performing centers. Of necessity, PBPs must accommodate multiple aspects of NICU culture. Successful PBP implementation requires a culture of change and progresses through recognizable stages of acceptance.[33] The specific change ideas NICUs may want to implement will depend on the specific types of alarms or alarming devices targeted for improvement. An example of possible PBPs and change ideas for QI work related to pulse oximetry alarms follows.

Pulse Oximeter Alarm Potentially Better Practices and Change Ideas

The Vermont Oxford Network (VON) iNICQ 2015 Quality Improvement Collaborative addressed medical device alarms and implementation of Joint Commission–mandated performance elements regarding alarm safety that must be met by accredited organizations.[32,34] Development of PBPs for this endeavor began in September 2014, when multidisciplinary teams from 220 VON member NICUs reviewed a comprehensive list of NICU medical devices for potential to harm patients, based on frequency of device use and consequences to the infant if the device's alarm was disabled or did not prompt a caretaker response. The results of this stakeholder survey focused the VON iNICQ 2015 QI Collaborative on the pulse oximeter as the device having the most impact on alarms and alarm safety in the NICU. Accordingly, 3 PBPs were developed by the Collaborative's 2015 Steering Committee for use by participating NICUs:

1. Apply the Joint Commission's alarm safety goals to SpO_2 monitoring by developing and implementing unit-based policies that describe the who, what, where, when, and how of alarm thresholds and parameters for oximeters.
2. Develop and implement unit-based policies to standardize staff response to alarm signals, and monitor and provide feedback regarding responses to oximeter alarms.
3. Improve the safety of supplemental oxygen therapy by using the full technical capabilities of the pulse oximetry monitoring to achieve desired SpO_2 stability while minimizing oximetry burden.

The PBPs addressed the Joint Commission alarm safety performance elements with respect to oximeter use in the NICU; however, participating NICUs were encouraged to prioritize and adapt them as warranted by local conditions. Several change ideas were suggested to help participating NICUs achieve these PBPs. For the first PBP, change ideas included developing patient or condition-specific alarms settings, such as alarm limits based on postmenstrual age groups, or creating parent education materials explaining the benefits and risks of oxygen and unit strategy for oximeter alarms. The second PBP might be implemented by revising unit policies to clarify preferred response to oximeter alarms, detailing standard stepwise assessment, and management of alarm conditions. Additionally, units could test systems that incorporate oximeter alarm frequency into nurse staffing models, to better maintain oxygen stability in such infants. The third PBP might be achieved through collaboration with biomedical engineering to educate NICU staff on current monitor capabilities, such as trend review, signal display averaging, and detailed alarm system functionality. Better understanding of the monitors might lead to creation of more appropriate default alarm settings, or even help use oximeter electronic SpO_2 trend data to refine clinical management.

Adapting Pulse Oximeter Alarm Potentially Better Practices Locally

Initial PBP implementation may produce intended improvement in an outcome or process but also result in unintended worsening of another depending on the local context. This dilemma may be successfully addressed through serial plan-do-study-act cycles using small tests of change and secondary interventions to fine-tune the initial implementation through use of balancing measures. For example, Ketko and colleagues[35] experienced increased oximeter alarm frequency after the implementation of narrowed SpO_2 alarms to avoid extreme high or low SpO2s and improve time in saturation target. Their multidisciplinary QI team responded by developing an alarm management bundle to decrease alarm frequency. Modification of their high-alarm algorithm and use of SpO_2 histograms resulted in increased time spent within the targeted saturation range and fewer high-SpO_2 alarms per day. Histogram technology was used to customize alarm limits to patients individually and an alarm frequency tool was used to avoid assigning more than 1 infant with frequent alarms to nurses.

MEASURES TO ACHIEVE IMPROVEMENT

Outcome Measures

Total alarm count

When implementing changes to address alarm fatigue, the most commonly used measure is total number of alarms per day. Many devices store a time-stamped alarm history, creating an easily collected source of QI data. Numerous studies and quality reports have used total alarm quantity as their primary outcome.[2,22,26,35–39] One team in a pediatric bone marrow transplant unit implemented a standardized cardiac monitor care process and noted a reduction in median number of alarms per patient per day from 180 to 40.[37] Another team working in a pediatric step-down unit implemented data-driven alarm settings and achieved reductions in heart rate alarms per patient per day, but respiratory rate alarms increased.[38] This serves as a reminder that, although total alarm counts may be more quickly or easily obtained, stratifying by alarm type might provide key information. One NICU team noticed a dramatic increase in oximeter alarms after narrowing alarm limits, which led them to develop an alarm management bundle intended to reduce alarm frequency.[35] Though data on total oximeter alarms were collected, this project primarily focused on the total number of high-SpO_2 alarms per monitored patient-day because many of the interventions focused on the high-alarm limit. A limitation of using this outcome is that details of the alarms, including need for intervention or provider response time, typically cannot be determined. Additionally, limited device storage capacity may require frequent data extraction.

Nonactionable alarm count

Nonactionable alarms, which capture clinicians' attention yet are not clinically significant, contribute heavily to alarm fatigue.[13,40] Reducing these alarms will have a direct impact on alarm fatigue without increasing risk to patients. Nonactionable alarms fall into 2 categories: false alarms and nuisance alarms. False alarms may be triggered by sensor noise or system malfunction, distracting providers when there is no alarm condition in the patient. Common examples include motion artifact and poor sensor adherence. Nuisance alarms reflect actual physiologic changes but do not require clinical action. These alarms often reflect vital signs that only briefly move outside the intended range but self-resolve within a clinically insignificant time period. For a QI initiative focused on reducing cardiac monitoring rates in adult units, trained clinical researcher staff classified alarms as true, false, or nuisance based on direct observations.[41] Their interventions reduced false alarm percentage (number of false alarms or total alarms) by half, yet the percentage of nuisance alarms was unchanged. Collecting data on nonactionable alarms will better enable teams to know if their changes lead to the desired improvement. However, classifying alarms as nonactionable, false, or nuisance alarms is generally time-intensive, so use of smaller or convenience samples may be more reasonable for QI.

Alarm priority

Alarm counts categorized into high, medium, or low priority may help determine which alarms are contributing most to a unit's alarm burden. High-priority alarms, such as apnea or very low SpO_2 or heart rate, should have limits set to reflect need for immediate attention, whereas medium-priority and low-priority alarms should sound when provider attention is less urgent.[12,42] In settings in which low-priority or medium-priority alarms contribute significantly to alarm burden, efforts to reduce these alarms may reduce alarm fatigue while maintaining patient safety through the high-priority alarms. In an adult ICU, implementation of a bundled intervention reduced total alarms by 88%, and the alarm reduction occurred only in medium-priority alarms as high-priority alarms were unchanged.[39] In an adult progressive care unit, an initiative that included changes in default alarm settings and retraining nurses to individualize certain alarm settings led to a 43% decrease in high-priority and medium-priority alarms.[2] Alarms of any priority should be set to actionable limits with appropriate alarm delays to optimize validity and proper response.

Response time and alarm duration

Alarm fatigue is difficult to measure directly, so a surrogate measure often used is alarm response time because a slow response may suggest a provider is desensitized or ignoring the alarm. Increased nonactionable alarms, whether false or nuisance, is associated with delayed nurse response times.[5,40,43,44] Because measured response time requires direct observation, the value of such data in QI work must be weighed against resources needed to accrue a meaningful number of measurements. A similar measure, which may be more easily obtained from devices' alarm history, is alarm duration. Because an initial response of nurses is to acknowledge the alarm and thus silence it, longer alarm duration generally should correlate to response time.[26] However, in situations in which alarm conditions may self-resolve, alarm duration would merely reflect patient condition and have little correlation with response time or alarm fatigue. In such cases, alarm duration data may be useful in determining appropriate alarm delay settings to avoid nuisance alarms.[17,37,45,46]

Clinician perception of alarm burden and alarm fatigue

To assess nurses' opinions and attitudes toward clinical alarms, many studies have used surveys or qualitative interviews.[22,35,43,47–49] Surveys may help in understanding current practices; developing change ideas; and, when used before and after change, assessing whether improvement occurred. Survey questions may assess for issues contributing to alarm recognition and response, actions taken in response to alarms, frequency of nuisance alarms, validity of alarms, monitor knowledge, and perceived unit noise level.[2,26,35,49]

Process Measures

Because process measures assess whether a change in the system is taking place, determining what to measure will depend on the project at hand and interventions put in place. Most commonly, measures focused on compliance with a system change will assist in determining if an improvement can be associated with the change implemented. Dandoy and colleagues[37] introduced a standardized cardiac monitor care process consisting of multiple components. They measured compliance not only with the complete bundle but also with individual bundle components. This enabled the team to evaluate which components were easily adopted versus those that needed increased compliance.

Balancing Measures

Alarms' purpose within the NICU is to detect physiologic deterioration requiring urgent attention. Therefore, it is important to ensure that necessary alarms are not missed or eliminated when implementing changes. This is particularly important when focusing on the reduction of high-priority alarms. To ensure interventions do not cause harm, an important balancing measure used is review of patient safety data or occurrence reports to determine if recognition and response to episodes of patient deterioration were delayed.[35,37] Although this measure would identify the most serious events, it may not evaluate for minor events. One concern of reducing alarms is that increased physiologic instability may be less readily recognized. Depending on the alarm type being addressed, the specific measure will vary. For instance, many alarm initiatives have focused on reducing pulse oximeter alarms, in which increased time with hypoxemia or hyperoxemia, determined by histogram trends or analysis of exported SpO_2 data, are important balancing measures.[35] Similarly, projects focused on reducing heart rate alarms may measure frequency of significant bradycardic events. Another potential balancing measure is long-term outcomes related to the intervention, such as tracking rates of ROP when addressing pulse oximeter alarms, although the time frame for responding to such measures is more prolonged.

DATA SOURCES

Monitor

Downloads or recordings directly from the alarming device are efficient ways to obtain alarm data.[50] Biomedical or clinical engineering or information technology support may be helpful to optimize device alarm data storage configuration and to understand electronic data export and analysis options.[26,36,39]

Third-Party Systems

Long-term, efficient alarm data collection and analysis may be enhanced through the use of clinical data warehouse or middleware systems. Such third-party systems may be customized to provide meaningful alarm information such as alarm counts by patient, alarm condition, alarm priority, alarm setting compliance, or alarm duration.[35,38,41,50]

Manual Data Collection

At times, data may need to be collected manually to determine the alarm type. This is particularly the case when designating an alarm as actionable or nonactionable. In this case, the use of direct observation, either by a team member or clinical staff, will be needed to classify each alarm. Given that this type of data collection is time-consuming, it is likely that smaller samples will need to be used.

Sustainability

On completion of a project in which notable improvements have been seen, it is important to consider how to sustain those changes. Interventions and the subsequent improvements are most easily sustained when new practices have become part of a culture change. Once the staff has adopted changes as part of their daily practice, there are a few additional ways to optimize sustainability. Updating relevant policies helps maintain consistency between clinical practice and documented guidelines. Training new personnel and periodically retraining others will contribute to a lasting culture change. Additionally, use of hard-wired changes in devices, through default alarm settings and alarm profiles, will promote standardization and sustainability.

SUMMARY

Alarm fatigue is a real safety concern in NICUs because the high alarm burden, coupled with a high proportion of nonactionable alarms, leads to a cry wolf phenomenon, causing missed alarms and patient harm. PBPs to address alarm fatigue include policies and staff training that clarify safe alarm practices, use of evidence-based and data-driven alarm settings to standardize response to alarms, and leveraging device alarm features to reduce nuisance and false alarms.

REFERENCES

1. Group TJCPSA. Medical device alarm safety in hospitals. Sentinel Event Alert 2013;(50):1–3.
2. Graham KC, Cvach M. Monitor alarm fatigue: standardizing use of physiological monitors and decreasing nuisance alarms. Am J Crit Care 2010;19(1):28–34 [quiz: 35].

3. Association for the Advancement of Medical Instrumentation [Internet]. Alarms Pose Challenges to Healthcare Facilities. Horizons. 2011. Available at: http://www.aami.org/publications/AlarmHorizons/articles/Alarms_Pose_Challenges_5.pdf. Accessed October 7, 2014.
4. ECRI Institute. Top 10 health technology hazards for 2013. Health Devices 2013; 41(11):342–65. Available at: https://www.ecri.org/Documents/Secure/Health_Devices_Top_10_Hazards_2013.pdf. Accessed October 7, 2014.
5. Bitan Y, Meyer J, Shinar D, et al. Nurses' reactions to alarms in a neonatal intensive care unit. Cogn Tech Work 2004;6(4):239–46.
6. Manzey D, Gerard N, Wiczorek R. Decision-making and response strategies in interaction with alarms: the impact of alarm reliability, availability of alarm validity information and workload. Ergonomics 2014;57(12):1833–55.
7. Getty D, Swets J, Pickett R, et al. System operator response to warnings of danger: a laboratory investigation of the effects of the predictive value of a warning on human response time. J Exp Psychol Appl 1995;1(1):19–33.
8. Bliss JP, Gilson RD, Deaton JE. Human probability matching behaviour in response to alarms of varying reliability. Ergonomics 1995;38(11):2300–12.
9. Bliss JP, Jeans SM, Prioux HJ. Dual-task performance as a function of individual alarm validity and alarm system reliability information. Proc Hum Factors Ergon Soc Annu Meet 1996;40(23):1237–41.
10. Bliss JP, Dunn MC. Behavioural implications of alarm mistrust as a function of task workload. Ergonomics 2000;43(9):1283–300.
11. Edworthy J, Hellier E. Alarms and human behaviour: implications for medical alarms. Br J Anaesth 2006;97(1):12–7.
12. Commission IE. IEC 60601-1-8:2006. Medical electrical equipment — Part 1-8: General requirements for basic safety and essential performance — Collateral standard: General requirements, tests and guidance for alarm systems in medical electrical equipment and medical electrical systems. Geneva (Switzerland): The International Electrotechnical Commission; 2006.
13. Paine CW, Goel VV, Ely E, et al. Systematic review of physiologic monitor alarm characteristics and pragmatic interventions to reduce alarm frequency. J Hosp Med 2016;11(2):136–44.
14. Lawless ST. Crying wolf: false alarms in a pediatric intensive care unit. Crit Care Med 1994;22(6):981–5.
15. Tsien CL, Fackler JC. Poor prognosis for existing monitors in the intensive care unit. Crit Care Med 1997;25(4):614–9.
16. van der Eijk AC, Horsch S, Eilers PH, et al. "New-generation" pulse oximeters in extremely low-birth-weight infants: how do they perform in clinical practice? J Perinat Neonatal Nurs 2012;26(2):172–80.
17. Cvach MM, Biggs M, Rothwell KJ, et al. Daily electrode change and effect on cardiac monitor alarms: an evidence-based practice approach. J Nurs Care Qual 2013;28(3):265–71.
18. Di Fiore J, Bloom J, Orge F, et al. A higher incidence of intermittent hypoxemic episodes is associated with severe retinopathy of prematurity. J Pediatr 2010; 157(1):69–73.
19. Schmidt B, Whyte R, Asztalos E, et al. Effects of targeting higher vs lower arterial oxygen saturations on death or disability in extremely preterm infants. JAMA 2013;309(20):2111–20.
20. Poets C, Roberts R, Schmidt B, et al. Association between intermittent hypoxemia or bradycardia and late death or disability in extremely preterm infants. JAMA 2015;314(6):595–603.

21. Lansdowne K, Strauss DG, Scully CG. Retrospective analysis of pulse oximeter alarm settings in an intensive care unit patient population. BMC Nurs 2016;15:36.
22. Sowan AK, Gomez TM, Tarriela AF, et al. Changes in default alarm settings and standard in-service are insufficient to improve alarm fatigue in an Intensive Care Unit: a pilot project. JMIR Hum Factors 2016;3(1):e1.
23. Mills B, Davis P, Donath S, et al. Improving compliance with pulse oximetry alarm limits for very preterm infants? J Paediatr Child Health 2010;46(5):255–8.
24. Brantley A, Collins-Brown S, Kirkland J, et al. Clinical trial of an educational program to decrease monitor alarms in a medical Intensive Care Unit. AACN Crit Care 2016;27(3):283–9.
25. Sink DW, Trzaski JM, Bellini S, et al. Modifiable Factors Associated With Oxygen Saturation Target Achievement (TA): A Prospective Multicenter Study. 2014;EPAS 2939.543.
26. Cvach MM, Frank RJ, Doyle P, et al. Use of pagers with an alarm escalation system to reduce cardiac monitor alarm signals. J Nurs Care Qual 2014;29(1):9–18.
27. van Pul C, V D Mortel HP, V D Bogaart JJ, et al. Safe patient monitoring is challenging but still feasible in a neonatal intensive care unit with single family rooms. Acta Paediatr 2015;104(6):e247–54.
28. Horbar JD, Rogowski J, Plsek PE, et al. Collaborative quality improvement for neonatal intensive care. NIC/Q Project Investigators of the Vermont Oxford Network. Pediatrics 2001;107(1):14–22.
29. Kilbride HW, Wirtschafter DD, Powers RJ, et al. Implementation of evidence-based potentially better practices to decrease nosocomial infections. Pediatrics 2003;111(4 Pt 2):e519–33.
30. Ohlinger J, Brown MS, Laudert S, et al. Development of potentially better practices for the neonatal intensive care unit as a culture of collaboration: communication, accountability, respect, and empowerment. Pediatrics 2003;111(4 Pt 2):e471–81.
31. Sharek PJ, Baker R, Litman F, et al. Evaluation and development of potentially better practices to prevent chronic lung disease and reduce lung injury in neonates. Pediatrics 2003;111(4 Pt 2):e426–31.
32. Hagadorn JI, Sink DW, Buus-Frank ME, et al. Alarm safety and oxygen saturation targets in the Vermont Oxford Network iNICQ 2015 collaborative. J Perinatol 2016;37(3):270–6.
33. Brown MS, Ohlinger J, Rusk C, et al. Implementing potentially better practices for multidisciplinary team building: creating a neonatal intensive care unit culture of collaboration. Pediatrics 2003;111(4 Pt 2):e482–8.
34. The Joint Commission [Internet]. National patient safety goals effective January 1, 2014. The Joint Commission Critical Access Hospital Accreditation Program. 2014. Available at: https://www.jointcommission.org/joint_commission_announces_2014_npsg. Accessed October 7, 2014.
35. Ketko A, Martin C, Nemshak M, et al. Balancing the tension between hyperoxia prevention and alarm fatigue in the NICU. Pediatrics 2015;136(2):e496–504.
36. Cvach MM, Currie A, Sapirstein A, et al. Managing clinical alarms: using data to drive change. Nurs Manag 2013;44(11 Safety Solutions):8–12.
37. Dandoy C, Davies S, Flesch L, et al. A team-based approach to reducing cardiac monitor alarms. Pediatrics 2014;134(6):e1686–94.
38. Goel V, Poole S, Kipps A, et al. Implementation of data drive heart rate and respiratory rate parameters on a pediatric Acute Care Unit. Stud Health Technol Inform 2015;216:918.

39. Sendelbach S, Wahl S, Anthony A, et al. Stop the noise: a quality improvement project to decrease Electrocardiographic nuisance alarms. Crit Care Nurse 2015;35(4):15–22 [quiz 11p following 22].
40. Bonafide C, Lin R, Zander M, et al. Association between exposure to nonactionable physiologic monitor alarms and response time in a children's hospital. J Hosp Med 2015;10(6):345–51.
41. Rayo M, Mansfield J, Eiferman D, et al. Implementing an institution-wide quality improvement policy to ensure appropriate use of continuous cardiac monitoring: a mixed-methods retrospective data analysis and direct observation study. BMJ Qual Saf 2016;25(10):796–802.
42. Chambrin MC. Alarms in the intensive care unit: how can the number of false alarms be reduced? Crit Care 2001;5(4):184–8.
43. Varpio L, Kuziemsky C, MacDonald C, et al. The helpful or hindering effects of in-hospital patient monitor alarms on nurses: a qualitative analysis. Comput Inform Nurs 2012;30(4):210–7.
44. Voepel-Lewis T, Parker ML, Burke CN, et al. Pulse oximetry desaturation alarms on a general postoperative adult unit: a prospective observational study of nurse response time. Int J Nurs Stud 2013;50(10):1351–8.
45. Gorges M, Markewitz BA, Westenskow DR. Improving alarm performance in the medical intensive care unit using delays and clinical context. Anesth Analg 2009; 108(5):1546–52.
46. Taenzer AH, Pyke JB, McGrath SP, et al. Impact of pulse oximetry surveillance on rescue events and intensive care unit transfers: a before-and-after concurrence study. Anesthesiology 2010;112(2):282–7.
47. Armbruster J, Schmidt B, Poets C, et al. Nurses' compliance with alarm limits for pulse oximetry: qualitative study. J Perinatol 2010;30(8):531–4.
48. Nghiem T, Hagadorn J, Terrin N, et al. Nurse opinions and pulse oximeter saturation target limits for preterm infants. Pediatrics 2008;121(5):e1039–46.
49. Sowan AK, Tarriela AF, Gomez TM, et al. Nurses' perceptions and practices toward clinical alarms in a transplant cardiac Intensive Care Unit: exploring key issues leading to alarm fatigue. JMIR Hum Factors 2015;2(1):e3.
50. Sowan AK, Reed CC, Staggers N. Role of large clinical datasets from physiologic monitors in improving the safety of clinical alarm systems and methodological considerations: a case from philips monitors. JMIR Hum Factors 2016;3(2):e24.